WILLIAM HARVEY LIBRARY

is due for return on or before the last date shown below

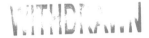

OXFORD MEDICAL PUBLICATIONS

Oxford Handbook of
Orthopaedics and Trauma

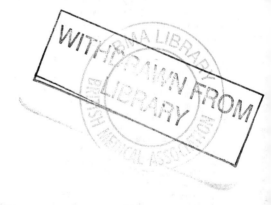

Published and forthcoming Oxford Handbooks

Oxford Handbook for the Foundation Programme 2e
Oxford Handbook of Acute Medicine 3e
Oxford Handbook of Anaesthesia 2e
Oxford Handbook of Applied Dental Sciences
Oxford Handbook of Cardiology
Oxford Handbook of Clinical and Laboratory Investigation 2e
Oxford Handbook of Clinical Dentistry 4e
Oxford Handbook of Clinical Diagnosis 2e
Oxford Handbook of Clinical Examination and Practical Skills
Oxford Handbook of Clinical Haematology 3e
Oxford Handbook of Clinical Immunology and Allergy 2e
Oxford Handbook of Clinical Medicine—Mini Edition 7e
Oxford Handbook of Clinical Medicine 8e
Oxford Handbook of Clinical Pharmacy
Oxford Handbook of Clinical Rehabilitation 2e
Oxford Handbook of Clinical Specialties 8e
Oxford Handbook of Clinical Surgery 3e
Oxford Handbook of Complementary Medicine
Oxford Handbook of Critical Care 3e
Oxford Handbook of Dental Patient Care 2e
Oxford Handbook of Dialysis 3e
Oxford Handbook of Emergency Medicine 3e
Oxford Handbook of Endocrinology and Diabetes 2e
Oxford Handbook of ENT and Head and Neck Surgery
Oxford Handbook of Expedition and Wilderness Medicine
Oxford Handbook of Gastroenterology & Hepatology
Oxford Handbook of General Practice 3e
Oxford Handbook of Genitourinary Medicine, HIV and AIDS
Oxford Handbook of Geriatric Medicine
Oxford Handbook of Infectious Diseases and Microbiology
Oxford Handbook of Key Clinical Evidence
Oxford Handbook of Medical Sciences
Oxford Handbook of Nephrology and Hypertension
Oxford Handbook of Neurology
Oxford Handbook of Nutrition and Dietetics
Oxford Handbook of Obstetrics and Gynaecology 2e
Oxford Handbook of Occupational Health
Oxford Handbook of Oncology 2e
Oxford Handbook of Ophthalmology
Oxford Handbook of Paediatrics
Oxford Handbook of Palliative Care 2e
Oxford Handbook of Practical Drug Therapy 2e
Oxford Handbook of Pre-Hospital Care
Oxford Handbook of Psychiatry 2e
Oxford Handbook of Public Health Practice 2e
Oxford Handbook of Reproductive Medicine & Family Planning
Oxford Handbook of Respiratory Medicine 2e
Oxford Handbook of Rheumatology 2e
Oxford Handbook of Sport and Exercise Medicine
Oxford Handbook of Tropical Medicine 3e
Oxford Handbook of Urology 2e

OXFORD MEDICAL PUBLICATIONS

Oxford Handbook of
Rheumatology

Published and forthcoming Oxford Handbooks

Oxford Handbook of
Rheumatology

THIRD EDITION

Alan J. Hakim
Consultant Physician and Rheumatologist,
Director of Strategy and Business Improvement,
Whipps Cross University Hospital NHS Trust,
London, UK

Gavin P.R. Clunie
Consultant Rheumatologist,
The Ipswich Hospital NHS Trust,
Ipswich, Suffolk, UK

Inam Haq
Senior Lecturer in Rheumatology and Medical Education,
Director of Undergraduate Studies,
Brighton and Sussex Medical School,
University of Brighton,
Sussex, UK

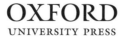

OXFORD
UNIVERSITY PRESS

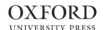

OXFORD
UNIVERSITY PRESS

Great Clarendon Street, Oxford OX2 6DP

Oxford University Press is a department of the University of Oxford. It furthers the University's
objective of excellence in research, scholarship, and education by publishing worldwide in

Oxford New York

Auckland Cape Town Dar es Salaam Hong Kong Karachi Kuala Lumpur
Madrid Melbourne Mexico City Nairobi New Delhi Shanghai Taipei Toronto

With offices in

Argentina Austria Brazil Chile Czech Republic France Greece
Guatemala Hungary Italy Japan Poland Portugal Singapore
South Korea Switzerland Thailand Turkey Ukraine Vietnam

Oxford is a registered trade mark of Oxford University Press
in the UK and in certain other countries

Published in the United States
by Oxford University Press Inc., New York

First published 2002
Second edition published 2006
Third edition printed 2011
Reprinted 2012

British Library Cataloguing in Publication Data
Data available

Library of Congress Cataloging in Publication Data
Data available

Typeset by Glyph International, Bangalore, India
Printed in China on acid-free paper through
Asia Pacific Offset

ISBN 978-0-19-958718-6

10 9 8 7 6 5 4 3 2

Foreword

The rheumatic diseases present in a variety of ways, many of the diseases are life-threatening and certainly severe and disabling and they cover almost the entire spectrum of clinical medicine. Patients, when asked what their major concern is in relation to rheumatic disease, inevitably mention pain and this is the focus of therapeutic intervention on which they would like us to concentrate. Doctors more readily concentrate on understanding pathology and trying to alter the process/pathogenesis.

The Oxford Handbook of Rheumatology is a relatively small but very practical textbook that covers all these aspects in appropriate detail. It starts with a full understanding of the anatomy of the problem, but very much answers questions in relation to why pain is perceived and how to treat it. It is a pragmatic, note-related approach to rheumatic disease and its treatment, ranging from the common to the very rare—with excellent cross-referencing between the different chapters and the way they deal with different aspects of the diseases.

Most rheumatology problems do not require the full intervention of specialist rheumatologists but are cared for in general practice by practice nurses, general practitioners with specialist interests, and the multi-disciplinary team. Those patients who require more specialist care are seen in hospital but still monitored by nurses and doctors many of whom who cover both primary and secondary care. Occasionally patients with most severe disease will be managed in hospital.

This small book, in addition to its practical, pragmatic approach, is soundly evidence-based and its approach and structure make it very readable and appropriate for trainees, specialists, nurses and general physicians. It is a book I would have been delighted to have when I started my career in medicine and I found many areas of interest and many new facts. It is a valuable resource for all those involved in rheumatic disease. It certainly should be on their bookshelves.

Professor David G I Scott
Consultant Rheumatologist,
Honorary Professor of Rheumatology
Chief Medical Advisor to the National Rheumatoid
Arthritis Society
Norfolk and Norwich University Hospital

Foreword from the previous edition

Rheumatic or musculoskeletal disorders can present in a number of familiar ways but sometimes are atypical and occasionally bewildering. They may appear insidiously or acutely and their impact ranges from a temporary nuisance, to a condition that is persistent and increasingly disabling, and sometimes a severe, even life-threatening illness.

Not only are they common, and increasingly so in an ageing population, they are often compounded by other disorders associated with ageing. But they affect people of all ages and especially those of working age in whom they are a major cause of sickness absence and curtailment of normal working life. Most do not call for specialist rheumatological care provided the General Practitioner and General Practitioner with a Special Interest are practiced in their diagnosis and treatment, and longterm care. Specialist referral is sought when the diagnosis is uncertain, the treatment ineffective, or a patient is acutely ill, which in some instances will lead to tertiarly referral.

This small book is up-to-date, based soundly on evidence and good clinical practice. It provides a compact but remarkably comprehensive vade mecum both for clinicians in training and trained clinicians who encounter patients with rheumatologic conditions in any guise, and specialists too. Notably, this new edition includes an important chapter on emergencies in rheumatology.

It is a book that I should have been glad to have by me from the beginning of my own career in rheumatology, and I commend it to clinicians today.

Carol Black
Professor Dame Carol Black, President,
Royal College of Physicians, and Professor of Rheumatology,
Royal Free & University College Medical School,
London

Preface

Rheumatic conditions are common both in general and hospital practice. Musculoskeletal symptoms are a primary feature of many multisystem illnesses, not only in the autoimmune joint and connective tissue diseases, but also metabolic, endocrine, neoplastic, and infectious conditions. Symptoms are also common in the context of injury, age-related change, and psychological distress. Many conditions in rheumatology are a major source of morbidity and mortality.

We have kept to the format of previous editions of this book, focusing first on history and physical signs in the differential diagnosis of rheumatic disease. The reader is then encouraged to consider diseases in more detail. There have been major advances in rheumatology, not least the introduction of biologic therapy. The third edition reflects this in being up-to-date with assessment, guidelines, and treatment options in 2010. We have also introduced a new section, Part 3.

Part 1 offers a practical guide to arriving at an appropriate differential diagnosis given the realistic presentation of rheumatic disease; for example, how to assess someone complaining of a pain in the elbow, knee pain, or of difficulty moving the shoulder, etc. The book suggests appropriate lines of enquiry for patients who present with characteristic patterns of abnormality such as widespread joint or muscle pain, or joint pains in association with a rash. The aim is to provide a guide for obtaining diagnostic information but also for discriminating good from bad information—where to lay emphasis in eliciting a history and examination signs. In most chapters in Part 1, text is laid out under the headings of Taking a history, Examination, and Investigations, with the subheadings indicating important considerations and areas of enquiry.

Part 2 lists a number of rheumatic conditions encountered in rheumatology and general practice. There is a focus on clinical features, specific findings of relevant investigations, and management. There is reference to childhood and adolescent rheumatic disease throughout. The aim is to provide a comprehensive, clinically orientated text. Some reference is made to disease epidemiology and pathophysiology. However, for more detail on the basic sciences the reader is referred to *The Oxford Textbook of Rheumatology*.

Part 3 is a rapid reference section on medication, injection techniques, and a chapter on rheumatological emergencies.

Acknowledgements

We would like to thank the editors of The Oxford Textbook of Rheumatology, Dr Philip Seo for his update of the text and authorship under the title of The Oxford American Handbook of Rheumatology, 2009, and the staff at Oxford University Press for their support and patience during the preparation of this latest edition.

Contents

Detailed contents

Editorial advisers

Symbols and abbreviations

📖	Cross-reference
α	Alpha
β	Beta
AAV	ANCA-associated vasculitides
AC	Adhesive capsulitis
ACA	Anticentromere antibody
ACE	Angiotensin-converting enzyme
AChA	Acrodermatitis chronicum atrophicans
AC(J)	Acromioclavicular (joint)
ACL	Anticardiolipin
ACR	American College of Rheumatology
ADM	Abductor digiti minimi
AKI	Acute kidney injury
ALP	Alkaline phosphatase
ALT	Alanine transaminase
AMA	Amyloid A
AML	Amyloid L
ANA	Anti-nuclear antibody
ANCA	Antineutrophil cytoplasmic antibody
AP	Anteroposterior
APB	Abductor pollicis brevis
APL	Abductor pollicis longus
ApL	Antipospholipid
APS	Antiphospholipid (antibody) syndrome
ARA	American Rheumatism Association
ARB	Angiotensin II receptor blockers
ARF	Acute renal failure
AS	Ankylosing spondylitis
AST	Aspartate transaminase
ASOT	Antistreptolysin O titre
ASU	Avocado/soybean unsaponifiable
ATN	Acetebular necrosis
ATN	Acute tubular necrosis
AZA	Azathioprine
BCP	Basic calcium phosphate (crystals)
bd	Twice daily

BLyS	B-lymphocyte stimulator
BMC	Bone mineral content
BMD	Bone mineral density
BMI	Body Mass Index
BSR	British Society of Rheumatology
BVAS	Birmingham Vasculitis Activity Score
C	Cervical (e.g. C6 is the sixth cervical vertebra)
CA	Coracoacromial
CAPS	Cryopyrin-associated periodic fever syndromes
CBT	Cognitive and behavioural therapy
CCP	Cyclic citrullinted peptide
CCS	Churg–Strauss syndrome
CHCC	Chapel Hill Consensus Conference
CINCA	Chronic, infantile, neurological, cutaneous, and articular syndrome
CIO	Corticocosteroid-induced osteoporosis
CK	Creatine kinase
CMC(J)	Carpometacarpal (joint)
CMP	Comprehensive metabolic panel
CMV	Cytomegalovirus
CNS	Central nervous system
COMP	Cartilage oligomeric matrix protein
COX	Cyclo-oxygenase
CPPD	Calcium pyrophosphate deposition (arthritis)
CREST	Calcinosis, Raynaud's, Esophageal dysmotility, Sclerodactyly, Telangiectasia (syndrome)
CRP	C reactive protein
CRPS	Complex regional pain syndrome
CS	Congenital scoliosis
CSS	Churg–Strauss syndrome
CT	Computed tomography
CTS	Carpal tunnel syndrome
CV(S)	Cardiovascular (system)
CWP	Chronic widespread pain
CXR	Chest radiograph
DAS	Disease Activity Score
dcSScl	Diffuse cutaneous systemic sclerosis
DEXA	Dual-energy X-ray absorptiometry
DIP(J)	Distal interphalangeal (joint)
DISH	Diffuse idiopathic skeletal hyperostosis
DLCO	Diffusion capacity for carbon monoxide

DM	Dermatomyositis
DMARD	Disease-modifying antirheumatic drug
DVT	Deep vein thrombosis
EA	Enteropathic arthritis
EANM	European Association of Nuclear Medicine
EBV	Epstein–Barr virus
ECG	Electrocardiogram
ECM	Erythema chronicum migrans
ECRB	Extensor carpi radialis brevis
ECRL	Extensor carpi radialis longus
ECU	Extensor carpi ulnaris
ED	Extensor digitorum
EDL	Extensor digitorum longus
EDM	Extensor digiti minimi
EDS	Ehlers–Danlos syndrome
EED	Erythema elevatum dictinum
EHL	Extensor hallucis longus
EI	Extensor indicis
ELMS	Eaton–Lambert myasthenic syndrome
EM	Erythema migrans
EMG	Electromyography
EN	Eythema nodosum
ENA(S)	Extractable nuclear antigen(s)
EPB	Extensor pollicis brevis
EPL	Extensor pollicis longus
ERA	Enthesitis-related arthritis
ESR	Erythrocyte sedimentation rate
ESSG	European Spondylarthropathy Study Group
EULAR	European League Against Rheumatism
FBC	Full blood count
FCR	Flexor carpi radialis
FCU	Flexor carpi ulnaris
FDA	Food and Drug Administration
FDL	Flexor digitorum longus
FDP	Flexor digitorum profundus
FDS	Flexor digitorum superficialis
FFS	Five Factor Score
FHB	Flexor hallucis brevis
FHH	Familial hypocalciuric hypercalcaemia
FJ	Facet joint
FM	Fibromyalgia

FMF	Familial Mediterranean fever
FPL	Flexor pollicis longus
FR	Flexor retinaculum
FVSG	French Vasculitis Study Group
GARA	Gut associated reactive arthritis
GBM	Glomerular basement membrane
GBS	Guillain Barré syndrome
GC	Gonococcal
GCA	Giant cell arteritis
GF	Glomerulonephritis
GFR	Glomerular filtration rate
GI	Gastrointestinal
GLA	Gamma linoleic acid
GOA	Generalized osteoarthritis
HA	Hydroxyapatite
HCQ	Hydroxychloroquine
HDCT	Hereditary disorder of connective tissue
HIV	Human immunodeficiency virus
HLA	Human leukocyte antigen
HPOA	Hypertrophic pulmonary osteoarthropathy
HPT	Hyperparathyroidism
HSCT	Haematopoietic stem cell transplantation
HSP	Henoch–Schönlein purpura
HTLV	Human T-cell leukemia virus
IBM	Inclusion-body myositis
IL	Interleukin
ILAR	International League of Associations for Rheumatology
im	Intramuscular(ly)
IMM	Idiopathic inflammatory myopathy
INR	International normalized ratio
IP	Interphalangeal
ISN	International Society for Nephrology
ITB	Iliotibial band
ITP	Immune thrombocytopenic purpura
iv	Intravenous
IVDU	Intravenous drug user
IVIG	Intravenous immunoglobulin
JCA	Juvenile chronic arthritis
JDM	Juvenile dermomyositis
JHS	Joint hypermobility syndrome

JIA	Juvenile idiopathic arthritis
JIO	Juvenile idiopathic osteoporosis
JPO	Juvenile polymyositis
JPSA	Juvenile psoriatic arthritis
JRA	Juvenile rheumatoid arthritis
JSpA	Juvenile spondyloarthropathy
KD	Kawasaki disease
KUB	Kidney ureter bladder
L	Lumbar (e.g. L5 is the fifth lumbar vertebra)
LAC	Lupus anticoagulent
LCL	Lateral collateral ligament
lcSScl	Limited cutaneous systemic sclerosis
LDH	Lactate dehydrogenase
LFTs	Liver function tests
LGL	Large granular lymphocyte
LH	Luteinizing hormone
LLLT	Low level laser therapy
LOPA	Late onset pauci-articular juvenile chronic arthritis
MAS	Macrophage activation syndrome
MCP(J)	Metacarpophalangeal (joint)
MCL	Medial collateral ligament
MCTD	Mixed connective tissue disease
MEN	Mycophenolate mofetil
MFS	Marfan's syndrome
MG	Myasthenia gravis
MMF	Mycophenolate mofetil
MMPI	Minnesota Multiphasic Personality Inventory
MND	Motor neuron disease
MPA	Microscopic polyangiitis
MPO	Myeloperoxidase
MR	Magnetic resonance
MRA	Magnetic resonance angiography
MRI	Magnetic resonance imaging
MSA	Myositis-specific
MTP(J)	Metatarsophalangeal (joint)
MTX	Methotrexate
MVP	Mitral valve prolapse
NCS	Nerve conduction study
NICE	National Institute for Health and Clinical Excellence (UK)
NMS	Neuromuscular scoliosis

NO	Nitrous oxide
NOMID	Neonatal onset multisystem inflammatory disease
NSAID	Non-steroidal anti-inflammatory drug
NSF	Nephrogenic systemic fibrosis
OA	Osteoarthritis
OI	Osteogenesis imperfecta
PAH	Pulmonary artery hypertension
PAN	Polyarteritis nodosa
PBC	Primary biliary cirrhosis
PCR	Polymerase chain reaction
PE	Pulmonary embolism
PET	Positron emission CT
PHP	Pseudohypoparathyroidism
PIN	Posterior interosseous nerve
PIP(J)	Proximal interphalangeal (joint)
PL	Palmaris longus
PLM	Polarized light microscopy
PM	Polymyositis
PML	Progressive multifocal leukoencephalopathy
PMN	Polymorphonuclear neutrophil
PMR	Polymyalgia rheumatica
po	Oral
PsA	Psoriatic arthropathy
PSA	Prostatic specific antigen
PTH	Parathyroid hormone
PV	Plasma viscosity
PVNS	Pigmented villonodular synovitis
qds	Four times daily
RA	Rheumatoid arthritis
RCT	Randomized control trial
REA	Reactive arthritis
RF	Rheumatoid factor
RNA	Ribonucleic acid
RNP	Ribonuclear protein
RP	Raynaud's phenomenon
RSD	Reflex sympathetic dystrophy (algo/osteodystrophy)
RSI	Repetitive strain injury
RS_3PE	Remitting seronegative symmetrical synovitis with pitting oedema
RTA	Renal tubular acidosis

sACE	Serum angiotensin converting enzyme
SAI	Subacromial impingement
SAMA	Serum amyloid A
SAP	Serum amyloid protein
SAPHO	Synovitis, acne, palmoplantar pustulosis, hyperostosis, aseptic osteomyelitis (syndrome)
SARA	Sexually transmitted reactive arthritis
s/c	Subcutaneous(ly)
SC(J)	Sternoclavicular (joint)
SCS	Spinal cord stimulation
SD	Standard deviation
SERM	Selective oestrogen receptor modulators
SI(J)	Sacroiliac (joint)
SIP	Sickness Impact Profile
SLE	Systemic lupus erythematosus
SNRI	Serotonin-norepinephrine re-uptake inhibitors
SpA	Spondyloarhthritis
SS	Sjögren's syndrome
SScl/Scl	Systemic sclerosis/Scleroderma
SSRI	Selective serotonin reuptake inhibitors
STIR	Short tau inversion recovery
SSZ	Sulfasalazine
T	Thoracic (e.g. T5 is the fifth thoracic vertebra)
TA	Takayusu's arteritis
TB	Tuberculosis
tds	Three times daily
TENS	Transcutaneous electrical nerve stimulation
TFTs	Thyroid function tests
TGF	Transferring growth factor
TIA	Transient ischemic attack
TM(J)	Temperomandibular (joint)
TNF(α)	Tumour necrosis factor (alpha)
tPA	Tissue plasminogen activator
TPMT	Thiopurine S-methyltransferase
TRAPs	Tumour necrosis factor-associated periodic syndrome
TSH	Thyroid stimulating hormone
U&E	Urea and electrolytes (in UK test includes creatinine)
UC	Ulcerative colitis
US	Ultrasound
UV	Ultraviolet

VDI	Vasculitis Damage Index
vs	Versus
VZIG	Varicella zoster immunoglobulin
WBC	White blood cell
WG	Wegener's granulomatosis
WHO	World Health Organization
WRD	Work-related disorder

Part I

The presentation of rheumatic disease

Evaluating musculoskeletal symptoms

Introduction

Pain is the most common musculoskeletal symptom. It is defined by its subjective description, which may vary depending on its physical (or biological) cause, the patient's understanding of it, its impact on function, and the emotional and behavioural response it invokes. Pain is also often 'coloured' by cultural, linguistic, and religious differences. Therefore, pain is not merely an unpleasant sensation; it is, in effect, an 'emotional change'. The experience is different for every individual; patients who think of themselves as having a 'high pain threshold' may have the hardest time coping.

In children and adolescents the evaluation of pain is sometimes complicated further by the interacting influences of the experience of pain within the family, school, and peer group. Stiffness is also common. It may be a manifestation of inflammation, reduced movement due to mechanical pathology including swelling, or used by an individual to describe reduced movement due to pain.

The GALS screen is a valuable quick assessment tool for identifying sites of reduced movement and function before entering in to a more detailed physical examination.

Localization of pain and pain patterns

- Adults usually localize pain accurately, although there are some situations worth noting in rheumatic disease where pain can be poorly localized (Table 1.1).
- Adults may not clearly differentiate between peri-articular and articular pain, referring to bursitis, tendonitis, and other forms of soft tissue injury as 'joint pain.' Therefore, it is important to confirm the precise location of the pain on physical examination.
- Pain may be well localized but caused by a distant lesion, e.g. interscapular pain caused by mechanical problems in the cervical spine, or right shoulder pain caused by acute cholecystitis.
- Pain caused by neurological abnormalities, ischaemic pain, and pain referred from viscera is harder for the patient to visualize or express, and the history may be given with varied interpretations.
- Bone pain is generally constant despite movement or change in posture—unlike muscular, synovial, ligament, or tendon pain—and often disturbs sleep. Fracture, tumour, and metabolic bone disease are all possible causes. Such constant, local, sleep-disturbing pain should always be investigated.
- Patterns of pain distribution are associated with certain musculoskeletal conditions. For example, polymyalgia rheumatica (PMR) typically affects the shoulder girdle and hips, whereas rheumatoid arthritis (RA) affects the joints symmetrically, with a predilection for the hands and feet.
- Patterns of pain distribution may overlap, especially in the elderly, who may have several conditions simultaneously, e.g. hip and/or knee osteoarthritis (OA), peripheral vascular disease, and degenerative lumbar spine all may cause lower extremity discomfort.

Table 1.1 Clinical pointers in conditions where pain is poorly localized

Diagnosis	Clinical pointer
Peri-articular shoulder pain	Referred to deltoid insertion
Carpal tunnel syndrome	Nocturnal paraesthesias and/or pain, often diffuse
Trochanteric bursitis	Nocturnal pain lying on affected side
Hip synovitis	Groin/outer thigh pain radiating to the knee

The quality of pain

Some individuals find it hard to describe pain or use descriptors of severity. A description of the quality of pain can often help to discriminate the cause. Certain pain descriptors are associated with non-organic pain syndromes (Table 1.2):

- Burning pain, hyperpathia (i.e., an exaggerated response to painful stimuli), and allodynia (i.e., pain from stimuli that are normally not painful) suggest a neurological cause.

Table 1.2 Terms from the McGill pain scale that help distinguish between organic and non-organic pain syndromes

Organic	Non-organic
Pounding	Flickering
Jumping	Shooting
Pricking	Lancinating ('Shooting')
Sharp	Lacerating
Pinching	Crushing
Hot	Searing
Tender	Splitting
Nagging	Torturing
Spreading	Piercing
Annoying	Unbearable
Tiring	Exhausting
Fearful	Terrifying
Tight	Tearing

- A change in the description of pain in a patient with a long-standing condition is worth noting, since it may denote the presence of a second condition, e.g. a fracture or septic arthritis in a patient with established RA.

Repeated, embellished, or elaborate description ('catastrophizing') may suggest non-organic pain, but be aware that such a presentation may be cultural.

Relieving and aggravating factors

In general mechanical disorders are worsened by activity and relieved by rest. This does not mean pain is not present at rest; in severe mechanical/degenerative disorders pain disturbs sleep. Patterns of pain distribution are associated with certain activities. In contrast, in inflammatory disorders pain may subside somewhat with activity.

Whether mechanical or inflammatory, pain is often worsened by excessive stressing/movement of the joint.

Individuals identify different relieving factors including hot/cold compress, supports, massage, etc.

Many individuals will have taken or be taking analgesics. It is important to understand which ones have been used, why they have been discontinued, and how effective they were. Was the frequency and dosage of analgesia correct and has there been good compliance with taking a medication before assuming inefficacy?

Changes in pain on examination

Eliciting changes in pain by the use of different examination techniques may be used to provide clues to the diagnosis:

- Palpation and comparison of active and passive range of motion can be used to reproduce pain and localize pathology. This requires practice and a good knowledge of anatomy.
- Many of the classic physical exam signs and manoeuvres have a high degree of inter-observer variability. Interpretation should take into account the context in which the examination is done and the effects of suggestibility.
- Palpation and passive range of motion exercises are performed while the patient is relaxed. The concept of 'passive' movement is the assumption that when the patient is completely relaxed, the muscles and tendons around the joint are removed as potential sources of pain; in theory, passive range of motion is limited only by pain at the true joint. This assumption has its own limitations, however, especially since passive movements of the joint will still cause some movement of the soft tissues. In some cases, e.g. shoulder rotator cuff disease, the joint may be painful to move passively because of subluxation or impingement due to a musculotendinous lesion.
- The clinician should be aware of myofascial pain when palpating musculotendinous structures, especially around the neck and shoulder regions. Myofascial pain is said to occur when there is activation of a trigger point that elicits pain in a zone stereotypical for the individual muscle. It is often aching in nature.
- Trigger points are associated with palpable tender bands. It is not clear whether trigger points are the same as the tender points characteristic of fibromyalgia.
- Local anaesthetic infiltration at the site of a painful structure is sometimes used to help localize pathology, e.g. injection under the acromion may provide substantial relief from a 'shoulder impingement syndrome'. However, the technique is reliable only if localization of the injected anaesthetic can be guaranteed. Few, if any, rigorously controlled trials have shown it to give specific results for any condition.

The assessment of pain in young children

The assessment of pain in young children is often difficult:

- Young children often localize pain poorly. Careful identification of the painful area is necessary through observation and palpation.
- A child may not admit to pain but will withdraw the limb or appear anxious when the painful area is examined.
- Observing a child's facial expression during an examination is very important, as is the parent's response.
- Quantification of pain often requires non-verbal clues, such as the child's behaviour. Pain rating scales are often helpful (Fig. 1.1).
- Turning the examination into a form of play may put the child at ease and assist with the examination. For example, asking the child to imitate your own movements may help you gauge range of motion.
- The trappings of clinic may make young children nervous, and removing a white coat or stethoscope from sight may also help place the patient at ease.

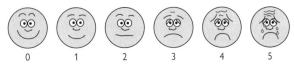

Fig. 1.1 Pain assessment in children—the faces rating scale.

Stiffness, swelling, and constitutional symptoms

Difficulty moving a joint may be a consequence of pain, swelling, stiffness, or all three. The added burden of a nerve or muscle pathology can make the symptom of stiffness more difficult to interpret:

- Stiffness is often worse after a period of rest. Short periods (less than 30 min) of stiffness that persist after mobilizing is not a meaningful observation. Stiffness lasting >30 min and often several hours after mobilizing is a typical symptom of inflammatory arthritis.
- Stiffness can occur in normal joints. Individuals typically click or crack their joints to stretch the tissues and gain relief.
- Stiffness may be a manifestation of tissue fibrosis; in tendons for example fibrosis may cause nodules to form that in their most extreme lead to locking or triggering (📖 Chapter 2, p 19).

Swelling may arise from a number of different sites. It is important to determine whether this is in the skin as a result of oedema, cellulitis, haematoma or varicosities, for example, whether it is tendon inflammation, synovial or bone tissue, or an effusion from synovial fluid or blood (haemathrosis).

Constitutional symptoms

Fatigue is a complex symptom experienced by many patients in association with systemic illness, anaemia, endocrinopathy or metabolic pathology, or as a consequence or disturbed sleep pattern.

Other constitutional symptoms include fever, excessive sweating, and weight-loss. These symptoms may also be a manifestation of other underlying diseases manifesting as arthritis (📖 Chapter 4, p 149).

Gait, arms, legs, spine—the GALS screen

Regional examination of the musculoskeletal system and the signs associated with musculoskeletal disorders is covered later (📖 Chapter 2, p 19). As an introduction to examination it is helpful to be familiar with the GALS screen,[1] designed to quickly identify the regions of the body functionally affected. Table 1.3 and Fig. 1.2, and Table 1.4 and Fig. 1.3 (reproduced with permission of Hodder Arnold) demonstrate this process in text and visual format.[2]

1 Doherty M, Dacre P, Dieppe P, Snaith M (1992). The 'GALS' locomotor screen. *Annals Rheumatic Disease* **51**,1165–9.
2 Hakim AJ (2010). Chapter 14. In *Chamberlain's Symptoms and Signs in Clinical Medicine*, 13e. Houghton A & Gray D. Hodder Arnold, London.

Table 1.3 Physical examination—general inspection
Standing the patient in the anatomical position, look at them from the front, rear, and side. At all times think about symmetry. The numbering in the table aligns with that in Fig. 1.2

Position	Observation
Front:	
1) Neck	Abnormal flexion (torticolis)
2) Shoulder	Muscle bulk across the chest
3) Elbow	Full (or hyper) extension
4) Pelvis	Level—tilted lower on one side may be leg length difference or spinal curvature (scoliosis)
5) Quadriceps	Muscle bulk
6) Knee	Alignment—bow-legged (varus deformity) or knock-kneed (valgus deformity)
7) Midfoot	Swelling, operation scars
	Loss of midfoot arch—flat feet
Rear:	
8) Shoulder	Muscle bulk across deltoid, trapezius, and scapular muscles
9) Spine alignment	Scoliosis (curvature to side). Operation scars (including neck)
10) Gluteal	Muscle bulk
11) Knee	Swelling
12) Calf	Muscle bulk, swelling
13) Hindfoot	Out-turning (eversion) of the heel associated with flat-foot.
	Achilles tendon swelling
Side	
14) Spine alignment	Cervical—normal lordosis; Dorsal/Thoracic—normal kyphosis; Lumbar—normal lordosis
15) Knee	Excessive extension—hypermobility

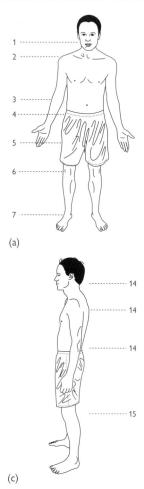

(a)

(c)

Fig. 1.2 Physical examination—general inspection (see Table 1.3 for description). Adapted from Houghton AR, Gray D. (2010) *Chamberlain's Symptoms and Signs in Clinical Medicine: An Introduction to Medical Diagnosis*, 13th edition. Hodder Arnold, London.

Measure lumbar flexion using Schöbers' test. With the patient standing upright make a horizontal mark across the sacral dimples and a second mark over the spine 10 cm above. The patient then bends forward as far as possible. Re-measure the distance between the marks. It should increase from 10 to >15 cm; less suggests restriction.

NB. Just looking at ability to bend forward and not at lumbar expansion is inadequate; the individual may have good range of hip movement giving false impression of lumbar mobility.

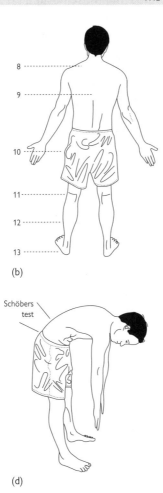

(b)

(d)

Fig. 1.2 *(Cont'd)*

Table 1.4 Physical examination screening tool—gait, arms, legs, and spine

Position	Observation	Command
Standing	**Gait:** smooth movement, arm swing, pelvic tilt, normal stride length, ability to turn quickly	'Walk to the end of the room, turn, and walk back to me'
	Lumbar spine:	
	Lumbar expansion	'Bend forward and touch your toes'
	Lumbar lateral flexion	'Place your hands by your side; bend to the side running your hand down the outside of your leg toward your knee ...'
	Hip: the Trendelenburg test. If the opposite side of the pelvis drops below the horizontal level this suggests weakness of the hip abductors on the weight-bearing leg	'Stand on one leg ... now the other.' Patient may not be able to do this if frail, has a neurological problem, unstable hypermobility, or a knee or ankle problem
Sitting facing you: **neck and thoracic spine**	**Neck:** smooth movement, no pain/stiffness	
	Forward flexion	'Bend forward chin to chest'
	Side flexion	'Bend sideways ear to shoulder'
	Extension	'Tilt head back'
	Rotation	'Turn head to the ..., chin to shoulder ... other side'
	Thoracic spine: smooth movement, no pain/stiffness 1) Lateral chest expansion 2) Rotation	'Fold your arms, turn body to the ...'
Sitting facing you: **hands, wrists, elbows, and shoulders**	**Hand, wrist, finger:** swelling deformity	'Place both hands out in front, palms down and fingers straight'
	Hand pronation: Observe palms and grip function	'Turn the hands over, palms up'—'make a fist'

Table 1.4 (Cont'd)

Position	Observation	Command
	Gently squeeze the MCP joints by compressing the row of joints together. Assess for pain. Feel for warmth. Look for operation scars	'Place palms of hands together as if to pray, with elbows out to the side'
	Wrist extension and flexion	'With the elbows in the same position place the hands back to back with the fingers pointing down'
	Elbows Look for nodules, rash	'Bend your elbows bringing your hands to your shoulders'
	Shoulders Abduction to 180 degrees	'Raise arms out sideways, hands above your head'
	Rotation	'Touch the small of your back'
Sitting facing you: hips, knees, and ankles	**Hips:** gently turn inward and outward looking for symmetry, restriction, pain	
	Knees:	
	Flex and extend, feeling the patella with palm of hand for 'crepitus' (grinding), and back of hand for warmth	
	Feel back of the knee, calf, and Achilles tendon for pain and swelling	
	Ankles and feet: gently squeeze the MTP joints of the toes by compressing the row of joints together. Assess for pain. Feel for warmth	'Turn your ankles in a circular motion' 'Now up and down' 'Wiggle your toes'

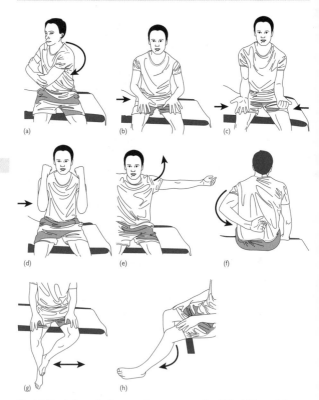

Fig. 1.3 Physical examination screening manoeuvres. See Table 1.4 for verbal commands. Adapted from Houghton AR, Gray D. (2010) *Chamberlain's Symptoms and Signs in Clinical Medicine: An Introduction to Medical Diagnosis*, 13th edition. Hodder Arnold, London.

Regional musculoskeletal conditions: making a working diagnosis

Introduction

This chapter aims to provide a guide to constructing an appropriate differential diagnosis in the patient who presents with regional musculoskeletal symptoms. It does not make reference to all possible diagnoses, only the most common. The section is divided into discussion of the neck, upper limb (shoulder, elbow, wrist), hand, thoracolumbar spine, lower limb (pelvis, groin, thigh, knee), and foot.

General considerations

- Findings from conventional clinical examination and imaging of the musculoskeletal system usually occur when the patient is at rest, and therefore only minimally symptomatic. Examination in the context of function (i.e. carrying, lifting, walking, bending, etc.) is not easy, although it is arguably more appropriate. Therefore, a thorough history utilizing a good depth of knowledge of functional anatomy is the best alternative and an invaluable way of obtaining good information about abnormal function and its causes.
- Time spent obtaining a detailed account of the onset of symptoms is often helpful whether or not the symptoms are of recent onset, or chronic, or obviously associated with trauma. Patients usually have a clearer concept of injury-induced disease and may try to rationalize the appearance of non-trauma-related symptoms by association with an event or injury.
- The term 'repetitive strain injury' is commonly used by the layperson to denote a diagnosis. It is not a diagnosis, merely a description of a likely mechanism by which injury has occurred. It is important to identify anatomically where the problem lies and to then enquire as to activities that may have induced or perpetuated the problem.
- With regard to the previous point always consider the possibility that the problem is a '**work-related disorder**' (WRD). A WRD may not just be musculoskeletal; consider the possibility of associated respiratory (asthma, fibrosis), dermatological (dermatoses), neurological (neuropathy, behavioural), psychosocial (anxiety, depression), and infective (sewage, carcasses, needlestick) pathologies. Examples of musculoskeletal WRD are given throughout this chapter.
- With children, it is important to obtain a history from both the child and a care provider. Second-hand information, even if provided by the mother, may be less reliable than direct information from someone who has the opportunity to observe the child during the day.
- Regional musculoskeletal lesions may be a presenting feature of a systemic disorder, such as an autoimmune rheumatic disease, malignancy, or infection. Clinical suspicion should guide the evaluation.

- Screening for disseminated malignancy, lymphoma, myeloma, and infection should at least include a FBC, metabolic screen, serum and urine protein electrophoresis with immunofixation, erythrocyte sedimentation rate (ESR), and c-reactive protein (CRP). Thereafter, tests should be directed specifically towards the clinical scenario.
- Weakness (as a symptom) may be due to a neuropathic or myopathic condition or it may be perceived according to the impact of other symptoms such as pain.

Neck pain

Background epidemiology

- About 10% of the adult population has neck pain at any one time, although many people do not seek medical help.
- About 1% of adult patients with neck pain develop neurological deficits, but overall levels of disability are lower than for patients with low back pain.
- Isolated neck pain in children and adolescents is unusual. More commonly, it accompanies thoracic spine pain or pathology.
- A continuum of radiological appearances exists in relation to age: intervertebral disc narrowing, marginal end-plate osteophytes, and facet joint changes. The appearances are often termed 'degenerative'; however, their correlation with the presence and severity of pain is poor.

Table 2.1 lists the major causes of neck pain in adults.

Functional anatomy

- The neck is the most mobile (37 separate articulations), but least stable part of the spine. There are seven vertebrae (C1–C7) and five intervertebral discs (C2/3–C6/7). The C5/6 disc is most often associated with radicular symptoms. If it occurs, cord compression is most likely in this region, although atlanto-axial (C1–C2) subluxation may produce the same picture, especially among patients with RA.
- Minor congenital abnormalities are not infrequent and increase the risk of degenerative changes.
- Nerve roots C2 and C3 cover sensation over the back of the head, the lower jaw line, and the neck.
- Nerve roots (C4–T1) leave the spine in dural root sleeves, traverse the intervertebral foramina and form the brachial plexus.
- Cervical nerves have a dermatomal representation (Fig. 2.1) and supply upper limb musculature in a predictable way.

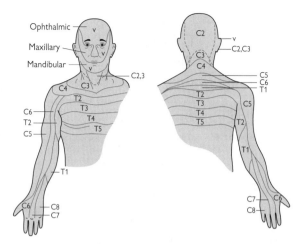

Fig. 2.1 Dermatomal distribution of the cervical and upper thoracic nerves reflecting the radicular pattern of nerve root lesions.

Table 2.1 The major causes of neck pain in adults

Soft tissue lesions (posture, psychogenic issues, and over-use as modifiers)	Neck strain
	Torticollis
	Myofascial pain
	Trauma [e.g. acute flexion—extension injury ('whiplash')]
	Cervicothoracic interspinous bursitis
Degenerative and mechanical lesions	Spondylosis
	Disc prolapsed
	Thoracic outlet syndrome
	Diffuse idiopathic skeletal hyperostosis (DISH)
Inflammatory conditions	Rheumatoid arthritis (📕 Chapter 5, p 233)
	Spondyloarthropathy (associated with fracture and inflammatory discitis) (📕 Chapter 8, p 281)
	Juvenile idiopathic arthritis (📕 Chapter 9, p 303)
	Polymyalgia rheumatica (PMR) (📕 Chapter 15, p 405)
	Myelitis

(Continued)

Table 2.1 *(Cont'd)*

Bone lesions	Traumatic fracture
	Osteomyelitis (e.g. TB)
	Osteoporosis (fracture) (☐ Chapter 16, p 431)
	Osteomalacia (bone disease or muscle pain)
	Paget's disease
Non-osseous infections	General systemic infection (general/cervical myalgias)
	Meningitis
	Discitis
Malignancy	Primary (rare) or secondary tumours (and pathological fracture)
	Myeloma, lymphoma, leukaemia
Brachial plexus lesions	Trauma
	Thoracic outlet syndrome (e.g. cervical rib)
Referred pain from	Acromioclavicular or temporomandibular joint
	Heart and major arteries (e.g. angina, thoracic aorta dissection)
	Pharynx (e.g. infection, tumours)
	Lung and diaphragm (e.g. Pancoast tumour, subphrenic abscess)
	Abdomen (e.g. gallbladder, stomach, oesophageal, or pancreatic disease)
	Shoulder (e.g. adhesive capsulitis) (☐ Chapter 2, p 19 and ☐ Chapter 19, p 517)

Taking a history

The site, radiation, and description of pain

- Nerve root (radicular) pain is usually sharp and reasonably well localized in the arms. It is often 'burning' and associated with paraesthesia and numbness. Nerve root irritation and compression by an intervertebral disc are common causes of radicular pain. However, in older adults and those who suffer recurrent bouts of pain it is usually due to encroachment of vertebral end-plate or facet joint osteophytes, or thickened soft tissue or fibrosis on the nerve leading to stenosis of the exit foramen.
- Pain from deep cervical structures is common. It often localizes poorly across the upper back. It can be referred to the upper arms, is typically described as 'heavy' or 'aching' and is more diffuse than nerve root pain.
- Muscle spasm often accompanies various lesions. It can be very painful.
- Pain from the upper cervical spine (C1–C3) can be referred to the temporomandibular joint (TMJ) or retro-orbital regions. Conversely, pain from both TMJ disorders and as a result of dental malocclusion can be referred to the neck.
- Pain from the lower neck may be referred to the interscapular and anterior thoracic wall regions. The latter may mimic cardiac ischaemic pain.
- Florid descriptions of the pain and of its extent and severity ('catastrophizing') are associated with prominent psychological modulators of pain.
- Evaluation of the shoulder joint is often necessary as pathology there often co-exists and symptoms around the shoulder often complicate neck evaluation.
- Occipital headache is a common manifestation.

Acute neck pain with trauma

Acute neck pain with trauma requires urgent assessment, even if there are no obvious neurological symptoms:

- Acute trauma requires urgent evaluation and consideration of fracture, spinal cord damage, and vertebral instability. About 80% of serious injuries occur from an accelerating head hitting a stationary object.
- An abrupt flexion injury may fracture the odontoid (this occurs less commonly with extension); however, fewer than one in five injuries at C1/C2 produce neurological deficit because of the wide canal at this level.
- If not traumatic or osteoporotic (the latter being relatively rare in the cervical spine), fractures may occur in bone invaded by malignancy.

New and/or associated symptoms

Ask about associated leg weakness, and new bladder or bowel symptoms. New onset acute neck pain with neurological features needs urgent evaluation. Neurological symptoms may also accompany chronic neck pain:

- Spinal osteomyelitis, meningitis, discitis (infection or inflammation), myelitis, and fracture may all present with acute or subacute neck pain. All may cause cord compression. Myelopathy due to spondylosis typically presents with a slowly progressive disability over weeks to months, although it can be acute, particularly if associated with central disc prolapse.

- Subacute pain, flaccid paralysis, and profound distal neurological signs may suggest myelitis, a condition caused mainly by infections and autoimmune diseases.
- Tinnitus, gait disturbance, blurring of vision, and diplopia associated with neck pain are all ascribed to irritation of the cervical sympathetic nerves.
- The vertebral arteries pass close to the facet joints just anterior to emerging nerve roots. Disruption of vertebral blood flow may cause dizziness in severe cases of neck **spondylosis**.

Previous trauma

Ask about previous trauma—it often precedes and influences chronic pain:

- Acute and occupational (chronic over-use) trauma is a common antecedent of chronic neck pain.
- **Cervical dystonia (torticollis)** can occur 1–4 days after acute trauma, it responds poorly to treatment, and can be long-standing. It may also complicate arthropathy, such as in RA or Parkinson's disease.
- Whiplash injury is associated with chronic myofascial pain.
- In some patients with chronic pain following (sometimes trivial) trauma, there may be dissatisfaction with the quality of care received at the time of the injury.
- Unresolved litigation associated with trauma correlates with the persistence of neck pain and reported disability.

Occupational and leisure activities

Some occupations and sports/activities are associated with recurrent neck pain:

- Neck pain (and early spondylosis) is prevalent in people whose occupations require persistent awkward head and neck postures, e.g. professional dancers.
- Although biomechanical factors may be an important influence in initiating and aggravating neck pain, there may also be an underlying genetic predisposition to OA and/or hypermobility.

Other points

Establish whether the pain started or varies with any non-musculoskeletal symptoms:

- Cardiac ischaemia, dyspepsia, or abdominal pain can result in referred pain to the neck (Table 2.1).

Examination

The neck is part of the functional upper limb and symptoms in the arms and legs may be relevant. Neurological examination of the arms is important:

- An adequate examination cannot be performed in a clothed patient. Despite the inconvenience, it is important to have the patient change into an examination gown to avoid missing potentially relevant clues.
- Inspection from front and back may reveal specific muscle wasting, or spasm and poor posture.
- Observing active movements reveals little if the patient has severe pain or muscle spasm. Inability to move the neck even small distances is

characteristic in advanced ankylosing spondylitis (AS) (📖 Chapter 8, p 281).

- Tenderness often localizes poorly in **degenerative disease**. Exquisite tenderness raises the possibility of a disc lesion, osteomyelitis, or malignancy (the latter two are rare).
- There may be 'trigger points' in neck stabilizer and extensor muscles. Activation of a trigger point elicits myofascial pain in a zone that is stereotypical for the individual muscle.
- Tender points (localized, non-radiating pain elicited by pushing with the thumb), notably at the occipital origin of the trapezius, the medial scapular border and the mid-belly of the trapezius, are features of fibromyalgia (FM) (📖 Chapter 18, p 489). It is not clear whether tender and trigger points are the same.
- Examination of passive mobility may be helpful primarily if it reveals gross asymmetry. The normal range of movement varies depending on age, sex, and ethnicity. Generally, at least 45° of lateral flexion and 70° of rotation should be achieved in a middle-aged adult. Global loss of passive mobility is non-specific and occurs with increasing age. The range of movement that might indicate hypermobility has not been established.
- Care should be taken if neck instability is a possibility (e.g. fracture, RA). Vigorous passive examination of forward flexion may exacerbate disc lesions.
- Examination of the shoulder is important to evaluate any referred pain or associated articular lesion (e.g. adhesive capsulitis) (see 📖 Shoulder pain, p 30 and 📖 Chapter 19, p 517).
- Neurological examination of upper and lower limbs is important in all cases where pain is referred to the arms and/or the legs if **cord compression** is a possibility: look for increased tone, clonus, pyramidal weakness, and extensor plantar response. Check for a cervicothoracic sensory level.

Investigations

Radiographs

Radiographs should be requested with specific objectives in mind:

- A lateral neck film may demonstrate soft tissue thickening in infection or synovium in RA (📖 Chapter 5, p 233), will document **spondylitis** (syndesmophytes, discitis and periosteal apposition in posterior elements associated with psoriasis), and the severity of spondylosis.
- Oblique views centred on the suspected level may show nerve root foramen stenosis from bony encroachment in patients with **radiculopathy**. There may be underlying OA (📖 Chapter 6, p 259).
- High cervical flexion and extension views and a 'through-the-mouth' (odontoid) view are useful to demonstrate odontoid pathology.
- In a patient with RA (📖 Chapter 5, p 233), if the distance between the anterior arch of the atlas and odontoid process is >3 mm on a lateral film taken in flexion, there is likely to be C1/C2 AP subluxation.
- On a lateral film superior odontoid subluxation in RA can be judged from a reduced distance from the antero-inferior surface of C2 to a line drawn between the hard palate and base of the occiput

(McGregor's line). The distance should be >34 mm in men and >29 mm in women. Lateral odontoid **subluxation** is best demonstrated with magnetic resonance (MR) imaging.

- Stepwise vertebral subluxation throughout the cervical spine demonstrated on a lateral film is characteristic of advanced RA.
- There may be only a few, but important signs of spinal infection, such as a soft tissue mass or isolated loss of joint space.

Magnetic resonance (MR) and computed tomography (CT)

- MR has largely superseded CT, arthrography, and CT-arthrography in assessing cervical spine/nerve, dural, vertebral, disc, and other soft tissue lesions in the neck.
- In many cases the relevance of some MR findings is still being established—patterns of signal abnormality do occur in asymptomatic people. The frequency of these effects increases with age.
- MR is the technique of choice for imaging disc prolapse, myelopathy (Plate 1), myelitis and for excluding infection or tumours. MR is used to help evaluate the need for, and plan, neurosurgical intervention in high cervical instability in RA patients.
- MR may show soft-tissue swelling around the odontoid in calcium pyrophosphate deposition (CPPD) disease (□ Chapter 7, p 269), but the diagnosis is best made with CT, which shows calcification around the odontoid and of adjacent ligaments ('crowned dens syndrome').
- In patients with the combination of unexplained radiographic signs and generalized symptoms MR is an important investigation. Cases of spinal infection such as tuberculosis (TB) or brucellosis and lymphoma and can be picked up (□ Chapter 17, p 473).

Isotope bone scan

- Scintigraphy has little role in diagnosing neck lesions.
- Despite improved image quality and tomographic images, the neck is poorly imaged on an isotope bone scan.

Treatment

Figure 2.2 shows the principles of treating mechanical cervical syndromes and the timing of MR scanning:

- Remember to review the diagnosis if pain is persistent despite treatment and symptoms seem disproportionate to the results or reports of imaging. In our experience, inflammatory sero-negative arthropathy-related neck pains are often mistaken for 'cervical spondylosis'. This may be because the clinician too readily assumes the latter diagnosis and/or radiologists misreport radiographs.

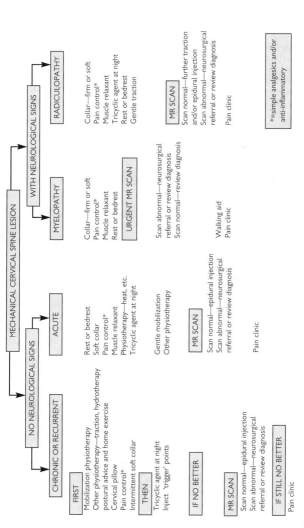

Fig. 2.2 The principles of treating mechanical neck syndromes and the timing of MR scanning.

Shoulder pain

Anatomy of the shoulder (Fig. 2.3)

- The glenohumeral joint is a ball and socket joint. The shallow glenoid cavity permits a wide range of movement. The circular fibrocartilagenous labrum sits on the glenoid, increases the articular surface area, and acts as a static joint stabilizer.
- Normal glenohumeral movements include depression, then glide and rotation of the humeral head under the coraco-acromial (CA) arch to enable elevation of the arm. As the arm elevates, there is smooth rotation and elevation of the scapula on the thoracic wall.
- Shoulder movements are a synthesis of four joints: glenohumeral, acromioclavicular (AC), sternoclavicular (SC), and scapulothoracic.
- Movements at AC and SC joints enable slight clavicular rotation, shoulder elevation/depression, and protraction/retraction.
- The rigid CA arch protects the glenohumeral joint from trauma and it, and the overlying deltoid, are separated from the capsule by the subacromial (subdeltoid) bursa.
- A cuff of muscles surrounds the glenohumeral joint capsule. These 'rotator cuff 'muscles are the supraspinatus, infraspinatus, teres minor, and subscapularis.
- The supraspinatus initiates abduction by depressing the humeral head, then elevating the arm alone for the first 10° of movement. The more powerful deltoid then takes over abduction. Infraspinatus/teres minor and the subscapularis externally and internally rotate the arm in the anatomical position respectively (Fig. 2.4).
- Production of powerful shoulder movements requires some degree of arm elevation as the larger muscles, such as the deltoid, latissimus dorsi (extensor), and teres major (adductor) work inefficiently with the arm in the anatomical position. The rotator cuff muscles act synchronously as joint stabilizers throughout the range of shoulder movement.
- The long head of biceps tendon originates above the glenoid usually attached to the labrum and runs within the glenohumeral joint capsule anteromedially in a bony groove.

Pain and shoulder lesions (📖 Chapter 19, p 517)

- Shoulder pain is common and may have its origin in articular or peri-articular structures or may be referred from the cervical or thoracic spine, thoracic outlet or subdiaphragmatic structures (Table 2.2).
- Shoulder lesions often produce pain referred to the humeral deltoid insertion (patient points to upper arm).
- Peri-articular disorders, mainly shoulder subacromial impingement (SAI) disorders, are the most common cause of shoulder pain in adults (>90% of cases).

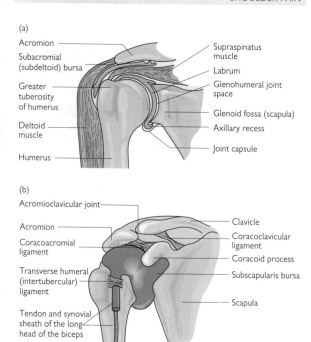

Fig. 2.3 (a) Major shoulder structures. (b) The relationship of the joint capsule to its bony surround and the coraco-acromial arch.

- Traumatic or inflammatory lesions of many different shoulder structures and conditions that result in neuromuscular weakness of the rotator cuff or scapular stabilizers may result in impingement pain.
- Pain from **subacromial impingement syndrome** is thought to be generated by the 'squashing' of subacromial structures between the greater tuberosity of the humeral head and the CA arch during rotation/elevation of the humeral head.

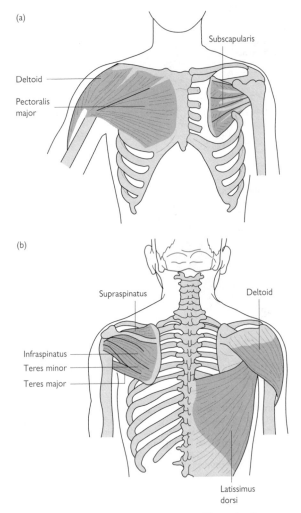

Fig. 2.4 The muscles of the shoulder: (a) anterior view; (b) posterior view.

Table 2.2 The most common causes of shoulder pain

Peri-articular lesions (often manifest as subacromial impingement pain)	Rotator cuff tendonitis/tears (very common age 40 years+)
	Calcific tendonitis
	Bicipital tendonitis
	Subacromial bursitis
	Enthesopathy-associated with SpA e.g. PsA
	Peri-articular muscle weakness
Articular lesions	Synovitis (glenohumeral or AC)
	OA (glenohumeral or AC)
	Glenohumeral instability (e.g. labral tears)
	Adhesive capsulitis ('frozen shoulder')
Neurologic	Cervical nerve root and radicular referred pain
	Neurological amyotrophy
	Spinal cord lesions: tumours, syringomyelia
Neurovascular	Complex regional pain syndrome (📖 Chapter 18, p 489)
Thoracic conditions (referred pain)	Mediastinal tumours
	Angina
Systemic and diffuse conditions	Polymyalgia rheumatica (📖 Chapter 15, p 405)
	Myositis (📖 Chapter 14, p 385)
	Chronic pain disorders (📖 Chapter 18, p 489)
	Polyarticular inflammatory arthritis
Bone disorders	Tumours
	Osteonecrosis (📖 Chapter 16, p 431)
	Paget's disease (📖 Chapter 16, p 431)
Subdiaphragmatic (referred pain)	Gallbladder disease
	Subphrenic abscess

Taking a history

When did the pain start?

Shoulder injuries are common, and may be acute or chronic (over-use).

- **Rotator cuff** lesions (inflammation, degenerative weakness, or tear) are often associated with activities and occupations that involve straining the arm in abduction or forward flexion. A history of an acute injury, however, is not always obtained. Subsequent calcification in the tendon following a supraspinatus injury can be asymptomatic or present with acute pain.

- Manual labour is a risk factor for rotator cuff lesions. There is typically no acute injury, but a history of repetitive movements over years that lead to injury.

- Athletes employed in throwing and racket sports are at risk of rotator cuff tendonopathy and labral tears. Rugby and American Football players are at risk of clavicle fracture, shoulder dislocation (and long-term instability), and disruption of the acromioclavicular (AC) joint.

- Pain from degenerative glenohumeral or AC joint arthritis might be a long-term sequelae of a bone or joint injury.

- The shoulder girdle is one of the most common sites for a chronic pain syndrome.

- **Myofascial pain** of the shoulder girdle is common and may mimic the symptoms of **cervical radiculopathy** and even reflux oesophagitis or ischaemic heart disease.

- Severe, persistent, sleep-disturbing pain of recent onset may be indicative of avascular necrosis, osteomyelitis, or bony tumours. Although uncommon in the shoulder region, these conditions should not be missed.

Where is the pain?

- Pain from the shoulder may be referred to the deltoid insertion.

- Well-localized pain may occur with AC joint arthritis (e.g. patient places a finger on the affected joint), but remember that referred C4 nerve root pain and pain from bone lesions of the distal clavicle is maximal in the same area.

- Glenohumeral articular and capsulitis pain is not well localized (e.g. the patient covers their shoulder with their hand).

- Pericapsular pain may be associated with SAI syndromes, but may also be myofascial (typically) or referred from the cervicothoracic spine.

- Bilateral shoulder pain should increase suspicion of the presence of an inflammatory polyarthritis such as RA (📖 Chapter 5, p 233), juvenile idiopathic arthritis (JIA) (📖 Chapter 9, p 303), psoriatic arthritis (📖 Chapter 8, p 281) or CPPD arthritis (📖 Chapter 7, p 269)—but these would be rare without other joint symptoms.

- Diffuse pain across the shoulder girdle muscles in those over 55 years of age raises the possibility of PMR (📖 Chapter 15, p 405). This pain is often associated with immobility and stiffness, particularly early in the day.

- A deep aching pain associated with stiffness is characteristic of **adhesive capsulitis (frozen shoulder).** The use of the term frozen shoulder is popular, but often incorrectly applied. It is a condition that is rare in patients under 40 years of age. The condition occurs in three phase: a painful phase, an adhesive ('frozen') phase, and a resolution phase. Phases often overlap and the duration varies but long-term limitation of shoulder movement remains in up to 15% of patients. It is associated with diabetes (📖 Chapter 4, p 193).

Does the pain vary?

Movement- or posture-related pain may be a clue to its cause:

- **Rotator cuff lesions** often present to rheumatologists with an SAI pattern of pain—that is, pain reproducibly aggravated by specific movements during each day such as reaching up (overhead) with the arm. Articular, bone, and adhesive capsulitis pain is more likely to be persistent.

- A history of recurrent bouts of shoulder pain in children and adolescents may suggest glenohumeral instability due to hypermobility or previous trauma, e.g. a labral tear. In an unstable shoulder, pain may result from synovitis, subchondral bone damage, or an SAI disorder. The frequency of recurrent anterior subluxation is inversely proportional to the age at which the initial dislocation occurs.

Are there spinal symptoms?

There is an association between neck conditions and shoulder pain. C4 nerve root pain is referred to the shoulder, adhesive capsulitis is associated with cervical nerve root symptoms (the nature of the link is unknown), and inflammatory neck lesions, such as CPPD and psoriatic spondylitis forms can be associated with bilateral shoulder pain referral and can mimic PMR.

Examination

Visual inspection

Inspect the neck, shoulders, and arms from the front, side, and back with the patient standing.

- Abnormality of the contour of the cervicothoracic spine could indicate muscle imbalance/spasm or might be associated with a nerve root origin of pain.

- Scapular asymmetry at rest is especially relevant when examining children and may indicate a congenital bony deformity. Subtle degrees of asymmetry are common and are not usually due to specific pathology, nor are they of consequence.

- Diffuse swelling of the whole shoulder may suggest a shoulder effusion/haemarthrosis or subacromial bursitis. In the elderly, **Milwaukee shoulder** should be considered. Swelling of the AC joint occurs with joint diastasis, arthritis and distal clavicular bone lesions.

- Arm swelling and skin changes distally could indicate a complex regional pain syndrome (📖 Chapter 18, p 489).

Elicit any tenderness

Eliciting tenderness of discrete shoulder structures is often unrewarding:

- Tenderness of the AC joint, humeral insertion of the supraspinatus tendon, and the long head of biceps tendon may be clues to pathology, but palpation will not be specific for diagnosis.

- An appreciation of trigger points associated with myofascial pain and tender points in fibromyalgia (📖 Chapter 18, p 489) is important in the interpretation of regional soft tissue tenderness.

Document bilateral shoulder movements

This aids diagnosis but also gives an indication of the level of functional impairment and can help in monitoring changes over time (Table 2.3). The movements are first tested actively (the patient does the movement) and then passively (the clinician supports the limb). Muscle strength can also be assessed while testing active movement.

- Observe arm elevation in the scapular plane from behind, noting symmetry of scapular movement, the pattern of pain during elevation, and the range of elevation. Hunching of the shoulder at the outset of arm elevation often occurs with an impingement problem. A painful arc may suggest a rotator cuff lesion. Inability to lift the arm suggests a rotator cuff tear or weakness, capsulitis, or severe pain, e.g. **acute calcific supraspinatus tendonitis**.
- Observe and compare internal rotation of shoulders, which can be judged by how far up the back the hand can reach. Poor performance may be due to rotator cuff weakness, weakness of the scapular stabilizing muscles, or pain (generally from shoulder impingement syndrome). This manoeuvre assumes normal elbow function.
- Observe the range of external rotation of the humerus from the front. Ask the patient to flex their elbows as if he were holding a tray and then rotate the arms outwards. Minor degrees of restriction caused by pain are not specific, but severe restriction is characteristic of adhesive capsulitis.
- Passive range of motion should be tested with two hands: one hand guides the movement, while the second rests on the shoulder. Many patients will subconsciously flex the spine to compensate for restricted range of motion at the shoulder; using both hands can help detect this and other abnormalities in movement at the joint.

Test for subacromial impingement

- Always compare the affected with the non-symptomatic side and make conservative judgments about muscle weakness if there is pain impeding voluntary effort.
- Most tests rely on their ability to narrow the distance between the humeral head and the CA arch, by driving the greater tuberosity under the CA arch as the humerus rotates (Fig. 2.5).
- Whether the tests are specific for lesions of the subacromial structures or for the site of **impingement** is unknown.

Movement of the glenohumeral joint

Move the glenohumeral joint passively in all directions by moving the upper arm with one hand and placing the other over the shoulder to feel for 'clunks', crepitus, and resistance to movement:

- If the humeral head can be slid anteriorly (often with a 'clunk') clearly without rotation in the glenoid it suggests instability.
- Grossly reduced passive shoulder movement (notably external rotation, with or without pain) is the hallmark of adhesive capsulitis.
- Pull down on both (hanging) arms. If the humeral head moves inferiorly (sulcus sign) there may be glenohumeral instability.

Table 2.3 Isolated muscle testing of shoulder girdle muscles

Muscle: nerve root, peripheral nerve, supply and muscle action	Muscle position	Isolated muscle test	Common pathology affecting muscle strength/bulk
Supraspinatus: C5/C6. Suprascapular nerve. Initial humeral abduction and stability of raised upper arm	From behind, seen and felt above the scapular spine at rest and when activated	Abduct arm from neutral against resistance	Tear or disuse following damage, e.g. after a fall, chronic over-use stress, or in athletes (throwing arm)
Infraspinatus: C5/C6. Suprascapular nerve. External rotation and stability of humeral head	From behind, seen and felt arising from medial scapular border passing laterally (below the scapular spine)	External rotation of arm in neutral, elbow supported and flexed at 90°	Tear or disuse following chronic damage
Serratus anterior: C5–C7. Long-thoracic nerve. Pulls the scapula forward on the thoracic wall (extends forward reach of arm)	Appreciated from behind when patient is pushing against a wall with arms outstretched in front, in that scapula remains fixed	Test by pushing wall with an outstretched arm or push-up. If paralysed there will be lifting and lateral excursion of the scapula	Damage to long-thoracic nerve from trauma. Patient may also have SAI
Deltoid: C5/C6. Axillary nerve. Flexion, extension but mainly abduction of humerus	Arises from the scapular spine and acromion, then swathes the shoulder inserting into the humerus laterally	Wasting may be obvious. Weakness in isometric strength of an arm abducted to 90°	Lesions of axillary nerve damaged by anterior shoulder dislocation (external rotation may also be weak from denervation of teres minor)

(a)

Painful arc
(active)

Action: Patient standing.
Slow arm abduction
(scapular plane).

**Positive
test:** Pain onset (maximal)
at (variable) angular
range.

(b)

Neer test
(passive)

Action: Patient sitting/standing.
Passive forward flexion.
Scapula fixed.

**Positive
test:** Pain at (variable) angle
of flexion.

(c)

Empty can
(active)

Action: Patient sitting/standing.
Active forward flexion
to 90° then internal
rotation—'can empties'.

**Positive
test:** Pain with flexion or
rotation of arm.

(d)

Kennedy–Hawkins
(passive)

FIX

Action: Patient sitting/standing.
Passive forward flexion (90°).
Fix elbow with hand.
Passive internal rotation.

**Positive
test:** Pain at some stage of
elevation or rotation.

Fig. 2.5 Tests useful for eliciting subacromial impingement.

Stress the acromioclavicular joint

Stressing the AC joint may reproduce the pain. This is conventionally done by compression or shear tests:

• These tests should not normally be painful. Although painful tests have not proved to be specific for AC pathology (pain from SAI may also be present), a positive test may provide a clue that the AC joint is arthritic, dynamically unstable, or that impingement of structures in the subacromial space under the AC joint is occurring.

• Hold the patient's arm in forward flexion (90°) and draw it across the top of the patient's chest. The resulting compression of the AC joint may produce pain. AC joint pain can also be elicited by passively elevating the arm through 180°, bringing the hand to the ceiling. Pain is experienced in the upper 10° or so of movement.

Shoulder examination with the patient supine

Examine the shoulders with the patient supine to test whether there is anterior cuff deficiency, glenohumeral joint laxity, or a labral tear: this is especially important in young adults and adolescents to identify an 'unstable shoulder'. Hold and support the upper arm held in slight abduction and external rotation (the elbow is flexed). Move the arm gently (cranially in the coronal plane) and apply gradual degrees of external rotation.

- Deficiency of anterior structures is suggested by patient apprehension that pain is imminent or that the shoulder will slip forward. With a labral tear there may be an audible or palpable 'clunk'.
- Pressure downward on the upper arm (taking the pressure off anterior shoulder structures by an anteriorly translocated humeral head) may relieve this apprehension or the pain associated with it (positive relocation test).
- An unstable shoulder identified with the above tests may denote previous traumatic injury (e.g. shoulder dislocation) or a hypermobility disorder.

Investigations

The optimum initial imaging for investigating undiagnosed shoulder pain is disputed. Some clinicians advocate management of shoulder problems based on history and examination alone. This is a practical approach to a common problem, since many problems get better in the short-term. The long-term sequelae of such management strategies, however, are unknown. Studies of shoulder pain primarily suggest that chronic shoulder problems are common, often despite initial improvement.

Radiographs

- The standard projection for screening purposes is anteroposterior (AP), although the AP axial–lateral view taken with the arm abducted may add information about the relationship of the glenoid and humeral head. Look for calcific deposits in soft-tissue basic calcium phosphate crystals: Milwaukee Shoulder (📖 Chapter 7, p 269).
- Supraspinatus outlet views are often used to assess acromial configuration and identify inferior acromial osteophytes in patients with SAI.
- If recurrent dislocation is suspected, associated humeral head defects may be identified by an AP film with internal humeral rotation or a Stryker view. Bilateral films distinguish anomaly (invariably bilateral) from abnormality.
- Bilateral AP AC joint views with the patient holding weights may identify, and grade degrees of, AC joint diastasis (separation). Distal clavicular erosion may be due to RA, hyperparathyroidism, myeloma, metastases, or post-traumatic osteolysis.
- Although characteristic patterns of abnormality are associated with SAI (Plate 2), minor age-related radiographic abnormalities are normal.

Other imaging: ultrasound, arthrography, CT arthrography, MR, isotope bone scan

- Ultrasound scoring systems for locating and grading rotator cuff tears now exist. The technique permits examination of the rotator cuff with the shoulder in different positions, but is highly operator dependent.
- Patterns of rotator cuff abnormality and subacromial impingement are well recognized with both arthrography and MR. However, there is no consensus about which of ultrasound, MR, or arthrography is most accurate for detecting rotator cuff tears.
- Children, adolescents, and young adults suspected of having unstable shoulders should have an MR examination, since detailed views of the humeral head, glenoid labrum, peri-articular glenohumeral soft tissues, and subacromial area are important.
- MR is the modality of choice in young adults when instability is diagnosed. Rotator cuff lesions and labral abnormalities are best assessed with MR. Enhancement with iv contrast may increase the chance of detecting a labral tear.
- No specific patterns of bone scan abnormality have been consistently recognized for isolated shoulder lesions, although a phase study may be diagnostic for complex regional pain syndrome in the arm.

Other investigations

- Local anaesthetic injection may help disclose the site of shoulder pain, although it is possible that by the time anaesthesia occurs the injected anaesthetic has spread to areas not intended as a target.
- Joint aspiration is essential if infection is possible. Fluid is usually aspirated easily from a grossly distended shoulder capsule. Haemarthroses can occur in degenerate shoulders (often in association with chondrocalcinosis), haemophilia, trauma, and pigmented villonodular synovitis.
- Electrophysiological tests (EMG/NCS) may confirm muscle weakness and help establish the presence of neuromuscular disease, e.g. myositis or neurological amyotrophy.
- Blood tests are required if looking for infection, inflammatory disease, etc.
- A normal creatine kinase (CK) and aldolase will rule out myositis in the majority of cases.
- Blood urea, electrolytes, creatinine, alkaline phosphatase, calcium, phosphate, thyroid function tests, and myeloma screen should be considered if metabolic bone or myopathic disease is considered.

Treatment (📖 Chapter 19, p 517 and 📖 Chapter 22, p 589)

- Physical therapy should play a focal part in encouraging mobilization of the joint, and early assessment is prudent. The following principles are recommended:
- Know whether there is an additional neck/spinal generated pain component (physical therapists are independent diagnosticians and some may erroneously aim therapy at cervicothoracic segments for individual shoulder lesions).

- Do not refer to physical therapy without knowledge of who will see the patient, and the approach that will be taken for instability and rotator cuff weakness.
- Simple analgesics are often necessary.
- Local steroid injections can be considered in the following situations:
  - tendonitis of the rotator cuff;
  - adhesive capsulitis (Plate 3);
  - AC joint pain;
  - subacromial bursitis (Plate 4).
- The principles of steroid injection and rehabilitation are dealt with in the last two sections of this chapter.
- There are several situations where local steroids should be avoided:
  - bicipital tendonitis (rest, analgesia, physical therapy);
  - the first 6 weeks of an acute rotator cuff tear;
  - when symptoms have become chronic and conservative therapy has not helped for a presumptive clinical diagnosis (This requires reassessment, imaging, and a diagnosis as surgery may be required).
- Surgical intervention may take the form of subacromial decompression arthroscopy, synovectomy of the SC joint and AC joint, or excision of the distal end of the clavicle.
  - subacromial decompression may be necessary for chronic rotator cuff tendonitis especially when imaging has shown inferior acromial osteophytes;
  - other interventions include repair of a rotator cuff or biceps tendon rupture and joint replacement (for pain relief rather than improvement in function mainly).
- Lithotripsy does not offer advantages over steroid injection and physical therapy for calcific supraspinatus tendonitis.

Pain around the elbow

Functional anatomy

- The humero-ulnar articulation is the prime (hinge) joint at the elbow. The radius also articulates with the humerus and allows forearm and hand supination/pronation, with the ulna at the elbow (Fig. 2.6).
- Normal extension results in a straight arm, but some muscular people lack the last 5–10° of extension and some (especially women) have up to an extra 10° of extension (hyperextension).
- Normal flexion is to 150–160° and forearm supination/pronation range is around 180°.
- Due to obliquity of the trochlea, extension is associated with a slight valgus that can be accentuated in women (up to 15°).
- Unilateral acute traumatic or chronic over-use lesions of the elbow are common. Bilateral symptoms may occur in these situations, but also consider the possibility of an inflammatory arthritis affecting the elbows or referred pain from the neck.

Pain may also be referred from proximal neurologic lesions in the arm, the shoulder or even from distal lesions such as carpal tunnel syndrome (CTS).

Taking a history

Is the pain exclusively located in the elbow or referred from elsewhere?

Establish whether the pain is associated with neck pain and whether it has neurogenic qualities or is associated with paraesthesias or numbness. There may be referral of pain from C6 or C7 nerve roots, shoulder lesions, or even from compression of the median nerve in the wrist.

Is there a history of acute or chronic (over-use) trauma?

- Pain at the lateral epicondyle 1–2 weeks after a weekend of 'home maintenance' might suggest lateral epicondylitis (tennis elbow) following excessive use of a screwdriver, for example.
- Other common sites of pain, where characteristic conditions related to over-use are recognized, include the medial humeral epicondyle (**'golfer's elbow'**) and the olecranon bursa (repetitive pressure/ friction). Although typically acute in onset, these conditions may develop insidiously.
- Fractures around the elbow and fractures/dislocations in the forearm are common. Dislocation of the radial head alone is rare and is usually associated with concurrent fracture of the ulna (radiographs may not easily identify the fracture). If not associated with fracture (and especially if recurrent), the condition may be associated with **generalized hypermobility** (📖 Chapter 16, p 431) or shortening of the ulna due to bone dysplasia.
- In children, a strong pull of the forearm or wrist (occurring primarily in pre-school children) can lead to a partial dislocation of the elbow (**'nursemaid's elbow'**), which can be corrected by supinating and flexing the forearm while supporting the radial head.

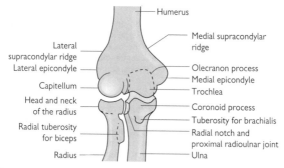

Fig. 2.6 Bony configuration at the (right) elbow (anterior view).

- In children, osteochondritis of the humeral capitellum can occur in mid to late childhood (**Panner's disease**), typically following repeated trauma.

Does the pain radiate distally?

- Forearm pain may be an additional clue to C6 or C7 radicular pain, but may also be due to the spread of musculoskeletal pain along the extensor group of muscles from lateral epicondylitis or from entrapment of the median nerve in the elbow region.
- Peritendonitis crepitans is pain, tenderness, and swelling in the forearm associated with occupational over-use. It is thought to be due to damage of the long wrist/hand flexors and extensors at the muscle–tendon junction.
- Diffuse pain in the forearm can occur as a result of over-use injury, particularly in musicians and typists, although there is overlap with regional pain syndromes.
- Pain around the forearm may also arise from inflammation at the wrist (see the next section) particularly in **De Quervain's tenosynovitis**.

Is there prominent stiffness with the pain?

- Stiffness is often non-specific but may denote inflammation such as synovitis of the joint or olecranon bursa and, therefore, raises the possibility of an autoimmune rheumatic or crystal deposition disease.
- In the middle aged and elderly, gout (📖 Chapter 7, p 269) of the olecranon bursa and surrounding soft tissues, particularly overlying the border of the ulna, is not uncommon and is often misdiagnosed as a cellulitis.

Ask about locking

Locking of the elbow either in flexion or supination/pronation may be due to loose intra-articular bodies. A single loose body is most commonly due to osteochondritis dissecans of the capitellum (e.g. in children with over-use throwing injury—**'Little League elbow'**) and multiple loose bodies are associated with OA or synovial chondromatosis.

Is the pain unremitting and severe?

This type of pain suggests bony pathology:

- Although non-fracture bone pathology is rare in the elbow region, local bony pain might suggest osteochondritis or avascular necrosis or, if part of a wider pattern of bony pain, metabolic bone disease.
- In the elderly and others at high risk for osteoporosis, supracondylar, and other fractures may occur with surprisingly little trauma.

Are there symptoms in other joints?

Ask about other joints, low back (sacroiliac) pains and risks for gout:

- Elbow synovitis alone is an uncommon presenting feature of adult RA.
- Elbow synovitis occurs in children presenting with JIA (📖 Chapter 9, p 303), but is rare (3%).
- Peri-articular enthesitis is a recognized feature of spondyloarthropathy (SpA) (📖 Chapter 8, p 281) and may mimic tennis elbow.
- The peri-articular tissue around the elbow is a moderately common site for gout.

Examination

Look for abnormality then palpate with the thumb. Observe the active, passive, and resisted active range of joint and related tendon movements, and consider examining for local nerve lesions. A complete assessment should include examination of the neck, shoulder, and wrist.

Visual inspection

Look for obvious deformity or asymmetry in the anatomical position:

- Up to 10° of extension from a straight arm is normal. More extension might suggest a hypermobility disorder.
- A child with an elbow lesion typically holds the extended arm close to the body, often in pronation.

Look for swelling or nodules:

- Swelling due to joint synovitis is difficult to see in the antecubital fossa unless it is florid: it is most easily seen (and more easily felt) adjacent to the triceps tendon insertion.
- The olecranon bursa, which may be inflamed, overlies the olecranon and does not as a rule communicate with the joint. Overlying erythema, although non-specific, may be associated with infection or gout.
- Nodules over the extensor surface or ulna border may be associated with RA (📖 Chapter 5, p 233).
- Psoriatic plaques are commonly found at the elbow extensor surface.

Observe active flexion and supination/pronation with the elbows held in 90° of flexion:

- Although the range of movement may be affected by extra-articular pain, loss of range usually implies an intra-articular disorder.

Palpate the lateral epicondyle of the humerus

- In **lateral epicondylitis (tennis elbow)** there is tenderness, which may extend a little distally. Resisted wrist and finger extension with the elbow in extension or passively stretching the tendons (make fist, flex wrist, pronate forearm, then extend elbow) may reproduce the pain.
- Lateral epicondyle tenderness may be due to inflammation of the radiohumeral bursa that lies under the extensor tendon aponeurosis.
- Note that tenderness of lateral and sometimes medial epicondyles can occur in chronic pain syndromes. In these cases, however, the relevant extensor or flexor tendon provocation tests are likely to be negative.

Palpate the medial humeral epicondyle

- Tenderness suggests traumatic **medial epicondylitis ('golfer's elbow'),** a regional or chronic pain syndrome, or enthesitis. Confirm the site of the pain by stretching the wrist flexors—supinate the forearm then passively extend both the wrist and elbow simultaneously. Resisted palmar flexion of the wrist or forearm pronation with elbow extension may also cause pain. Tasks that rely on this repetitive movement are often the provoking cause.
- Consider osteochondritis of the medial humeral epicondyle as a cause of persistent pain following an injury. The 8–15-year-old age group is at particular risk as this is a site of secondary ossification.

Passively flex and extend the elbow joint

Passively flex and extend the joint and note the range of movement and 'end-feel' (the feel of resistance at the end of the range of passive joint movement):

- 'End-feel' may tell you whether there is a block to full flexion or extension from a bony spur or osteophyte (solid end-feel) or from soft tissue thickening/fibrosis (springy, often painful).
- Note any crepitus (often associated with intra-articular pathology) and locking (may have loose bodies in the joint).

Supinate and pronate the forearm

Passively supinate and pronate the forearm supporting the elbow in 90° of flexion with your thumb over the radioulnar articulation:

- There may be crepitus or instability/subluxation associated with pain. Instability might suggest a tear or damage to the annular ligament (due to trauma or chronic/aggressive intra-articular inflammation).

Test peripheral nerve function if there are distal arm symptoms

- Given its course around the lateral epicondyle, the integrity of the radial nerve should always be tested when a lateral elbow lesion is suspected.
- The **median nerve** runs in the antecubital fossa and may be affected in traumatic elbow lesions. It is particularly susceptible where it runs between the two heads of pronator teres (from medial epicondyle and the coronoid process of the ulna) and separates into anterior interosseous and terminal median nerve branches.

- The **ulnar nerve** lies in the groove behind the medial epicondyle. Bony or soft tissue abnormality in this area may affect nerve function and lead to reduced sensation in the little finger and weakness in the small muscles of the hand, the flexor carpi ulnaris (FCU), the extensor carpi ulnaris (ECU), or the abductor digiti minimi (ADM). The median and ulnar nerves are dealt with in more detail in the later sections on wrist and hand disorders.

Investigations

Radiographs and other imaging

- Standard AP and lateral radiographs are the most straightforward way of imaging the elbow initially. CT or MR may then be needed if the diagnosis is still obscure and referred pain can be ruled out.
- Look for periosteal lesions and **enthesophytes** (new bone spurs at clear entheses like the triceps insertion). Periosteal apposition and enthesophytes are typical in psoriatic arthritis (📖 Chapter 8, p 281).
- A lateral radiograph may identify displacement of the anterior fat pad associated with a joint effusion (**sail sign**).
- Dislocations of the radial head and associated ulna fractures in children are easily missed. To make this diagnosis a high degree of suspicion and further imaging are often needed.

Needle arthrocentesis/olecranon bursocentesis

- Arthrocentesis/bursocentesis with fluid sent for microscopy and culture should always be done in suspected cases of sepsis. Fluid should be sent for polarized light microscopy in cases of bursitis that may be due to gout. Serum urate is worth requesting but may not be raised in acute gout.
- Examination of fluid for crystals should always be considered in cases of mono-arthritis in the elderly or patients on dialysis.

Electrophysiology

If nerve entrapment is suspected and there is some uncertainty after clinical examination then electrophysiological tests may provide useful information. Testing can help identify the degree and likely site of nerve damage and can help to discriminate between a peripheral and nerve root lesion.

Treatment

- The management of fractures is beyond the scope of this text.
- Epicondylitis is best managed early on with rest, splinting, analgesia, and local steroid injections. The efficacy of physical manipulation has not been proven, although there are theoretical reasons why ultrasound therapy could be of value (e.g. it passes through the myofascial planes and concentrates near bone). Resistant cases may benefit from surgery—a 'lateral release'.
- Steroid injections (Plate 5) may be of value in the following situations:
  - lateral or medial epicondylitis (hydrocortisone);
  - inflammatory arthritis (usually long acting steroid);
  - olecranon bursitis;
  - ulnar nerve entrapment.

The principles of steroid injection are dealt with later (📖 Chapter 22, p 589):

- Surgical procedures include excision of nodules and bursae, transposition of the ulnar nerve, synovectomy, excision of the head of the radius, and arthroplasty.
- Arthroplasty in inflammatory arthritis is best reserved for intractable pain and should be undertaken by an experienced surgeon. Lesser procedures such as proximal radial head excision can be effective to improve pain and function if forearm pronation and supination are poor.
- Radiation synovectomy of the elbow (Y-90 or Re-186) for inflammatory arthritis, pigmented villonodularsynovitis (PVNS), or synovial chondromatosis (📖 Chapter 18, p 489) requires ultrasound guidance (see EANM guidelines www.eanm.org).
- There are case reports for the utility of autologous blood injection for lateral epicondylitis.

Wrist pain

Functional anatomy of the wrist

- The wrist includes radiocarpal (scaphoid and lunate) and intercarpal articulations. The ulna does not truly articulate with the lunate, but is joined to it, the triquetrum, and the radius (ulnar side of distal aspect), by the triangular fibrocartilage complex.
- The intercarpal joints are joined by intercarpal ligaments and are most stable when the wrist is in full extension. Anterior carpal ligaments are stronger than posterior ones and are reinforced by the flexor retinaculum. Wrist and finger flexor tendons, the radial artery, and the median nerve enter the hand in a tunnel formed by the carpal bones and the flexor retinaculum (carpal tunnel).
- Flexion (70°), extension (70°), radial and ulnar deviation (about 20° and 30° from midline, respectively) occur at the wrist but supination/pronation of the wrist and hand is due to radiohumeral movement at the elbow.
- Flexor carpi radialis (FCR) and ulnaris (FCU) are the main flexors of the wrist, although palmaris longus (PL) also helps (Fig. 2.7). All arise from the medial humeral epicondyle.
- All carpal extensors arise from the lateral humeral epicondyle (Fig. 2.7).
- Radial deviation (abduction) occurs primarily when radial flexors and extensors act together. Ulnar deviation (adduction) occurs primarily when ulnar flexors and extensors act together.

Taking a history

Table 2.4 details the major diagnoses for painful conditions of the wrist and hand.

Determine the exact location of the pain

- Pain localizing only to the wrist most likely comes from local tissue pathology. Cervical nerve root pain as a result of a C6, C7, or C8 lesion and pain from peripheral nerve lesions is likely to be located chiefly in the hand.
- Pain at the base of the thumb, aggravated by thumb movements, in middle and old age is typical of OA (□ Chapter 6, p 259) of the trapezium-first metacarpal joint. Pain in this area might also be due to tenosynovitis of thumb tendons.

Trauma history

- Injury/post-injury conditions are common. A history of trauma is important.
- Common fractures in adults are: scaphoid and base of the first metacarpal (**Bennett's**), and head of the radius (**Colles'**).
- Distal radioulnar physeal injuries may occur in children.
- Post-traumatic chronic wrist pain following injuries may be due to ligamentous injury and chronic carpal instability or **osteonecrosis** (lunate).

(a)

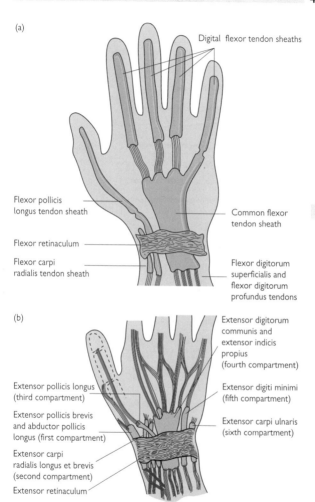

Digital flexor tendon sheaths

Flexor pollicis
longus tendon sheath

Flexor retinaculum

Flexor carpi
radialis tendon sheath

Common flexor
tendon sheath

Flexor digitorum
superficialis and
flexor digitorum
profundus tendons

(b)

Extensor digitorum
communis and
extensor indicis
propius
(fourth compartment)

Extensor pollicis longus
(third compartment)

Extensor pollicis brevis
and abductor pollicis
longus (first compartment)

Extensor carpi
radialis longus et brevis
(second compartment)

Extensor retinaculum

Extensor digiti minimi
(fifth compartment)

Extensor carpi ulnaris
(sixth compartment)

Fig. 2.7 Flexor (a) and extensor (b) tendon sheaths crossing the wrist. Flexor carpi radialis (FCR) inserts into the second and third metacarpals. Flexor carpi ulnaris (FCU) inserts into the pisiform, hamate, and fifth metacarpal. Extensor carpi radialis longus (ECRL) inserts into the base of the second, extensor carpi radialis brevis (ECRB) into the third, and extensor carpi ulnaris (ECU) into the fifth metacarpal, respectively.

Table 2.4 Painful conditions of the wrist and hand: major diagnoses

Articular disorders	Inflammatory arthritis (e.g. RA, JIA)
	Degenerative arthritis*
	Crystal arthritis
	Ligamentous lesions*
	Carpal instability (e.g. lunate dislocation)
Peri-articular disorders	De Quervain's tenosynovitis
	Tenosynovitis of common flexor/extensor tendon sheath
	Flexor pollicis tenosynovitis
	Distal flexor stenosing tenosynovitis (trigger finger or thumb)*
	Ganglia*, subcutaneous nodules, tophi
	Diabetic cheiro-arthropathy
	Dupuytren's contracture*
Bone pathology	Fracture*
	Neoplasia
	Infection
	Osteochondritis (lunate—Kienböck's; scaphoid—Prieser's) (□ Chapter 16, p 431)
Neurologic	Median nerve entrapment (carpal tunnel* or at pronator teres)
	Anterior interosseous nerve syndrome
	Ulnar nerve entrapment (cubital tunnel or in Guyon's canal in wrist)
	Posterior interosseous nerve entrapment
	Radial nerve palsy
	Brachial plexopathy
	Thoracic outlet syndrome
	Cervical nerve root irritation or entrapment*
	Reflex sympathetic dystrophy (□ Chapter 18, p 489)
	Spinal cord lesions, e.g. syringomyelia

*Common conditions.

- Unusual or florid pain descriptors suggest a **regional pain syndrome** (e.g. reflex sympathetic dystrophy). Following trauma, regional pain syndromes are not uncommon in children, adolescents, or young adults.

Are there features to suggest synovitis?

- Pain due to wrist joint synovitis may be associated with 'stiffness' and be worse at night or in the early morning. Stiffness 'in the hand' may have various causes, but these will include multiple tendon/small joint synovitis, diabetic cheirarthropathy, or even scleroderma (☐ Chapter 13, p 363).
- Wrist synovitis occurs commonly in adult RA and in children with both systemic and rheumatoid factor positive JIA. It occurs in 5% of oligo-articular JIA cases (☐ Chapter 5, p 233 and ☐ Chapter 9, p 303).
- In the elderly, wrist synovitis may be due to calcium pyrophosphate dihydrate (CPPD) crystals (☐ Chapter 7, p 269).

The quality of the pain

- Although primary bone pathology is rare, local bony pain (unremitting, severe, sleep disturbing) might suggest avascular necrosis in those at risk or, if part of a wider pattern of bony pain, metabolic bone disease (e.g. physeal pain in children with rickets) (☐ Chapter 16, p 431).
- Radicular pain may be burning in quality and is typically associated with numbness and paraesthesia. Such neurogenic pain is commonly due to nerve root irritation or compression.

Other joint/musculoskeletal symptoms

- Wrist and extensor tendon sheath synovitis is a common presenting feature of adult RA. Other joints may be affected.
- CPPD arthritis commonly involves the wrist, and can mimic RA in its joint distribution and presentation in the elderly.
- Wrist synovitis and enthesitis occurs in SpA. Pain may be considerable, although swelling is minimal. There may be inflammatory-type symptoms of spinal pain and enthesitis elsewhere.

Ask specifically about job/leisure activities

- Repetitive lateral and medial wrist movements with thumb adducted can cause tenosynovitis of the abductor pollicis longus (APL) or the extensor pollicis brevis (EPB), commonly called **De Quervain's tenosynovitis**.
- If there is no obvious history of trauma, tendonitis may be a presenting feature of a systemic autoimmune rheumatic disease or even gonococcal infection in adolescents and young adults.
- Over-use pain syndromes may occur as a result of repetitive activity. The term **'repetitive strain injury'** is controversial as discussed in the Introduction to ☐ Chapter 2, p 19. Objective assessment of pain, location of swelling, etc., from the outset is invaluable in assessing the response to treatment. Lack of objective findings (if imaging is normal) suggests a regional pain disorder.

Examination

Visual inspection

Inspect the dorsal surface of both wrists looking for swelling, deformity, or loss of muscle bulk (Plate 6):

- Diffuse swelling may be due to wrist or extensor tendon sheath synovitis.
- A prominent ulna styloid may result from subluxation at the distal radioulnar joint owing to synovitis or radioulnar ligament damage.
- Prominence ('squaring') of the trapezoid–first metacarpal joint commonly occurs in OA of this joint.
- Loss of muscle bulk in the forearm may be due to a chronic T1 nerve root lesion or disuse atrophy.

Flexion/extension range tests for major wrist lesions

- The normal range of both flexion and extension in Caucasian adults is about 70°. Synovitis invariably reduces this range.
- When wrist synovitis is present, swelling on the dorsum of the wrist may become more apparent. Substantial common flexor or extensor tendon swelling will probably also block the full range of wrist movement.
- There is normally an additional 20° of flexion and extension to the active range with passive movement.
- Elicited pain and crepitus are unlikely to be specific for any type of lesion but may draw your attention to the anatomical site of the lesion.

Examine the dorsum of the wrist in detail

- Note any abnormal excursion of the ulnar styloid associated with pain and/or crepitus suggesting synovitis.
- Post-traumatic carpal instability, particularly scapulolunate dissociation, is relatively common. The latter is demonstrated by eliciting dorsal subluxation of the proximal scaphoid pole by firm pressure on its distal pole as the wrist is deviated radially from a starting position with the forearm pronated and the wrist in ulnar deviation. Note any gap between scaphoid and lunate, and any associated tenderness.
- Note any tenderness or thickening of the common extensor tendon sheath and tendon sheath of APL and EPB.
- Tenderness at the base of the thumb may be due to wrist synovitis, carpal or carpometacarpal OA, tenosynovitis, a ganglion, or a ligament lesion.
- **Finkelstein's test** for De Quervain's tenosynovitis may be used to elicit APL/EPB tendon pain. With the thumb adducted and opposed, the fingers are curled to form a fist. Passive ulnar deviation at the wrist stretches the abnormal tendons and elicits pain. Although it is a sensitive test, it is not specific for tendon pain.
- In adults, protrusion of the thumb out of the fist on the ulnar side of the hand during the first part of this test is unusual and suggests thumb, and perhaps general, hypermobility.

Test the integrity of the tendons

Many muscles/tendons that move both the wrist and digits originate at the elbow; therefore, the quality of information gained from isolated tendon resistance tests (either for pain or strength) may be affected by pain elsewhere around the wrist, wrist deformity, or elbow lesions. Interpret findings cautiously. Useful information might be obtained by passive movement of a tendon, rather than by resisted active movement, and also by feeling for thickening or crepitus of the tendons.

Investigation and treatment

The investigation and treatment of wrist conditions is covered in the following section on symptoms in the hand.

Symptoms in the hand

Symptoms in the hand are a common presenting feature of some systemic conditions, and localized neurological and musculoskeletal lesions are common, especially in adults. Detailed knowledge of anatomy is beyond the scope of this text. Functional anatomy is important and the more common abnormalities are summarized below.

Functional anatomy of the hand

The long tendons

- Digital power is provided primarily by flexor and extensor muscles arising in the forearm. Their action is supplemented and modified by small muscles in the hand. Precise movements of the hand are mainly due to small muscles.
- Powerful digital flexors (Fig. 2.7): flexor digitorum superficialis (FDS), flexor digitorum profundus (FDP), and flexor pollicis longus (FPL).
- FDS flexes proximal interphalangeal joints (PIPs) and, more weakly, metacarpophalangeal joints (MCPs)/wrist.
- FDP flexes distal interphalangeal joints (DIPs) and, increasingly weakly, PIPs, MCPs/wrist.
- FPL flexes (at 90° to other digits) mainly the PIP, but also the whole thumb in a power grip (see below).
- Powerful digital extensors (Fig. 2.7): extensor digitorum (ED) arises from the lateral epicondyle splitting at the wrist to insert into each digital dorsal expansion (digits two to five) that attaches to all three phalanges (Fig. 2.8). The fifth digit has an additional tendon, extensor digiti minimi (EDM) that also arises at the lateral epicondyle.
- APL abducts the thumb at the MCP, provided the wrist is stable.
- EPB and EPL extend the thumb.
- Extensor indicis (EI) arises from the ulna posterior border distal to EPL and joins the index finger ED tendon.
- The muscles of the thenar eminence (Table 2.5) act synchronously. All except adductor pollicis (ulnar nerve, C8/T1) are supplied by the median nerve from C8/T1 nerve roots. All three muscles are supplied by the ulnar nerve (C8/T1).

The intrinsic muscles

- The longitudinal muscles of the palm (four dorsal and four palmar interossei and four lumbricals) all insert into digits.
- Palmar interossei, from metacarpals 1, 2, 4, and 5, insert into dorsal tendons.
- Each dorsal interosseous arises from origins on two adjacent metacarpals. The muscles abduct the second and fourth fingers and move the middle finger either medially or laterally.
- The four lumbricals (Fig. 2.9 and Table 2.6) arise from tendons of FDP in the palm passing to the lateral side of each MCP inserting into the dorsal expansions.
- The interossei combine with lumbricals to facilitate fine control of flexion and extension of MCPs and PIPs.

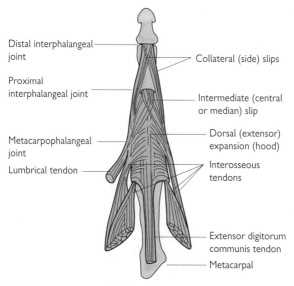

Fig. 2.8 Extensor expansion of a finger.

Table 2.5 Muscles of the thenar eminence

Muscle	Origin	Insertion
Abductor pollicis brevis	Flexor retinaculum, scaphoid, and trapezium	Thumb proximal phalanx and dorsal expansion
Flexor pollicis brevis	Flexor retinaculum, trapezium, trapezoid, and capitate	Thumb proximal phalanx (base of radial side)
Opponens pollicis	Flexor retinaculum and tubercle of the trapezium	First metacarpal (lateral border)
Adductor pollicis	Capitate, bases of second/third metacarpals and distal third metacarpal	Thumb proximal phalanx (medial side)

Grip
- For power, the wrist extends and adducts slightly, and the long digital flexors contract.
- A modified power grip, the hook grip, is used to carry heavy objects like a suitcase. The thumb is extended out of the way and extension at MCPs accompanies flexion at PIPs/DIPs.

- More precision in the grip can be obtained using varying degrees of thumb adduction, abduction, and flexion. The thumb can be opposed with any of the four other digits depending on the shape of the object to be held and the type of manipulation required.

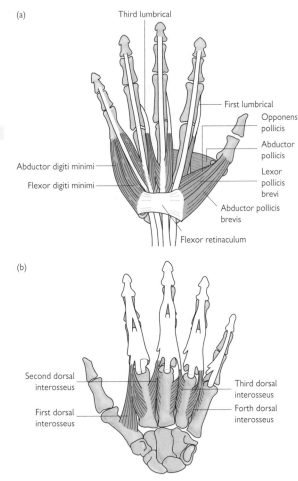

Fig. 2.9 (a) Lumbrical muscles and muscles of the thenar and hypothenar eminences. (b) Dorsal interossei.

Table 2.6 Muscles of the hypothenar eminence

Muscle	Origin	Insertion
Abductor digiti minimi	Flexor retinaculum (FR), pisiform, and pisohamate ligament	Base of the fifth proximal phalanx and dorsal expansion
Flexor digiti minimi Brevis	Flexor retinaculum and Hook of hamate	Base of the fifth proximal phalanx
Opponens digiti minimi	Flexor retinaculum and Hook of hamate	Medial side of the fifth metacarpal

Taking a history

A history of acute or over-use trauma with subsequent localized symptoms requires a straightforward application of anatomical knowledge, precise examination, and judicious choice of imaging techniques for diagnosis. However, there are more subtle or less easily delineated patterns of symptoms in the hand, particularly when pain is diffuse or poorly localized.

Is the pain associated with immobility or stiffness?

- Stiffness may be associated with joint or tendon synovitis but is not specific. Prompting may provide more accurate localization of symptoms.
- If unilateral, especially on the dominant hand, be suspicious that diffuse hand pain may be due to a regional pain syndrome.

Is stiffness local or diffuse?

- Patterns of joint involvement in autoimmune rheumatic disease and polyarticular arthritis are summarized in 📖 Chapter 3, p 149.
- If localized in the palm, there may be **Dupuytren's contracture** (associated with diabetes). If diffuse, there may be thickening of soft tissue from a systemic process, e.g. hypothyroidism, scleroderma, diabetic cheiro-arthropathy, or disorders of mucopolysaccharide metabolism (the latter especially in infants, although Fabry's syndrome can present in adulthood associated with acroparasthesias and palmar telangiectasia).
- Stiffness due to an upper motor neuron lesion (an interpretation of increased tone) is unlikely to be confined to the hand and is likely to be associated with weakness. The pattern of symptoms over time should give a clue to its aetiology.

Are there neurologic qualities to the pain or characteristics typical of a common nerve lesion?

- 'Burning' or 'deep' episodic pain varying with head, neck, and upper spinal position is typical of cervical nerve root pain. Ask about occupation and other activities that are associated with neck problems, the relationship with sleep posture, and frequent headaches.

- Pain on the radial side of the hand waking the patient at night and often relieved, at least partially, by shaking the hand is typical of median nerve entrapment in the wrist. However, pain in this condition is often poorly localized at initial presentation. Remember other lesions that produce pain in the area around the thumb base: trapezoid–first metacarpal joint OA, tenosynovitis of APL/EPB (De Quervain's) or EPL, referred pain from a C6 nerve root lesion, and ligament lesions (e.g. ulnar collateral ligament of first MCP—**'skier's thumb'**).

Tingling/pins and needles/numbness
Make sure both you and the patient understand what you each mean by these terms:
- Symptoms usually denote cervical nerve root or peripheral nerve irritation/compression, although they can reflect underlying ischaemia.
- Tingling in the fingertips of both hands, however, is recognized to occur commonly in patients diagnosed with fibromyalgia.
- Symptoms associated primarily with specific positions of the whole arm may be due to thoracic outlet compression of neurovascular structures.

Pain arising from bone
Pain in the hands arising from bones may be difficult to discriminate. Radiographs will often lead to confirmation of the diagnosis:
- The most common tumour in the hand is an enchondroma. It is usually painless. If they are painful, then one should suspect infarction or malignant change.
- Secondary metastases and malignant bone tumours in the hand are rare, but must be ruled out in children, adolescents, and young adults with persistent localized bone pain.
- Paget's disease of hand bones can occur, but is relatively rare.
- Digital bone pain from osteomalacia/rickets occurs, but is unusual at presentation.
- Digital pain may rarely be due to sarcoidosis, hyperparathyroid bone disease, thyroid acropathy, hypertrophic (pulmonary) osteoarthropathy (HO), or pachydermoperiostitis. Look for clubbing.

Ischaemic pain?
A history suggestive of ischaemic pain in the hands is rare in rheumatologic practice. Persistent ischaemic digital pain is a medical emergency:
- Digital vasomotor instability [e.g. **Raynaud's phenomenon** (RP); 📗 Chapter 13, p 363] is episodic, triggered by cold and emotion, and characterized by digital colour changes: white/blue then red.
- Pain from vasculitis is likely to be persistent and associated with a purpuric rash, nail-fold infarcts, or splinter haemorrhages.
- Ischaemic pain associated with cervicothoracic posture or prolonged arm elevation manoeuvres may be due to a lesion of the thoracic outlet.
- Pain may be due to thromboembolism (e.g. antiphospholipid syndrome), infective endocarditis, or thrombo-arteritis obliterans (**Buerger's disease**).

'Swelling'

Examination is more reliable than a history:

- Apart from isolated lesions, such as **ganglia**, patients' description of soft tissue or joint swelling may be unreliable and should be substantiated by examination. Nerve lesions can give the impression that swelling is present (think what a dentist's local anaesthetic does for your lip!). Patients with **carpal tunnel syndrome**, for example, frequently complain of the hand swelling at night.

'Weakness'

Ask about trauma, neck, and median nerve entrapment symptoms:

- Acute tendon injuries are common industrial accidents. Chronic occupational over-use may also lead to rupture.
- If weakness is profound and there has been no obvious trauma, the cause is likely to be neuromuscular.
- If not associated with pain, weakness is more likely to be neurological than musculoskeletal in origin.
- Weakness associated with pain may be due to a neurological or musculoskeletal lesion, the latter situation often due to an inability to use the hand (or part of it) because of pain or an alteration in biomechanical function as a result of deformity, which may only be slight.
- True weakness associated with stiffness is associated with myelopathy or even motor neuron disease. A detailed history of the progression of symptoms is important and neurologic examination should be thorough.

Trigger finger

This may denote **stenosing tenosynovitis** of a digital flexor tendon. Damage to the tendon and its sheath can result in a fibrous nodule attached to the tendon that moves and catches under the proximal annular ligament just distal to the MCP. It may not be painful. This most commonly affects the middle and ring fingers, and is prevalent among professional drivers, cyclists, and those in occupations requiring repeated use of hand-held heavy machinery.

Examination

The sequence below is comprehensive, but should be considered if a general condition is suspected. Often an examination only needs to be more specifically directed.

Inspection of the nails and fingers

- Pits/ridges and **dactylitis** are associated with psoriatic arthritis (Plate 7 and 📖 Chapter 8, p 281).
- Splinter haemorrhages may be traumatic, but are associated with infective endocarditis or **vasculitis** (📖 Chapter 15, p 405).
- Obvious cuticle damage and punctate cuticle erythema (dilated capillary loops) are features of secondary Raynaud's phenomenon or scleroderma (Plate 8).
- Peri-ungual erythema is associated with a number of autoimmune rheumatic and connective tissue diseases.
- Multiple telangiectasias are associated with limited cutaneous systemic sclerosis (📖 Chapter 13, p 363).

- Diffuse finger thickening (dactylitis) may be due to gross tendon thickening (e.g. SpA or sarcoid), or connective tissue fibrosis/thickening (scleroderma, cheiro-arthropathy). Bony or soft-tissue DIP or PIP swelling should be discriminated.
- A shiny/waxy skin appearance, often pale, may indicate scleroderma.
- Scattered, tiny, non-blanching dark red punctate lesions are typical of cutaneous skin vasculitis.
- Erythematous or violacious scaly papules/plaques over MCPs or PIPs may suggest dermatomyositis (📖 Chapter 14, p 385).

Note any diffuse swelling of the hand
- Diffuse soft-tissue/skin swelling, may occur in association with RA, **RS₃PE syndrome**, JIA, reflex sympathetic dystrophy -CRPS1 (Plate 9), and scleroderma.
- RS₃PE (remitting seronegative symmetric synovitis with pitting oedema), which presents mainly in adults in their 70s, may be a distinct type of non-erosive polyarticular/tendon synovitis, but may be associated with other, often haematological, conditions.
- Swelling associated with -CRPS1 may be localized or diffuse (Plate 9). Skin may be shiny and later there is often a dark red or blue mottled appearance.
- Typical skin appearances are critical to making a clinical diagnosis of scleroderma. The skin may be initially puffy, but later shiny and tight and, with progression, atrophic with contractures.

Note any muscle wasting
Wasting may be due to a degree of chronic denervation (e.g. the thenar eminence in CTS), disuse atrophy (e.g. painful polyarthropathy, joint hypo-mobility), or catabolism of muscle (e.g. polymyositis, RA). In the elderly there may be age-related muscle loss ('sarcopenia').

Note any deformity of digits
- Deformities tend to occur with long-standing polyarticular joint disease, e.g. OA, severe RA, and psoriatic arthritis.
- Isolated deformities may be due to previous bone or tendon trauma, severe neurological lesions and Dupuytren's contracture. A **mallet finger** (loss of active DIP extension) is due to rupture of the distal extensor tendon expansion usually due to direct trauma.

Inspect the palm and dorsum of the hand
- Palmar erythema is not specific, but is associated with autoimmune disorders of connective tissue and joints.
- Check for Dupuytren's contracture (fascial thickening on ulnar side).
- On the dorsum of the hand, ganglia and swelling of the common extensor tendon sheath are usually easily noted. Swelling of the extensor tendon sheath is commonly associated with RA in adults.

Palpation of joints and nodules
Palpation of joints and nodules is best done using thumb pads with the patient's wrist supported:
- Swelling should be noted for site, consistency, tenderness, and mobility. Osteophytes and exostosis are peri-articular or at sites of pressure, may be tender, but are always fixed (Plate 6d).

- **Ganglia** are hard and usually quite mobile (can occur anywhere).
- **Rheumatoid nodules** (occur anywhere, but typically on the dorsum of the hand and the extensor surface of the elbow) and tophi (usually distal) are rubbery, hard, relatively fixed, but may be moved (Plate 6a).
- Synovitis is often represented by soft ('boggy'), often springy, swelling around a joint. It may be tender and warm but this is not invariable.
- Synovitis in a single joint may be due to autoimmune rheumatic disease, OA, infection, or foreign-body synovitis (e.g. rose thorn synovitis).

Palpate tendons in the palm or on the volar aspect of the phalanges
- Thickening, tenderness, and crepitus suggest **tenosynovitis**, but tenosynovitis can be hard to spot if it is mild. Tethering and thickening of tendons in the palm associated with excessive digital flexion when the hand is at rest and a block to passive finger extension suggests chronic flexor tenosynovitis (take care to note any contributory joint damage).
- Passive tendon movement by gently flexing/extending a proximal phalanx may disclose palpable tendon nodules, crepitus and tenderness.

Discriminate Dupuytren's contracture from flexor tendonopathy
Dupuytren's contracture typically involves the fourth and fifth fingers (40% bilateral). It is common in males aged 50–70. The fascia extends to the second phalanx, thus, if severe, the condition causes fixed flexion of MCPs and PIPs. It is associated with epilepsy, diabetes, and alcoholism, and usually is not painful.

Investigation of wrist and hand disorders
Radiographs
- An AP view of the hand and wrist is a useful screening investigation to characterize a polyarthropathy and diagnose traumatic and metabolic bone lesions (Table 2.7).
- Radiographs may reveal soft tissue swelling around joints compatible with a diagnosis of synovitis.
- Radiographs are insensitive for identifying erosions in early autoimmune joint disease.
- An oblique view of the hand may add information about joint erosions if an erosive MCP arthritis is considered.
- Lateral and carpal tunnel views of the carpus can be obtained by varying the degree of X-ray projection angle; however, unless searching for evidence of fracture these views are rarely needed.

Further imaging: US, MR, and isotope bone scan
- In experienced hands, US can be a useful way of looking for early synovitis and patterns of abnormality in association with median nerve entrapment.
- MR may demonstrate a torn or avulsed triangular cartilage in patients with a post-traumatic painful wrist or with carpal instability.
- MR images of the carpal tunnel are especially useful in confirming median nerve compression/tethering and soft tissue wrist pathology, particularly when symptoms recur after carpal tunnel release surgery.
- MR can provide valuable information about the degree and distribution of inflammatory disease in joints and tendons, particularly in children and patients where history and examination are difficult.

- MR is more sensitive than radiography in identifying joint erosions in RA. Choosing MR over US depends on availability and sonographer experience.
- Isotope bone scan is not specific for any single condition, but in young adults (after closure of epiphyses and before OA is likely) it may be useful for disclosing patterns of inflammation at and around joints. ^{99m}Tc-labelled human immunoglobulin may be more specific for detecting patterns of synovitis in children and adults.

Table 2.7 Some conditions/features that may be diagnosed on simple AP hand/wrist radiographs

Bone conditions	Fractures (e.g. scaphoid, base of first metacarpal)
	Tumours
	Metabolic bone diseases (e.g. rickets, hyperparathyroidism)
	Avascular necrosis (e.g. post-traumatic—lunate, sickle cell disease)
	Sarcoidosis (📖 Chapter 18, p 489)
Specific features	Cartilage damage (joint space loss and subchondral bone changes)
	Articular erosions
	Osteophytes
	Infection (cortex loss, patchy osteolysis)
	Calcium deposition in joint (e.g. triangular ligament chondrocalcinosis)
	Soft tissue swelling (e.g. over ulnar styloid in wrist synovitis)
	Peri-articular osteoporosis (associated with joint inflammation)
	Carpal dislocation (e.g. lunate displacement in chronic carpal pain)
Polyarticular/overall patterns of radiological abnormality	OA (distribution of osteophytes and subchondral bone changes)
	RA, JIA (e.g. deformities, erosion appearance/distribution)
	Psoriatic arthritis (e.g. deformities, erosion appearance—DIPs)
	CPPD arthritis/gout (e.g. erosion appearance in gout) (📖 Chapter 7, p 269)

Laboratory investigations
- *FBC, ESR, CRP:* The characteristic, although non-specific, picture in patients with a systemic inflammatory condition such as RA or polyarticular JIA, is mild anaemia with normal red cell indices, high or high normal platelets, and increased acute phase response. Lymphopenia frequently accompanies autoimmune disease. Neutrophils are raised in infection, with steroids, and in systemic JIA or adult Still's disease (📖 Chapter 9, p 303).
- Blood urea, electrolytes, creatinine, and urate will detect hyperuricaemia and renal impairment associated with gout (📖 Chapter 7, p 269). Blood calcium, phosphate, albumin, vitamin D, alkaline phosphatase, and PTH will screen for metabolic bone disease (📖 Chapter 16, p 431).
- Rheumatoid factor (RF) and anticyclic citrullinated peptide (CCP) are useful for diagnosing rheumatoid arthritis. Antinuclear antibody (ANA) and a screen of extractable nuclear antibodies (ENAs) may be helpful for the evaluation of a number of disorders, including SLE and scleroderma.
- In children with JIA, a positive ANA is associated with a risk of uveitis.
- Other investigations to consider: serum angiotensin converting enzyme (sACE) for sarcoidosis, glycosylated haemoglobin in diabetics, serum, and urinary protein electrophoresis for myeloma.

Other investigations
- Neurophysiology (EMG/NCS) is a useful adjunct to clinical examination in diagnosis of upper limb neuropathies.
- Joint/bursa fluid aspiration is mandatory in suspected cases of sepsis and should be sent for culture and microscopy. Crystal arthropathy should also be considered.

Treatment of wrist and hand disorders

Treatment for specific diseases is considered in Parts 2 and 3. Management of the soft tissue lesions in the hand and wrist, like elsewhere, combines periods of rest and splinting with active physical therapy, avoidance of repetitive activity, and analgesia. In most cases, the condition will resolve spontaneously, but severe or persistent pain and disability may warrant input from a hand occupational therapist, local steroid injections, or occasionally surgical soft tissue decompression.
- Conditions that respond to local steroid therapy include:
  - tenosynovitis e.g. De Quervain's;
  - tendon nodules and ganglia;
  - flexor tenosynovitis (and trigger finger);
  - Dupuytren's contracture;
  - carpal tunnel syndrome;
  - synovitis: radiocarpal and radioulnar at the wrist, MCPs and PIPs, first carpometacarpal.
- The accuracy of needle placement is likely to be improved by US guidance; however, greater efficacy from such an approach over blind injection has not yet been shown.
- The principles of steroid injection are dealt with in 📖 Chapter 22, p 589.

- Functional evaluation (from a physical and occupational therapist) is likely to be of use in cases of polyarthropathy. Early use of splints, orthotics, and exercises may lead to greater functional ability and a decrease in symptoms.
- Surgical options for the hand and wrist may include:
  - fusion or resection of the carpal bones;
  - ulna styloidectomy and wrist synovectomy (RA);
  - tendon repair and transfer operations (RA);
  - synovectomy of joints and/or tendons (RA);
  - fusion of small joints;
  - PIP/MCP replacements;
  - Dupuytren's release/fasciectomy;
  - carpal tunnel release;
  - trapeziectomy for thumb CMC joint OA.

Many of these procedures primarily reduce pain; function may not be restored.

Upper limb peripheral nerve lesions

Background

- Upper limb peripheral nerve lesions are common. Most are entrapment neuropathies. Occasionally, nerve trauma may present to primary care providers or rheumatologists with (primarily) regional muscle weakness.
- Although not specific for its diagnosis, the **triad of pain, paraesthesia, and weakness is suggestive of nerve entrapment**. Features may be considered more specific for nerve entrapment if there is a history of acute or over-use trauma proximal to the distribution of the symptoms.
- Lesions may characteristically occur in association with specific activities, occupations, or sports (e.g. ulnar neuropathy in cyclists).
- Accurate diagnosis relies on demonstration of the anatomic lesion. Useful in this respect is knowledge of likely sites of entrapment or damage and, in the case of entrapment, the ability to elicit a positive Tinnel's sign (i.e. percussion over the site of entrapment eliciting sensory symptoms in the appropriate nerve distribution).
- Always compare examination findings in both upper limbs.
- Neurophysiologic examination (NCS) is an adjunct to clinical diagnosis. It should not be relied on to make a diagnosis in the absence of good clinical assessment.
- MR techniques and their interpretation are becoming increasingly more sophisticated in identifying patterns of abnormality in these disorders.

The long thoracic nerve

- Entrapment is in the differential diagnosis of painless shoulder weakness. The nerve origin is at C5–C7, and its course runs beneath the subscapularis and into the serratus anterior.
- Muscle paralysis is often painless and implies loss of the last 30° of overhead arm extension, disrupted scapular rhythm, and scapula winging. Winging is demonstrated by inspection from behind with the patient pressing against a wall with an outstretched arm.
- Damage to the nerve occurs typically from an anterior direct blow or brachial plexus injury. Damage sometimes occurs after carrying heavy backpacks (e.g. army recruits) or after surgical resection of a cervical rib.
- It can also occur spontaneously after infection. There is no specific treatment.

The suprascapular nerve

- The nerve origin is at roots C4–C6; its course is lateral and deep to the trapezius, through the suprascapular notch, terminating in the supraspinatus and posteriorly in the infraspinatus. It carries pain fibers from the glenohumeral joint and AC joint.
- Impingement of the nerve at the suprascapular notch should be considered in a patient complaining of shoulder pain despite a normal examination and imaging tests.
- Injury to the nerve often gives diffuse shoulder pain, although painless paralysis of the muscles can occur.

- Injury is often thought to occur from repeated stretching of the nerve at the notch. Weightlifters are prone to bilateral injury and volleyball players prone to dominant side injury.
- Compression by ganglia or tumours occurs and can be confirmed by MR.

Ulnar nerve

The ulnar nerve originates from C8 and T1. It lies along the medial side of the brachial artery in the upper arm, then above the medial humeral epicondyle where it passes posteriorly, piercing the medial intermuscular septum. It then runs behind the elbow in a groove between the olecranon and medial epicondyle, covered by a fibrous sheath and arcuate ligament (cubital tunnel). Following the line of the ulna in the flexor compartment of the forearm, branches supply the flexor digitorum profundus (FDP) and the flexor carpi ulnaris (FCU). The nerve enters the hand on the ulnar side dividing into superficial (palmaris brevis and skin over the medial one and a half digits) and deep (small muscles of the hand) branches:

- Lesions are usually due to entrapment.
- The ulnar nerve is occasionally damaged in the relatively exposed cubital tunnel (**cubital tunnel syndrome**) resulting in pain and paraesthesia along the medial forearm, wrist, and fourth/fifth digits. Damage may occur from direct trauma, compression, or recurrent subluxation. The Tinnel test at the elbow may be positive and there might be sensory loss over the palmar aspect of the fifth digit.
- There are a number of sites where entrapment of the ulnar nerve may occur around the wrist, either proximal to the volar carpal ligament or beneath it or the pisohamate ligament. External compression, acute or recurrent trauma, and ganglia are the usual causes. Symptoms have been noted in cyclists, users of pneumatic or vibrating tools, and in avid videogame players. Entrapment of the purely sensory cutaneous branch can occur from excessive computer mouse use.
- Motor weakness may be most evident by observing general muscle wasting in the hand (hypothenar eminence, interossei, adductor pollicis) and flexion deformity of the fourth and fifth digits—the latter caused by third and fourth lumbrical weakness (Plate 10).
- Flexion of the wrist with ulnar deviation (FCU) and thumb adduction may be weak (adductor pollicis weakness will be evident if you ask the patient to 'run the thumb across the base of the fingers' as normally it can sweep across touching the skin).
- Froment's sign also signifies weakness of the adductor pollicis, and is demonstrated by a weakness in holding paper between the thumb and the index finger when both are in the sagittal plane.
- Discrimination of a wrist site from an elbow site of nerve entrapment is helped by the site of a positive Tinnel test, preservation of power of wrist flexion/medial deviation (FCU) in a wrist lesion, and electrophysiology.
- Rest, analgesia, and occasionally local steroids are helpful. A review of posture, repetitive activity, and a biomechanical assessment with changes in activities and technique are recommended. Surgical decompression may also be necessary.

Radial nerve

The nerve origin is at roots C5–C8, and its course runs anterior to sub-scapularis then passes behind the humerus in a groove that runs between the long and medial heads of triceps. It then winds anteriorly around the humeral shaft to lie between brachialis and brachioradialis. In the flexor compartment of the arm it divides at the level of the lateral epicondyle into superficial branch (cutaneous/sensory) and the posterior interosseous nerve (PIN), which runs through the supinator muscle into the forearm to supply the extensor compartment muscles:

- Entrapment needs to be considered in those cases of shoulder or upper arm trauma, where subsequent presentation includes arm and wrist weakness.
- Compression of the radial nerve in the upper arm causes stiffness in the dorsal arm and forearm, weakness of the wrist, and little finger extension. The triceps is usually unaffected as nerve supply to the muscle leaves the radial nerve proximally.
- Transient compression of the nerve at the site of the medial head of triceps has been described in tennis players.
- Compression can occur as the nerve pierces the lateral intermuscular septum just distal to the radial head and also where the PIN pierces the supinator.
- At this lower site, compression is often a consequence of trauma, may be associated with a positive Tinnel test and local tenderness, and the pain may be reproduced by extreme passive forearm pronation combined with wrist flexion. Symptoms may mimic those of lateral epicondylitis. Surgical exploration may be necessary to confirm a diagnosis.

Median nerve

The nerve origin is from C6–T1 nerve roots. Its course from the brachial plexus runs together with the brachial artery in the upper arm (supplying nothing) then enters the forearm between the two heads of pronator teres (from medial humeral epicondyle and coronoid process of the ulna). It runs deep in the forearm dividing into median and anterior interosseous branches. The median branch enters the hand beneath the flexor retinaculum on the radial side of the wrist. All pronator and flexor muscles in the forearm (except FCU and the medial half of FDP) are supplied by the two branches. The median supplies sensory nerves to the radial side of the hand:

- Entrapment syndrome at the wrist is very common; **carpal tunnel syndrome** (CTS).
- In the rare **pronator syndrome**, trauma, swelling, or masses between the two pronator heads can cause entrapment giving lower arm pain, paraesthesias, and weakness of forearm pronation. There is local tenderness and reproduction of pain from resisted forearm pronation or wrist flexion.
- Pain in CTS is often present at night and relieved by exercising the hand. Daytime symptoms can persist. Pain can be referred up the arm even to the shoulder. Sensory symptoms are confined to the radial three and a half digits.

- Clumsiness is a common early feature of CTS.
- Symptoms reproduced by a positive Tinnel's sign (percussion over the volar aspect of the wrist) and Phalen's manoeuver (volar aspect of the wrist rested on the back of a chair and the hand allowed to fall loosely under gravity, held for 1 min) indicates nerve compression.
- A severe or chronic lesion is associated with sensory testing abnormality (Fig. 2.10) and motor weakness of the abductor pollicis brevis (APB), opponens pollicis, and the first and second lumbricals.
- Nerve conduction studies are indicated if the diagnosis is uncertain, the condition is progressive, motor neuron disease is suspected (thenar muscle wasting marked/progressive with minimal sensory symptoms), dual pathology is suspected, surgical decompression is being considered, and in cases of surgical failure. False negative results occur in 10% of cases.
- MR appears to be more sensitive than US for detecting abnormalities involving the median nerve in or around the carpal tunnel.
- Aetiology of CTS is debated, but probably multifactorial. The following are associated: Colles' fracture, trauma, carpal OA, diabetes, inflammatory joint/tendon disease (e.g. RA, scleroderma), ganglia, menopause and pregnancy. Hypothyroidism, acromegaly, amyloid, and benign tumours are also associated with CTS.

Treatment of carpal tunnel syndrome

- Night splinting may be curative, especially early in the condition.
- NSAIDs are helpful if there is underlying inflammatory disease.
- Local steroid injections are of value. If partial remission is achieved consider repeating the injection (Plate 11).
- Surgical decompression is indicated when there is failure of conservative therapy, progressive/persistent neurological changes, or muscle atrophy/weakness.
- Failure of surgical release of the carpal tunnel requires further consideration of underlying causes such as a ganglion or other soft tissue lesion. Reconsider also whether there really is a mechanical/local or perhaps a more subtle cause (e.g. mononeuritis or peripheral neuropathy, entrapment at the pronator or nerve root lesion).

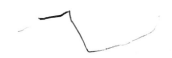

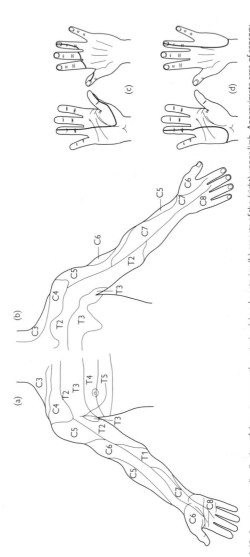

Fig. 2.10 Approximate distribution of dermatomes on the anterior (a) and posterior (b) aspects of the (right) upper limb. Approximate area of sensory change in lesions of the median (c) and ulnar (d) nerves.

Thoracic back and chest pain

Background

- The thoracic segment (T1–T12) moves less than the lumbar and cervical spine. Segmental movement in any direction is about 6°. However, given the number of segments this can add up to appreciable mobility overall. Less segmental movement results in reduced frequency of problems overall (only 6% of patients attending a spinal clinic have thoracic spine problems).
- Ribs (1–10) articulate posteriorly with vertebrae at two points: the articular facet of the rib head with the costovertebral facet on each vertebral body and the articular facet of the rib tubercle with the costotransverse facet on each vertebral lateral process. These are both synovial joints. Ribs 11 and 12 do not have costotransverse joints.
- The ribs, each continuous with its costal cartilage, articulate anteriorly by a synovial joint with the manubrium (1–2), sternum (2–7), each costal cartilage above (8–10), or do not articulate (11/12—'floating ribs').
- A massive block of spinal extensor muscles is responsible for maintaining the body against gravity. Some extend over some distance (e.g. the spinalis thoracis from the upper thoracic to the mid-lumbar spinous processes).
- Dermatomes are circumferential and extend from T2 at the clavicles to T10 at the umbilicus. However, up to five nerve roots may contribute innervation of any one point in a truncal dermatome.

Taking a history

The interpretation of cardiac, oesophageal, or pleural chest pain as musculoskeletal in origin is a common occurrence. It may result in missing a serious condition (Tables 2.8 and 2.9):

- A review of the patterns of quality and radiation of cardiac and oesophageal pain in the clinical context should always be considered.
- Pleuritic pain is common. Chronic pulmonary emboli may be underdiagnosed and have serious consequences. Any inflammatory, infective, or infiltrative pleural lesion will be painful.
- Lesions confined to pulmonary parenchyma do not produce pain.
- Pericardial pain can be misinterpreted as musculoskeletal or pleuritic.
- Mediastinal abnormalities can produce pain that is often referred.

The interpretation of neurogenic or musculoskeletal chest pains as cardiogenic, oesophageal, or pleural is a common occurrence and may lead to unnecessary investigations. Take a good history:

- Thoracic spine lesions can result in referred anterolateral chest pain.
- Costovertebral and costotransverse joint dysfunction is relatively common and is generally age-related, but can occur in anyone with spinal deformity. It may produce thoracic spine pain alone or result in an extensive pattern of radiation of pain over the back, lateral, and anterior chest wall.

Table 2.8 Characteristics of chest pain from non-neurological and non-musculoskeletal pathology

Process	Characteristics of pain
Angina	Gradual onset often related to exercise, a heavy meal, or emotion. Squeezing, strangling, or constriction in chest, can be aching or burning in nature. Commonly substernal, but radiates to any of anterior chest, interscapular area, arms (mainly left), shoulders, teeth, and abdomen. Reduces with rest and sublingual nitrates
Myocardial infarction	Similar to above regarding quality and distribution. Longer duration. Less easily relieved
Pericardial inflammation	Sharp or steady substernal pain. Can be referred to shoulder tip, anterior chest, upper abdomen, or back. Often has a pleural component and is altered by change in position—sharper more left-sided when supine but eased by leaning forward
Aortic dissection	Acute onset with extremely severe peak. Felt in centre of chest or back. Lasts for hours
Pleuritic inflammation	Common. Sharp, knife-like, superficial. Aggravated by deep inspiration, sneezing, or coughing. If accompanied by haemoptysis consider pulmonary embolism
Mediastinal conditions	Empyema or surgical emphysema may be intense and sharp and radiate from substernal to shoulder area. Associated with crepitus. Mediastinitis and tumour pain resembles pleural pain. May have constant feeling of constriction/oppression
Peptic disease	Penetrating duodenal ulcers can cause intense, persistent mid-thoracic back pain
Oesophageal reflux	Persistent retrosternal burning is typical. Often post-prandial, when lying or at night/early morning. Oesophageal spasm can be similar to angina and can cause mid-thoracic back pain, but reflux symptoms often co-exist

- Lower cervical spine lesions can refer pain to the anterior chest wall.
- Many painful chest conditions are associated with radiation of the pain down the left arm. This pattern is not specific for myocardial ischaemia.
- Lower cervical pain may be referred to the interscapular region.
- Interscapular pain may also be associated with mechanical lumbar disorders. Unlike infection, tumours, and fracture, referred pain is eased or abolished by changes in position or posture.

Table 2.9 Painful neurological and musculoskeletal conditions of the thoracic spine and chest wall

Thoracic vertebral disease	Osteoporotic or pathological fracture
	Tumours, e.g. osteoid osteoma, metastasis
	Osteomyelitis
	Page's disease
	Osteomalacia, rickets
	Costovertebral joint dysfunction
Nerve irritation	Root irritation/compression from disc prolapse or osteophyte at exit foramen, from structure distal to exit foramen, or from neuroma
Biomechanical/ degenerative	Scoliosis (non-structural compensatory, structural)
	Diffuse idiopathic skeletal hyperostosis (DISH)
	Calcium pyrophosphate dihydrate disease (of ligamentum flavum)
Herpes-Zoster of intercostal nerve	
Chest wall/superficial lesions	Rib fracture
	Other rib lesions, e.g. tumours, fibrous dysplasia, osteomalacia
	Costochondritis/enthesitis (e.g. PsA)
	Intercostal muscle tear/strain
	Mastitis or fibrocystic disease of the breast
	Myofascial pain and fibromyalgia
	Parietal pleural inflammation/infection/infiltration
Spondyloarthropathy (e.g. ankylosing spondylitis)	Spinal inflammation
	Acute discitis
	Chronic indolent discitis
Scheuermann's osteochondritis	In adolescents only

If there is thoracic back pain alone and it is acute and/or severe consider osteoporotic fracture, tumours, and infection:
- Osteoporotic vertebral collapse is common in post-menopausal women. An acute, non/minimal-trauma-associated severe pain is typical. Fractures occur in many other situations, e.g. AS or a neoplastic bone lesion.
- Spinal infections should not be missed. The most common are *Staphylococcus aureus*, *Brucella*, and *Mycobacterium tuberculosis* (🕮 Chapter 17, p 473).

Ask about the quality of pain
- Musculoskeletal pain (local or referred) generally associates with specific movements, positions, or postures, and is reproducible.
- Pain that increases with coughing, sneezing, or deep inspiration, is suggestive of pleural lesions. Rib and intercostal lesions or costovertebral joint dysfunction may also cause this sort of pain.

Ask about other symptoms and risk factors
- The pain from a fracture/lesion (osteoporotic, malignancy, infection) is often localized and extreme, waking the patient at night.
- Acute or chronic thoracic spine lesions may be associated with cord compression. Ask about recent change in sphincter function and progressive lower limb stiffness or heaviness.
- Risks for **osteoporosis** (📖 Chapter 16, p 431).
- Systemic symptoms of fever (osteomyelitis).
- Bone pain elsewhere (metastases, **osteomalacia, Paget's disease**).
- Spinal pain in adolescence (for an adult with kyphosis/spinal pain).
- A positive family history is recognized in idiopathic juvenile scoliosis, osteoporosis, and generalized osteoarthritis (📖 Chapter 6, p 259).
- Depression and anxiety are important modulators of pain. However, although thoracic back and chest pains may be psychogenic, it is unwise to settle on this diagnosis without excluding musculoskeletal conditions and diseases of viscera that can cause referred pain.

Examination

Visual inspection
Observe the patient (who has undressed down to their underwear) from the back and front. Look for deformity, asymmetry, swellings, and note the respiratory pattern:
- Any **scoliosis** should be noted. Non-structural scoliosis is frequently due to posture, severe back or abdominal pain, leg length discrepancy, and, rarely, can be psychogenic. Structural scoliosis may be due to various lesions at any age (See 'Spinal Disorders in Children and Adolescents,' 📖 Chapter 2, p 19).
- There is a normal mild thoracic kyphos; however, marked kyphos in adults (particularly post-menopausal women) might suggest multiple osteoporotic vertebral fractures or degenerative disc disease. A loss of normal kyphosis (flat spine) may be seen in spondylitis or possibly severe muscle spasm.
- Loose folds of skin on the back might denote multiple vertebral fractures.
- Costochondral swelling occurs in some cases of **costochondritis or rickets** ('rickety rosary') in children. Look for synovitis of costosternal or sternoclavicular joints (which is found with spondyloarthropathy).

Palpation
Palpate over the vertebrae, paravertebral joints, and back musculature with the patient prone. Palpate the anterior chest wall:
- Spinal osteomyelitis may be associated with obvious skin swelling and erythema, exquisite focal tenderness, and extensor spasm. Tumours may give similar signs, though skin erythema is not likely.

- Costotransverse joints may be tender (4–5 cm from midline). Discomfort at any costovertebral joint and its referred pain can be elicited by individual rib manipulation (downward pressure on the rib lateral to its vertebral joints when the patient is prone).
- Identify any trigger points that reproduce myofascial pain in back muscles.
- Tender swelling of the sternoclavicular, costomanubrial, or sternocostal joints may suggest **spondylarthropathy or SAPHO** (synovitis, acne, pustulosis (palmoplantar), hyperostosis, and (aseptic) osteomyelitis).
- Inflammation of costal cartilages is often associated with painful swelling and tenderness. Rib and intercostal lesions should be easily discriminated from referred pain by eliciting local tenderness.

Check thoracic spinal movement

Movements of the thoracic spine should be checked. Ask the patient to sit on the couch with their arms folded in front of them. Guided by movements of the spinous processes, gauge the range of thoracic spine movement:

- Approximate normal ranges of movement in the above position are extension 30°, lateral flexion 30°, flexion 90°, and rotation 60°.
- Scoliosis is often associated with rotation that is accentuated on flexion.
- Abnormal mobility will not be specific for any underlying condition, but may draw attention to the major affected spinal segment. Painful segments are 'guarded' and may appear hypomobile.
- Spondylitis may become obvious if there is extensive spinal hypomobility.
- Chest expansion should be measured from forced expiration to complete inspiration measuring at expansion, with a tape, at the level of the xiphisternum. Normal young adult chest expansion should measure at least 3 cm.

Other examination

- Given the range of serious conditions causing chest pains, a full medical examination is important and should always be considered.
- Neurological examination of the legs should be considered in anyone who is at risk of spinal cord compression. Look for increased tone, weakness, and brisk reflexes.
- Breast and axillary lymph node examination should be done.

Investigations

Radiographs

- Lateral view radiographs generally provide more information about thoracic spine lesions than anteroposterior views; however, together, both views should confirm osteoporosis, degenerative disease (e.g. previous **Scheuermann's osteochondritis**, ochronosis, DISH), and Paget's disease (📖 Chapter 16, p 431).
- Look for vertebral squaring (in AS) and either marginal or non-marginal **syndesmophytes** as in psoriatic spondylitis (Plate 12) or other SpA (📖 Chapter 8, p 281).
- Discriminate **enthesitis from DISH** at the corners of vertebrae by the presence of erosions with bone reaction (enthesitis) compared with bone proliferation alone (DISH). Enthesitis, associated with chronic spondylodiscitis, is part of the SpA spectrum of diseases.

- Normal radiographs do not exclude malignancy.
- Bone lesions can be well characterized by CT (e.g. osteoid osteoma).

MR
- MR is important in discriminating tumour from infection.
- Disc lesions, spinal canal, and cord are well visualized with MR.
- Fat suppressed or gadolinium-enhanced MR sequences may be necessary to detect enthesitis or spondylodiscitis associated with SpA.

Isotope bone scan
- A bone scan is a sensitive test for infection and malignancy.
- In suspected cases of (previously undiagnosed) malignancy, it is more sensitive than radiographs, can often confirm the lytic or sclerotic nature of a lesion, and will identify any other skeletal sites of disease.
- It is a useful investigation in patients with malignancy who present with back pain. A lack of additional lesions strongly suggests against a single spinal abnormality being malignancy-related.
- Tomography can detect abnormality in the pars interarticularis, facet joint, and disc/vertebral body.
- Bone scan sensitively identifies rib and, in most cases, inflammatory intercostal lesions. If solitary the differential diagnosis is of a metastasis, primary malignant or benign bone tumour, healed rib fracture, fibrous dysplasia, Paget's bone disease, hyperparathyroidism, or infection.

Other investigations to consider in patients with chest pain
- CXR, then consider pulmonary ventilation/perfusion scan and spiral CT to evaluate for pulmonary embolism.
- CT of the chest in patients with unexplained pleural pain.
- ECG and an exercise stress test for patients with possible cardiac ischaemia.
- Transthoracic echocardiography to show thickened pericardium or an effusion associated with pericarditis.
- Upper gastrointestinal endoscopy in suspected cases of peptic ulceration.
- Diagnostic trial of a proton pump inhibitor in cases of reflux oesophagitis.

Treatment

For treatment of thoracic and chest wall lesions see the next section on low back pain and also 📖 Chapter 20, p 525.

Low back pain and disorders in adults

Epidemiology

- The lifetime prevalence of back pain is 58% and the greatest prevalence is between 45 and 64 years of age.
- Most recent statistics report in the order of 12 million primary care consultations and over 2.4 million adult specialist consultations annually in the UK for low back pain (population 64 million). Low back pain is the fifth most common reason for all physician visits in the United States.
- Two per cent of the workforce in the United States is compensated for back injuries every year.
- Estimated annual cost to the National Health Service, UK, is £500 million with over £5 billion lost annually due to absence from work. The financial health care and indirect employment costs of low back pain in the United States are estimated to be more than $24 billion.

Lumbar and sacral spine anatomy

- There are normally five lumbar vertebrae. Anomalies are not uncommon at the lumbosacral junction.
- The transition between the mobile lumbar spine (flexion, extension, and lateral flexion) and fixed sacrum together with high weight-loading combine to make the region highly prone to damage.
- The facet joints are sharply angled, effectively reducing rotation in lumbar segments.
- The sacroiliac joints (synovial) are held firmly by a strong fibrous capsule and tough ligaments. The amount of normal movement (essentially rotation) is normally inversely proportional to age.
- The spinal cord ends at L1/L2. Nerves then run individually, are normally mobile in the spinal canal, and together are termed the cauda equina.
- Each nerve exits its appropriate lateral intervertebral exit foramen passing initially superior and then laterally to the disc, e.g. L4 from L4/L5 exit foramen. However, in the spinal canal each nerve descends immediately posterior to the more proximal intervertebral disc before it exits. Thus, for example, L4 root symptoms can occur from either lateral herniation of the L4/5 disc or posterior herniation of the L3/L4 disc (or from both).
- Facet joint innervation is from posterior primary rami, each of which supplies the corresponding joint at its level, one higher and one lower.

Basic principles of assessment

- Low back pain can arise from damage or inflammation of the thoracic or lumbar spines or from the posterior pelvis. Pathology in retroperitoneal abdominal and pelvic viscera can result in referred pain to the low back.
- A simple way of categorizing back pain is to consider its cause to be mechanical, inflammatory, neurologic, referred, or due to bone pathology (Table 2.10).

- Over 90% of episodes of low back pain in adults are mechanical, self-limiting, and do not require investigation.
- Indicators for further investigation include age >55 years, stiffness, focal pain, pain that disturbs sleep, nerve root symptoms, and chronic persistent (>6 weeks) pain.
- The low back is often a focus for those who may use pain (consciously or unconsciously) as a protective device in the face of domestic, emotional, or occupational stress. These stresses commonly influence the description and impact of pain but rarely act alone in causing pain—there is usually some underlying organic pathology.

Table 2.10 Common and/or serious causes of low back pain in adults

Mechanical/degenerative (very common)	Hypermobility (📖 Chapter 16)
	Facet joint arthritis
	Disc disease (annular tear, internal disruption, prolapse)
	Scoliosis/kyphosis
	Spinal stenosis
	Sacroiliitis
Inflammatory (common)	AS (📖 Chapter 8)
	Sacroiliitis (e.g. AS, brucellosis)
Infection (rare)	Osteomyelitis (e.g. *Staphylococcus aureus*, TB, brucellosis) (📖 Chapter 17)
Bone disease (common)	Osteoporotic fracture (📖 Chapter 16)
	Paget's disease
	Osteomalacia
Neoplasia (rare)	Secondary metastases
	Multiple myeloma
Other	Sickle cell crisis
	Renal disease (e.g. tumours, infection)
	Gynaecological disease
	Fibromyalgia (📖 Chapter 18, p 489)

Taking a history

Differentiate whether the pain is likely to be primarily mechanical or inflammatory, due to bone pathology or referred:

- The site and extent of the pain does not easily discriminate the cause. All disorders may be associated with mechanical deformity and/or muscle spasm that may cause pain in a more diffuse distribution (Plate 13).
- Generally, pain due to mechanical lesions is often acute in onset, while patients with pain from inflammatory lesions often present after symptoms have been present for some time.
- Inflammatory pain is often associated with morning stiffness that can last for several hours and is eased by movement. Mechanical lesions tend to worsen with use. Many 'mechanical' or 'degenerative' lesions may have an inflammatory component, e.g. internal disc disruption causing discogenic pain.
- Intrinsic bone pathology often causes severe, unremitting, focal pain. Sleep is disturbed. Pain does not ease substantially with movement.
- About 3% of patients presenting with back pain have non-musculoskeletal causes. A significant proportion of women have pelvic conditions such as ovarian cysts or endometriosis. Pain may be cyclical.
- For those aged over 55 with no previous similar episodes of pain increase suspicion of an underlying neoplastic lesion. Investigation is required.
- Associated systemic symptoms are common in osteomyelitis and may be present if a malignancy has disseminated.

Ask about pain radiation and symptoms in the legs

- Progressive neurological leg symptoms suggest a worsening/expanding lesion such as a tumour, infection/vertebral collapse, Paget's disease, or lumbosacral **spinal stenosis**.
- Pressure on the cauda equina sufficient to cause a disturbance in perineal sensation and/or bowel/bladder paralysis is a neurosurgical emergency (**cauda equina syndrome**; 📖 Chapter 20, p 525).
- Leg pain caused by nerve root irritation/compression is often clearly defined and sharp, often accompanied by numbness or paraesthesias. The most commonly involved nerve roots are L4, L5, or S1. Pain generally radiates to below the knee and often, but not always, to the heel and big toe.
- Sciatic nerve entrapment at the piriformis muscle can produce identical radicular symptoms to L5 or S1 nerve root entrapment.
- Neurological symptoms in the distribution of the femoral nerve (primarily anterior thigh musculature) might suggest a high lumbar nerve root lesion (L1–L3, for example).
- Disc prolapse is the most common cause of nerve root pain, but bony encroachment at the nerve root exit foramen by vertebral end-plate or facet joint osteophytes, and/or soft tissue thickening or fibrosis can cause similar pain (foramenal stenosis).
- Annular disc tears and internal disruption (i.e. microfractures in vertebral end-plates) can cause a pattern of pain, termed discogenic pain, characterized by low back and referred buttock/posterior thigh pain aggravated by movement.

- Generally, all mechanical lesions of the lumbar spine can result in referred pain around the pelvis and anterior thighs. However, pain from lumbar facet joints and probably other segmental structures can be referred to the lower leg.
- Aching in the back and posterior thighs after standing is typical of, but not specific for, spondylolisthesis. There are often added spasms of acute pain, especially if there is segmental instability.
- The symptoms of spinal stenosis are often relieved by sitting bent slightly forward, since the spinal canal dimensions increase in this position.
- **Sacroiliitis** (Plate 2) often causes referred pain to the buttocks and back of thighs. It occurs commonly in spondyloarthropathy (◻ Chapter 8, p 281).
- Sacroiliac pain can occur in multiparous women—the condition may be associated with hypermobility.

Note the description of the pain

- Pain may be 'severe' whatever the cause; however, note whether the patient's descriptors of it suggest non-organic influences.
- Sharp, lancinating leg pains suggest nerve root irritation/compression (radicular pain), whereas leg pain referred from other structures within a lumbar segment is generally deep and aching. The distribution may be similar (see above). More persistent, rather than episodic, radicular pain may denote stenosis of the nerve root exit foramen.
- A description of bilateral buttock/leg pain that worsens on walking is consistent with spinal stenosis, especially in those with normal peripheral pulses and no bruits.
- A change in the description of pain in someone who has an established diagnosis may be important, e.g. subacute, severe, unremitting localized pain in a patient with AS who normally has mild inflammatory pain might reflect a superadded **discitis;** or, acute severe unremitting sleep-disturbing pain in an elderly woman with known chronic mechanical pain associated with OA might suggest osteoporotic fracture.
- Florid descriptions of the pain and its severity are associated with psychological modulators of pain.

Previous back pain and trauma, occupation, and family history

- **Scheuermann's disease** (which is associated with irregular vertebral endplates) causes spinal pain in adolescence. It is a risk for spinal degeneration and kyphosis in adults.
- Previous trauma may have caused pars interarticularis fractures (an antecedent of spondylolisthesis), vertebral fracture (risk of further mechanical damage), or ligament rupture (subsequent segmental instability).
- It is generally accepted that the high prevalence of disc disease among manual workers at a relatively young age provides some evidence for a causal relationship.
- It is often the case that patients with chronic pain following (sometimes trivial) trauma may be dissatisfied with the quality of care received at the time of the injury. Be aware that many believe, and there is some evidence to support this, that the way in which spinal pain is handled at its onset significantly influences its subsequent course.

- Sacroiliitis is an early part of brucellar arthritis (20–51% of patients). Poor animal- or carcass-handling hygiene or ingestion of infected foodstuffs/milk can lead to infection. Spondylitis is a late feature and is characterized by erosions, disc infection, and abscesses.
- A positive family history of low back pain might, in context, suggest SpA (sacroiliitis), hypermobility ([Chapter 16, p 431), or generalized osteoarthritis ([Chapter 6, p 259).

Examination

Inspect the undressed patient from the side and behind

- Note the fluidity of movement when the patient is undressing.
- Check the skin for redness, local swelling, and skin markings. Redness and swelling occasionally accompany osteomyelitis.
- Lipoma, hairy patches, *café-au-lait* patches, or skin tags often reflect underlying structural nerve or bone abnormality, e.g. spina bifida, diastematomyelia, neurofibromatosis.
- Skinfolds often suggest an underlying significant structural change, such as osteoporotic fracture or spondylolisthesis.
- Note any deformity: hyperlordosis (associated with L5/S1 damage and weak abdominal musculature), prominent thoracolumbar kyphosis (multiple disc degeneration or vertebral fractures), scoliosis (degenerative, compensatory muscle spasm for unilateral pain).
- Look from the side. A gentle lordotic curve is normal. Flattening suggests muscle spasm or fusion in SpA. With major **spondylolisthesis**, a step between spinous processes can sometimes be seen.

Observe active movements while the patient is standing

Lumbar forward flexion ('... with your legs straight, slowly reach down to try and touch your ankles ...'), lateral flexion ('... with your legs and back straight, tip sideways and run your hand down your leg towards your knee ...') and extension ('... with your legs straight, slowly bend backwards ...'). ([Chapter 1, p 3). Note: flexion can be mediated by the hip joints; extension can be affected by slight pelvic tilt and body sway. Ask what can be achieved normally and what is painful:

- Abnormal movements are not specific for any condition though they may help to localize a problem.
- Pain in extension is characteristic of retrospondylolisthesis, facet joint arthritis, or impinging spinous processes. May be relieved by flexion.
- Failure of the spinous processes to separate in a patient who manages good forward flexion would be consistent with permanent spinal stiffness, e.g. AS, with flexion mediated by the hip joints.
- Forward flexion can be measured using the modified **Schöber's test**. When erect, mark the skin at the point midway between the posterior superior iliac spines (Venus' dimples) and again 10 cm above and 5 cm below. Measure the increase in distance between the outer marks at full forward flexion—in a young adult this is normally more than 6 cm.
- Ask the patient to stand on one foot then lift onto their toes a few times. Weakness might imply an L5 nerve root entrapment (gastrocnemius/soleus).

Table 2.11 Testing muscle strength in the lower limbs (patient supine unless otherwise stated). Weakness may denote nerve root entrapment

Muscle or muscle group	Nerve roots	Test[*]
Hamstrings (knee flexion)	L5, S1, S2	Ask patient to flex the knee to 45°, hold patient's ankle and ask them to bend the knee further against your hold
Iliopsoas (hip flexion/internal rotation)	L1, L2, L3	Ask patient to lift the leg with a bent knee, hold up the upper leg and resist your push. Try to push the leg down and slightly outwards
Quadriceps femoris (hip flexion, knee extension)	L2, L3, L4	Hold the patient's relaxed upper leg above the couch (grasped underneath above the knee). The lower leg should drop loosely. Ask them to straighten the lower leg against your resistance
		From patient standing test repetitive squatting for more subtle weakness
Tibialis anterior (ankle dorsiflexion), Tibialis posterior (ankle inversion and dorsiflexion)	L4, L5	With the knee straight ask the patient to pull back their foot (show them first) against your pull. Resist dorsiflexion
		Standing or walking on heels tests for more subtle weakness. Note: if the hind foot rests in valgus or the patient significantly everts the foot during dorsiflexion, the test may also recruit peroneal muscles (L5, S1)
Extensor hallucis longus	L5, S1	Ask the patient to pull their big toe back against your finger (at the base)
Gastrocnemius and soleus (ankle plantar flexion)	S1, S2	Ask the patient to point their toes. Resist the movement by pressing against the ball of the foot
		Standing or walking on the toes tests for more subtle weakness

[*] Compare sides. Score according to scale, for example: 0 = no muscle contraction; 1 = contraction visible; 2 = active movement, gravity eliminated; 3 = active movement against gravity; 4-/4/4+ = active movement against slight/moderate/strong resistance; 5 = normal power.

Table 2.12 Principal combinations of signs used for identifying lumbar nerve root lesions

Nerve root	Paraesthesias and sensory change	Muscle weakness	Tendon reflex changes
L2	Upper thigh: anterior, medial, and lateral surfaces	Hip flexion and adduction	None
L3	Anterior surface of lower thigh	Hip adduction and knee extension	Knee jerk possibly reduced
L4	Anteromedial surface of lower leg	Knee extension, foot dorsiflexion, and inversion	Knee jerk decreased
L5	Anterolateral surface of lower leg and dorsum/medial side of foot/toe	Hip extension and abduction. Knee flexion. Foot/toe dorsiflexion	None
S1	Lateral border and sole of foot. Back of heel and calf	Knee flexion. Plantar flexion and eversion of foot	Ankle jerk decreased

Examination of the prone patient

Ask the patient to turn to lie prone. Palpate low back and over sacrum:

- Diffuse tenderness may be due to muscle spasm.
- Superficial tenderness over the spinous processes or interspinous interval might suggest interspinous ligament disruption or impinging processes.
- Paravertebral bony tenderness may suggest facet joint arthritis.
- Costovertebral angle (CVA) or loin tenderness could indicate renal pathology.
- Tenderness over the SI joints is not specific for sacroiliitis.
- A positive femoral stretch test reproduces L1–L4 (especially L3) radicular pain in the anterior or medial part of the thigh. Flex the patient's knee to 90° and passively extend the hip.

Other examination

- In suspected cases of spinal stenosis or cauda equina syndrome, it is essential to check for sensory loss in the sacral nerve dermatomes. Also check anal sphincter tone by rectal examination (S5).
- In suspected cases of spinal stenosis, the patient can be asked to walk until limited by pain then re-examined. If there is any ischaemia of the cauda equina or of a nerve root (from foraminal stenosis) nerve root signs may become more obvious.

Investigations

- There are two important initial steps in investigating low back pain. First deciding whether radiographs will help. Secondly, although relatively rare in practice, the possibility of infection, malignancy, and cauda equina compression always needs to be considered. Simple radiographic views are insensitive indicators of these conditions and, in most cases, are not specific although most radiologists would agree they are desirable in addition to CT or MR. Laboratory tests are mandatory in all suspected cases of inflammation, infection, and malignancy.

Radiographs—decision-making in requesting them

(Table 2.13, see also Table 2.16)

- Lumbar spine radiographs are not always helpful. Remember that nine out of ten cases of back pain in the primary care setting are mechanical and self-limiting. Features on a plain radiograph of the lumbar spine correlate poorly with the presence or pattern of pain.
- Spondylosis is common, age-related, and often isn't symptomatic.
- Children, athletes, and young adults with back pain need prompt radiographic investigation. Failure to detect and treat a pars interarticularis fracture may lead on to a spondylolysis. Abnormalities are more readily appreciated in these age groups as the frequency of age-related degenerative changes in the spine is low.
- Obtaining radiographs to help in the management of patients is a different issue to obtaining them to aid diagnosis and one that requires careful thought, e.g. is the patient likely to perceive that they have received suboptimal care if a radiograph is not requested?

Table 2.13 Commonly reported patterns of radiographic abnormality in adults, the interpretation, and suggested reaction

Radiographic abnormalities	Lesion suggested	Sensible further action
Lumbosacral anomalies	Risk for future back pain	May not be clinically significant. Risk for low back pain (esp. if hypermobile)
Generalized osteopenia	Osteoporosis	Measurement of bone density. Rule out secondary causes, e.g. myeloma
Narrowed disc space, marginal vertebral end-plate osteophytes or both	Intervertebral disc disruption	MRI if persistent symptoms or signs of same level nerve root entrapment, spinal or nerve root exit foramen stenosis
Localized lucent or sclerotic lesion, loss of cortex	Tumour, infection, or fracture	Discuss case with radiologist. MRI or CT may be advised. A bone scan may be helpful. Initiate appropriate laboratory tests immediately
Facet joint OA	Facet joint syndrome	Consider whether there is associated spinal/nerve root exit foramen stenosis (?radicular symptoms) or symptoms suggestive of spondylolisthesis. CT or MRI is then likely to be appropriate
Pars interarticularis defect	Spondylolysis/spondylolytic	Probable prior fracture. Further oblique film centered on suspected level or CT should confirm. Association with symptoms or signs of disc disease or spondylolisthesis suggests an unstable segment. Flexion and extension lateral view radiographs may show instability. MRI helpful for imaging soft-tissues including nerves
Short lumbar pedicles	Spinal stenosis	Consider MRI if symptoms suggest spinal stenosis
Mixed patchy sclerosis and lucency in entire (enlarged) vertebra(e)	Paget's disease	Neurological leg symptoms suggest spinal/exit foramen stenosis or vascular 'steal'

- Spondylolysis may be seen on a lateral view, but is seen better on oblique views. Oblique views may also show pedicle stress fractures in athletes.
- Spondylolisthesis may be identified and graded by a lateral film. Flexion and extension views may be helpful in delineating subtle cases, and instability (spondylolytic).
- General osteopenia is a risk factor for low bone mass; however, it is not a sensitive indicator of low bone mass.
- Look for vertebral squaring (in AS), non-marginal syndesmophytes (in other SpA, such as psoriatic), or flowing syndesmophytes (in DISH).
- Consider obtaining an AP view of the pelvis. Established (but not early) sacroiliitis can be ruled-out. A further 'coned' view is often helpful.
- Sacroiliitis (peri-articular osteoporosis, erosion, sclerosis of bone, widening joint space) occurs in all types of SpA. It can be unilateral.
- Sclerosis of the SI joint on the lower iliac side alone suggests osteitis condensans ilii. Joint space is normal and joint margin well defined.
- Patterns of metabolic bone disease, Paget's disease and hip pathology are usually readily identifiable on a pelvic film.

Isotope bone scan
- A bone scan is a sensitive test for infection or malignancy. It is a useful investigation in patients with previously diagnosed malignancy who present with back pain, especially in those who have had no previous skeletal metastases. A lack of additional lesions strongly suggests against a single spinal abnormality being malignancy-related.
- It is not specific for the various degenerative lesions, but can help localize the site of a lesion.
- Bone scan SI joint appearances in sacroiliitis can be unreliable.

CT or MR?
The choice of imaging depends largely on likely clinical and radiographic differential diagnosis:
- For spondylolytic spondylolisthesis, CT shows the exact site of pars' defects. The usual appearance is of sclerotic irregular edges.
- Nerve impingement can be shown by CT or MRI.
- Intervertebral disc prolapse, both posterior and posterolateral, can be shown by either technique. Prolapse material is of similar CT density and MR signal to the disc, and well-defined against epidural fat.
- Changes in the normal disc signal pattern are associated with age-related disc degeneration. Discogenic pain has been associated with MRI abnormalities classified according to Modic.
- On T_2-weighted MR, disc material is usually of higher signal than 'scar' (e.g. fibrosis from a previous lesion), in which signal decreases with aging. Recent scarring enhances immediately, but old scarring does so only slowly. This discrimination requires gadolinium-enhanced MR.
- CT or MR shows early sacroiliitis in AS when X-rays are normal.

- The shape and outline of the spinal canal are ideally shown on CT, but are also seen with MR. It is difficult for MR to distinguish fibrous structures from sclerotic or cortical bone, though it shows intrathecal content more readily which is an advantage in identifying intradural tumours.
- Spondylodiscitis (part of SpA), if chronic, may be difficult to discriminate from degenerative disc/vertebral end-plate disease. Fat-suppressed or gadolinium-enhanced sequences may show high signal at the anterior disc vertebral end-plate junctions.

Screening for infection, malignancy, or metabolic bone disease
- In cases where the history and examination suggest a mechanical condition, but where the clinician wishes to be more confident of excluding an inflammatory condition, an ESR and CRP are suggested.
- A raised ESR would point towards further laboratory investigation.
- An infection screen should include an FBC for anaemia and leukocytosis, CRP, blood, and urine cultures. If spinal tuberculosis is suspected a plain CXR should be taken and serial (over 3 days) early morning urine samples taken.
- Serum and urine protein electrophoresis (with immunofixation) are essential tests in the 'work-up' for myeloma. Urea and creatinine are also important as hypercalcaemia, and acute renal impairment have prognostic significance in this condition.
- Routine blood tests may point to an underlying metabolic bone disorder such as Paget's disease or osteomalacia. These tests are normal in post-menopausal osteoporosis.
- If osteoporosis is diagnosed (☐ Chapter 16, p 431) a screen for secondary causes should include ESR (and if raised, serum, and urine protein electrophoresis), calcium, phosphate, sex hormones, but also serum 25-hydroxyvitamin D, parathyroid hormone (PTH), thyroid function tests (TFTs), and liver function tests (LFTs).

Treatment (☐ Chapter 20, p 525)
- An important therapeutic intervention in the case of acute pain is to take the patient seriously, take a positive view, and in the absence of sinister signs, e.g. nerve root pain, urge early mobility.
- Analgesics and muscle relaxants can be used in the short term, initially regularly, then as required.
- Physical therapy with graded-activity programmes may be of value, certainly early in disc disease or spondylosis.
- **Cord compression** due to bone collapse from a tumour is an acute emergency and should be discussed immediately with an oncologist or radiation oncologist, and a spinal orthopaedic or neurosurgeon.
- Cases with disc prolapse failing to respond to conservative therapy, or cases where there is ongoing or **rapidly progressive neurological deficit**, should be referred for surgery.
- Available surgical techniques for acute or persistent disc disease include decompression procedures (e.g. nerve root decompression and partial facetectomy), prosthetic intervertebral disc replacement, intradiscal thermocoagulation, and intradiscal steroid injections, although evidence for long-term efficacy is lacking for all these procedures.

- Surgery for **spinal stenosis** is useful for relieving leg neurogenic features, but not indicated if there is no significant neurological compromise. Surgery is not usually done if the only effect of spinal stenosis is back pain.
- In chronic back pain, aerobic exercises combined with behavioural methods may be more effective than exercise alone and can help motivate the patient. Methods may also incorporate psychological and social assessment and management.
- The common treatments available for chronic back pain include:
  - analgesics and muscle relaxants;
  - anti-epileptics/antidepressants for neuropathic pain;
  - local anaesthetic/steroid injections;
  - acupuncture;
  - transcutaneous electrical nerve stimulation (TENS);
  - physical therapy;
  - ergonomic advice;
  - multidisciplinary programs—counseling; cognitive therapy; education; relaxation; corsets and belts.
- Timely surgery for structural scoliosis (more common in JIA than the general population) can lessen spinal curvature.

Spinal disorders in children and adolescents

Background

- Common conditions in adults such as degenerative back pain and intervertebral disc disease are rare in childhood or adolescence.
- In hospital series up to 85% of referred children have identifiable causes (Table 2.14) though spinal hypermobility in the context of generalized hypermobility and fibromyalgia has not been adequately addressed.
- Not all presentations are with pain. Some children present with either deformity or neurological symptoms.
- A diagnosis must be firmly established or at least rigorously sought because serious disease can present with few symptoms.

Table 2.14 Cause of childhood back pain. Experience of an orthopaedic clinic (a review of 233 referrals)

Cause of back pain	Frequency (%)
Non-specific (i.e. no cause found) Consider 'Hypermobility'	32
Scoliosis	21
Spondylolysis/listhesis (non-trauma)	11
Scheuermann's disease	7
Infection	6
Tumours, e.g. osteoid osteoma	4
Psychogenic	4
Dic prolapse	3
Inflammatory, e.g. spondyloarthropathy	3
Trauma (excluding strains)	2
Limb length inequality/biomechanical	2
Renal pain	<1
Rickets	<1
Congenital anomalies	<1

Taking a history

Keep an open mind as to whether a history from the child, parents, or primary care-giver provides the most useful information. There are merits in consulting all of them.

Severity, distribution, and quality of pain

- Pain may be mild even though there is a serious underlying disorder.
- If the pain occurs, or initially occurred, during sport, consider **pars interarticularis fractures**, spondylolytic **spondylolisthesis** or **Scheuermann's disease** (vertebral epiphyseal osteochondritis; 📖 Chapter 16, p 431).
- Persistent pain, unrelieved by rest and disturbing sleep, requires consideration of a bone, bone and/or disc infection, or osteoporotic fracture [steroid-related or juvenile idiopathic osteoporosis (JIO)].
- JIO is rare, occurs between 6 and 13 years of age and is more common in boys. The main differential diagnosis is **osteogenesis imperfecta** (📖 Chapter 16, p 431).
- Although uncommon, neurological symptoms, such as burning pain, paraesthesias, and weakness in the legs, suggests nerve root irritation.
- Spinal stiffness in a child (typically between 2 and 6 years of age) associated with irritability and a diffusely tender back may be due to infective **discitis** (although organisms are only found in 50%). In an older child or adolescent (typically 10–15 years of age) and with a less striking history, immobility-related stiffness could represent juvenile enthesitis-related arthritis (ERA).

Conditions where pain may be absent

Spinal conditions are not always associated with pain. Occasionally, a child may present with back deformity or neurological symptoms in the legs alone:

- The history may be non-specific and, for example, in a very young child, nothing more than a refusal to walk.
- Scheuermann's disease commonly presents in teenagers with a painless thoracic **kyphosis**. Pain is more likely to be present if the chondritis is thoracolumbar, rather than thoracic. The condition is often asymptomatic.
- **Spinal dysraphism** (bony abnormality—usually spina bifida, associated with neural anomaly—invariably cord tethering) and spinal cord tumours can often present with neurological leg symptoms/signs alone without back pain. Symptoms may be mild initially.
- Scoliosis is usually pain-free. Pain with scoliosis usually indicates significant underlying pathology. The differential is wide (Table 2.15).
- The most frequent single cause of a **scoliosis** in schoolchildren (40%), found from radiographic screening, is pelvic tilt due to **leg length discrepancy**.

Past developmental, medical, family, and social history

- Ask about milestones in musculoskeletal development. Abnormality or delay might suggest spinal dysraphism or neuromuscular conditions.
- Osteoporosis may be evident from previous fragility fracture—axial or appendicular—or may be intimated from risk factors, e.g. steroid use.
- Previous low back trauma may have been pars interarticularis fractures preceding (the current) vertebral slip or disc prolapse.

- Irradiation therapy is a cause of scoliosis.
- Ask about previous TB or immunization against it in patients you think are at risk of **TB osteomyelitis.**

Table 2.15 Causes of scoliosis in children and adolescents

Structural scolioses (vertebral rotation, vertebral structural change, and loss of normal spinal flexibility)	Idiopathic: infantile (0–3 years); juvenile (3–10 years); adolescent (>10 years)
	Neuromuscular
	Congenital: failure of vertebral formation, segmentation, or both
	Neurofibromatosis
	Heritable disorders of connective tissue, e.g. osteogenesis imperfecta
	Trauma: fracture; surgical (e.g. post-laminectomy); irradiation
	Spondyloepiphyseal dysplasia
	Metabolic bone disease
	Lumbosacral anomalies (e.g. spondylolytic spondylolisthesis)
	Cervicothoracic anomalies [e.g. cervical fusion (Klippel–Feil)]
	Rheumatoid arthritis
	Extraspinal contractures (e.g. post-empyema, post-burns)
Non-structural scolioses (lateral spinal curvature, but no vertebral rotation)*	Postural
	Nerve root irritation associated
	Abdominal pain associated (e.g. appendicitis, renal pain)
	Associated with local inflammation
	Spinal infection
	Spinal tumours
	Secondary to leg length discrepancy
	Related to soft-tissue contractures around the hip
	Psychogenic

* It is characteristic of non-structural scolioses that if the underlying cause is successfully dealt with, the scoliosis resolves.

- Torticollis may be associated with chronic squint, previous trauma (which may be associated with a psychogenic component) and neuroleptic drugs. It can be a sign of an underlying neurological or inflammatory lesion or occurs because of an underlying structural anomaly.
- A history of a heritable disease of connective tissue can often be elicited from the family of a child with structural scoliosis.
- A history of back pain is sometimes elicited from families of children with non-specific back pain. Joint dislocation and multiple soft-tissue musculoskeletal injury (especially over-use) in family members raises the possibility of general hypermobility (**joint hypermobility syndrome** or other heritable connective tissue disease, e.g. **Marfan syndrome** (☐ Chapter 16, p 431)).
- The existence or child's perception of social disharmony at home or school is likely to be more important in influencing the impact of back pain, rather than a cause of it. Nevertheless, in children with non-specific spinal pain or fibromyalgia, social conflict resulting in stress and anxiety may be very important in generating symptoms.

Examination

It is best, and certainly ultimately more informative, to undertake the examination only when the child is comfortable with the situation, with their modesty and dignity preserved, and with consent to go ahead after a reassurance that the examination will be stopped if it is painful. With younger children there may be 'an examinable moment', usually after the child has gained confidence in the surroundings and with the situation. Observing the young child while playing is a considerate way of starting the examination.

Age-related variations in biomechanical development and gait patterns

- Walking while holding a hand or furniture develops by 12 months and normally independent walking by 18 months.
- Until 3 years the stance is broad-based in relation to pelvic width, the knee may not fully extend and the ankle may be plantar flexed at foot-strike.
- Climbing stairs is usually done using alternate feet by age of 3 years.
- Tiptoe walking is not abnormal at first, but should disappear by 2 years. If this pattern remains, consider spasticity, **tethered cord**, or muscle weakness.
- Flat feet up to age 5 are normal (a consequence of the distribution of fat and paucity of muscle development). Only investigate if symptomatic.
- Leg alignment often concerns parents. Up until 2 years of age it is normal to have genu varum. From 2–5 years mild genu valgum may occur (see 'Knee' later in ☐ Chapter 2, p 19). Angles of >10° or asymmetry may be associated with underlying disease.
- Regression of motor development is a clue to the presence of disease.

Observation

Observe children unclothed to underwear if possible; initially at play then look from behind. Look for weakness, scoliosis, kyphosis, and swellings.
- The main cause of spinal asymmetry will be scoliosis (Table 2.15).
- Localized soft tissue swelling may denote soft tissue extension of a spinal tumour.
- An 'apparent' kyphosis associated with scoliosis is usually a result of spinal rotation.

- In children with neck pain look for a short neck (rule out *Klippel–Feil*) or asymmetric scapulae (Sprengel's deformity: a higher, **hypoplastic scapula**).
- Adolescent kyphosis may be due to Scheuermann's disease or fractures. Unless there has been steroid use, the former is more likely.
- Note any skin markings, such as *café-au-lait* spots, skin indents (lumbar area), and lumbosacral hair. They may be markers of bony abnormality.
- Note any muscular weakness. With truncal weakness [e.g. DM, (📖 Chapter 14, p 385)] the child may have to roll over before getting up from a supine position. Hip girdle weakness may be present in a child unwilling to squat and unable to stand from squatting without exhibiting **Gower's sign** (unable to stand up from the floor without using hands to push off).

Examine the gait pattern

- Look for asymmetry and a limp.
- Back or leg pain from any cause can give rise to a limp. Also, limp may be the only feature of a serious underlying neurological or bony deformity.
- Asymmetry of shoulder height, transverse posterior skinfolds, pelvic tilt, and arm swing may be a clue to spinal pathology.

Spinal examination with the child standing

Examine the whole spine while the child is standing. The immature spine is usually far more flexible than an adult's:

- Ask about the presence and site of neck or low back pain during forward flexion, extension, and lateral flexion (and rotation for neck). Experienced examiners should be able to detect significantly limited movements.
- Palpate along the line of (lumbar) spinous processes. An inward step may be caused by spondylolisthesis.
- Palpate any swellings. Lipoma are painless. Soft tissue tumours may be, but are not necessarily, tender and fixed.

Examine the sitting patient

Examine the child who is sitting on the couch, legs hanging over the side:
    This is the best way to elicit pain from posterior vertebral structure pathology in thoracic or lumbar segments (e.g. pars osteoid osteoma, pars fracture). Combine extension and rotation movements. Ask if the pain is worse on one side than the other.

Examine the supine patient

Examine the child or adolescent when supine. Look for leg length discrepancy, lower leg asymmetry, and do a neurological examination:

- Measure and determine actual or apparent leg length discrepancy.
- True leg length discrepancy is a cause of non-structural scoliosis. Apparent leg length discrepancy/pelvic tilts can occur to compensate for scoliosis caused by spinal lesions.
- Different foot or leg sizes/appearances are a non-specific sign of spinal dysraphism.
- Hip and sacroiliac examination should be done routinely in children with low back pain. Tests for dural irritation and neurologic examination are essential (see section on 'Low back pain and disorders in adults,' 📖 Chapter 2, p 19).

- Although limb pain, weakness, and other neurological symptoms occur, the majority of children with intradural tumours have none of these features. A normal examination does not rule out serious pathology.

Examine the prone patient

- Palpate over the spinous processes, interspinous spaces, paracentrally between spinous processes (over facet joints), and in the sacroiliac area.
- Diffuse tenderness may only be a reflection of muscle spasm and its extensive mechanical effect. Where there are isolated areas of tenderness feel for skin warmth, as this may be a site of infection.

Investigations

Radiographs

- Radiographs have a characteristic appearance in certain cases of bone tumour but may also, in some cases, be normal (Table 2.16).
- A normal isotope bone scan rules out most serious pathology.
- A widened interpedicular distance on an AP film is a sign of meningomyelocele, spinal dysraphism, or an intraspinal mass.
- Posterior vertebral scalloping on a lateral radiograph is seen in lumbar or cervical spines, and is most commonly associated with lesions occurring in childhood and most commonly due to **spinal tumours, neurofibromatosis, osteogenesis imperfecta, Ehlers–Danlos syndrome,** and **Marfan syndrome** (📖 Chapter 16, p 431).
- Spondylolysis/pars fractures may be visible on lateral X-rays, but are best characterized by oblique films (Plate 13). Associated internal disc derangement or radiculopathy is best characterized using MR.
- Appearances of **Scheuermann's disease** (juvenile kyphosis, associated with multiple irregular vertebral endplates, with anterior ring epiphyseal fragmentation and vertebral wedging) are an occasional incidental X-ray finding.
- Radiographs of the neck may show a degree of cervical spine fusion (**Klippel–Feil** syndrome). Suspect hypermobility in non-affected segments and investigate C1/C2 with MR if there are high cervical pain or myelopathic symptoms.
- Isotope bone scan can detect spinal bony abnormalities; a negative test rules out most subtle lesions, e.g. osteoid osteomas.
- Consider SI joint radiographs and MR in patients with prominent immobility-related low back pain and stiffness (commonly due spondyloarthropathy-related conditions).

Investigating scoliosis

- The cause of painful scoliosis must be determined. Consider MR or CT of any localized area of pain. Idiopathic scoliosis is asymptomatic and is a diagnosis of exclusion.
- Mild idiopathic scoliosis (5–10°) can be determined on a postero-anterior thoracolumbar radiograph and is relatively common in the school population (7%). A scoliosis of > 20° occurs in 1 in 500 people and is three to four times more common in girls than boys.
- In 10–20% of those with a trunk inclination of >5°, the scoliosis progresses at least a further 5°. Most have a non-progressive scoliosis.

Table 2.16 Radiographic features of spinal tumours in children (see also Table 20.7)

Tumour type	Notable clinical features and radiological appearances
Osteochondroma	Has the appearance of an exostosis
Osteoid osteoma	Radiographs often normal. Bone scan will localize lesion and CT sharply define it
Osteoblastoma	Lytic with central ossification on radiograph. Can metastasize
Aneurysmal bone cyst	Lucent lesion with central trabeculae on radiographs. MR important to document soft-tissue expansion
Langerhans cell histiocytosis (eosinophilic granuloma)	Either solitary, polyostotic, or associated with systemic illness. Lytic lesion can cause solitary vertebral collapse, even collapse of adjacent bones. Used to be called histiocytosis X
Myeloma	Rare in children. Lytic lesions on radiographs. Distribution of lesions can be shown with isotope bone can, but use as adjunct to radiographs
Ewing's sarcoma	Age 5–20 usually 'Moth-eaten' destruction of bone on radiograph
Lymphoma	Sclerotic ('ivory') vertebra on film
Osteosarcoma	Mixed lytic/sclerotic appearance on radiographs
Metastases	Most likely are from leukaemia or neuroblastoma
Intra- and extramedullary tumours	Delay in diagnosis common. Up to 50% have abnormal films: widened spinal canal, pedicle erosions, scalloping of vertebral bodies. MR usually characterizes the lesion

Laboratory investigations

Laboratory investigations should be sought if infection, inflammation or malignancy is considered (see section on low back pain and disorders in adults).

The management of various spinal disorders in adults and children is included in 📖 Chapter 20, p 525.

Pelvic, groin, and thigh pain

Anatomy

Anatomy of the pelvis and hip region

- The bony pelvis consists of two inominate bones (ilium above the acetabulum and ischium below it) that articulate with each other at the anterior symphysis pubis and posteriorly with the sacrum at the SI joints.
- SI joints are initially synovial but become fibrous with age. A few degrees of rotation can be demonstrated in children and young adults.
- Strong ligaments stabilize the posterior pelvis through sacroinominate, lumbo(L5)–sacral, and lumbo(L5)–iliac attachments.
- The symphysis pubis is a cartilaginous joint and normally does not move.
- When standing, weight is transferred through the head of the femur. The femoral head is stabilized in the acetabulum by the acetabular labrum and strong pericapsular ligaments.
- The ligamentum teres crosses the hip joint and carries blood vessels to the head of the femur in children and young adults. In old age, blood supply is largely via vessels that enter the femoral neck.
- Two bursae are found at the insertion of the gluteus maximus: one separates it from the greater trochanter, the other separates it from the vastus lateralis.
- The ischial bursa separates gluteus maximus from the ischial tuberosity and can become inflamed from over-use.

Anatomy of pelvic musculature

- Three groups of muscles move the hip joint: the gluteals, the flexor muscles, and the adductor group.
- The major gluteal group muscles are:
  - gluteus maximus (L5, S1/2): arises mainly from ilium and sacrum, projects down posteriolaterally and inserts into the posterior femur and the lateral tensor fasciae latae. It extends and externally rotates the hip (the hamstrings also extend the hip);
  - gluteus medius (L4/5, S1): lies deeper and more lateral. It inserts into the lateral greater trochanter and abducts and internally rotates the hip;
  - piriformis, obturator internus, and quadratus femoris arise deep in the pelvis and insert into the posterior greater trochanter. All externally rotate the hip.
- The major hip flexor, psoas major (L2/3), is a massive muscle that arises from the lateral part of the vertebrae and intervertebral discs (T12–L5) and lateral processes of the lumbar vertebrae. It runs anteriorly over the iliac rim, across the pelvis, under the inguinal ligament, and inserts into the lesser trochanter. The iliacus (L2–L4) arises from the 'inside' of the iliac blade, passes under the inguinal ligament medially to the lesser trochanter. Both flex, but the psoas also internally rotates the hip.

- The psoas is enveloped in a fascial sheath. Retroperitoneal or spinal infections that track along soft tissue planes sometimes involves the psoas sheath and can cause inflammation in the psoas bursa, which separates the muscle from the hip joint.
- All adductor muscles arise from the pubis or ischiopubic rami. The adductor longus and gracilis are the most superficial; they arise from the pubis and insert into the femoral shaft and pes anserinus ('goose's foot') below the knee, respectively. The adductor magnus (L4/5) is the largest of the deeper adductors; it inserts into the medial femoral shaft.
- Adductors stabilize movement around the hip towards the end of the stance phase of the gait. Body weight is transferred onto one leg during this action and, therefore, adductors need to be strong, especially for running.

Functional anatomy of the hip

- With a flexed knee the limit of hip flexion is about 135°.
- Hip extension (at 30°), internal rotation (at 30–35°), and external rotation (at 45–55°) is limited by strong, pericapsular ligaments.
- Abduction is limited to 45–50° by contact between the greater trochanter and acetabular labrum rim. Adduction is limited to 20–30° with a fixed pelvis (Plate 14). These are adult ranges.
- Greater femoral neck anteversion (angle of the neck compared to the distal femur) allows greater internal rotation of the hip (and reduced external rotation). Tibial torsion can compensate but this and hip anteversion results in a toe-in gait. Femoral neck retroversion (if the angle is posterior to the femoral intercondylar plane) allows greater external rotation of the hip, usually resulting in a toe-out gait.
- Normally infants have more anteversion than older children or adults (30–40° at age 2 compared with 8–15° at age >18).

Neuroanatomy

- The femoral nerve is formed from L2–L4 nerve roots and supplies mainly muscles of the quadriceps group and some deeper hip adductors.
- With contributions from L4–S3 roots, nerves from the plexus converge at the inferior border of the piriformis to form the sciatic nerve. This is at a foramen formed by the ilium (above and lateral), sacrum (medial), sacrospinous ligament (below), and sacrotuberous ligament (posteromedial).
- In about 10% of people the sciatic nerve divides before exiting the pelvis. In some a branch exits above the piriformis muscle. Nerve entrapment and trauma at this site may give rise to **piriformis syndrome**, and may benefit from physical therapy.

Taking a history

Age

Age is a risk factor for some conditions:

- **Congenital hip dislocation** is common (prevalence 1:500), more so in girls than boys (8:1). It should be considered in toddlers if there is delay in motor milestones or pain on 'weight-bearing'.
- The most common cause of hip pain in children aged 2–12 years is transient synovitis (which is unilateral and self-limiting). The differential diagnosis includes **Legg–Calvé–Perthes' disease** [osteonecrosis of the femoral head (📖 Chapter 16, p 431)], and Lyme or post-streptococcal arthritis.
- Legg–Calvé–Perthes' disease (age 3–12 years) is four to five times more common in boys, and bilateral in 10–20% of cases.
- Slipped capital epiphysis is rare in children younger than 8 or older than 16 years old. It is associated with obesity and endocrine disorders (4% are hypothyroid).
- Unless there has been previous hip disease (e.g. osteonecrosis, synovitis), trauma, or a long-standing biomechanical abnormality (e.g. **epiphyseal dysplasia, HDCTs**, hip osteoarthritis (OA) is uncommon in adults less than 55 years old.
- Paget's disease of bone is rare in adults over 50 years old.

Distribution and type of bone and soft tissue pain

- All mechanical lesions of the lumbar spine can result in referred pain around the pelvis and thighs. It is often bilateral, localizes poorly, and is aching in nature.
- Lateral pelvic pain is often referred from the lumbosacral spine. If pain localizes (i.e. the patient points) to the greater trochanter, it may be due to **trochanteric bursitis, enthesitis, or meralgia paraesthetica** (lateral femoral cutaneous nerve syndrome, see Table 2.17).
- Hip joint pain is felt in the groin, but it can be located deep in the buttock when ischial bursitis and sacroiliac pain should also be considered. It may be referred distally to the anteromedial thigh and knee.
- Groin pain on weight-bearing suggests hip pathology such as synovitis, osteonecrosis or OA, but it is not specific. Tendonitis of the adductor longus, osteitis pubis, a femoral neck stress fracture (4% of all stress fractures), osteoid osteoma, or psoas bursitis can give similar symptoms.
- Bone pathology typically gives unremitting pain. Sleep is often disturbed.
- Pain from deep musculoskeletal pelvic structures is typically poorly localized, although can be severe. If the pain appears to be 'catastrophic' consider pelvic bone disease (tumours, infection, Paget's disease, osteomalacia, osteoporotic fracture) (📖 Chapter 16, p 431 and 📖 Chapter 17, p 473), or an unstable pelvis (chronic osteitis pubis with diastasis/laxity of the symphysis pubis and sacroiliac joints).
- **Enthesitis and osteitis pubis** associated with spondyloarthropathy (SpA) (📖 Chapter 8, p 281) are probably under-recognized.

Table 2.17 Patterns of pain around the proximal leg and their major causes

Pattern of pain	Causes
Pain in buttock and posterior thighs	Referred pain from: lumbar spine, e.g. facet, OA, spondylolisthesis; SI joint inflammation; lower lumbar nerve root irritation; sciatic nerve entrapment (piriformis syndrome)
	Localized pain: ischial bursitis/enthesitis or fracture; coccidynia
	Diffuse muscular pain/stiffness: myositis or PMR
	Paget's or other bone lesion of sacrum
Lateral pelvic pain	Referred from lumbosacral spine
	Trochanteric bursitis/enthesitis
	Gluteus medius tear
	Lateral hip joint pain, e.g. osteophyte
Groin pain	Hip disease, e.g. OA, osteonecrosis, synovitis
	Psoas bursitis
	Adductor tendonitis, osteitis pubis
	Pelvic enthesitis
	Paget's disease (pelvis or femur)
	Femoral neck or pubic ramus fracture
	Hernia
Anterior or medial pain	Referred from: lumbar spine, e.g. facet OA, thigh spondylolisthesis; upper lumbar nerve root; hip joint, femoral neck, psoas bursa
	Myositis, PMR, diabetic amyotrophy
	Meralgia paraesthetica (anterolateral)
	Adductor tendonitis, osteitis pubis
	Ischaemia (claudication)
	Lymph nodes

- Aching in the back of the legs after standing is found with spondylolisthesis (i.e. anterior displacement of a vertebra).
- Sacroiliac pain and stiffness radiates to the buttocks and posterior thighs.

Pain in a muscular distribution
- Diffuse pain in the buttocks and thighs occurs in **polymyalgia rheumatica** (PMR). It is often sudden or subacute in onset, associated

with stiffness, and may give similar symptoms to those caused by sacroiliitis but invariably occurs for the first time in a much older age group.

• Pain is not characteristic of an autoimmune myositis (📖 Chapter 14, p 385). When it does occur, it is unlikely to be confined to pelvic musculature or to be unilateral, but should be considered where acute or subacute onset diffuse pelvic girdle/thigh pain accompanies weakness.

Quality and distribution of nerve pain

• Nerve root pain is often clearly defined and sharp. It may be burning in quality and is often accompanied by numbness or paraesthesias. L5 or S1 lesions generally cause pain below the knee, but can also cause posterior thigh pain. L1–L3 root lesions can cause pain in the anteromedial thigh.

• Pain with paraesthesia on the anterolateral part of the thigh may be due to entrapment of the lateral cutaneous nerve of the thigh under the lateral part of the inguinal ligament (i.e. **meralgia paraesthetica**). Symptoms may be referred to this area with L2 or L3 nerve root lesions, since this is where the nerve originates (Fig. 2.12).

• Diabetics with uncontrolled hyperglycaemia are at risk of diabetic amyotrophy. Acute unilateral or bilateral thigh pain with muscle wasting occurs. It should not be misdiagnosed as PMR (in which weakness or wasting do not occur) or inflammatory myopathy.

• Footballers are at risk of adductor tendonitis (often an adductor apophysitis) and osteitis pubis owing to substantial mechanical forces placed on pelvic structures during running and kicking.

• Although hip fractures are usually obvious, they can also present subacutely in a patient who continues to walk; this is particularly common among the elderly, who may develop stress fractures of the hip.

Previous trauma, low back, and musculoskeletal problems

• Previous trauma or disease causing permanent deformity of any lumbosacral or hip joint structure can be considered a risk factor for further trouble (Table 2.18).

• Multiparity is a risk factor for osteitis pubis, sacroiliac, and pelvic pain.

• Trochanteric bursitis may co-exist with referred back pain.

• Tears of the gluteus medius can occur at its greater trochanter insertion and give similar symptoms to those caused by bursitis.

• Historically, tailors were at risk of ischial bursitis because of sitting on the floor continually crossing and uncrossing their legs, which causes friction irritation of soft tissues overlying the ischial tuberosity.

Examination

The reader is referred to the sequence of examination for the low back, including the sacroiliac and lower limb neurologic examination (📖 Chapter 2, p 19). Always consider lower spinal, muscle, or neurological pathology when assessing weakness and pain around the pelvis.

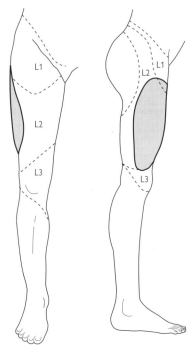

Fig. 2.12 The approximate areas within which sensory changes may be found in lesions of the lateral cutaneous nerve of the thigh (hatched area) and high lumbar radiculopathy (broken line). Shaded area-sensory symptoms distribution from meralgia paraesthetica.

Observation and palpation

For observation and palpation the patient should be supine on a couch:

- Look for leg length (Plate 15) discrepancy (hip disease, scoliosis) and a leg resting in external rotation (hip fracture).
- Psoriasis over the knees may be associated with sacroiliitis.
- Swelling in the groin may be a hernia (reducible, moves with cough), lipoma (soft/non-tender/diffuse), a saphenous varix, or lymphadenopathy (hard/rubbery and invariably mobile). A hip joint effusion cannot be felt.
- Tenderness over the hip joint in the groin is not specific for joint pathology: the joint is deep, muscles and psoas bursa overlie it.
- If the groin is very tender with slight touch, consider hip fracture or infection. Hyperpathia (and allodynia) is consistent with complex regional pain syndrome (☐ Chapter 18, p 489).
- Numbness over the anterolateral thigh suggests meralgia paraesthetica (Fig. 2.12).

Table 2.18 Risk factors for painful pelvic or hip lesions

Risk factor	Pelvic/hip pathology
Mechanical abnormality of the low back	Referred pain
	Trochanteric bursitis
Mechanical abnormality of the hip (e.g. Perthes', slipped epiphysis, epiphyseal dysplasia, Paget's)	Hip OA
	Hypermobility/dislocation
Corticosteroid use	Osteoporotic fracture
	Osteonecrosis of the femoral head (Plate 16)
Autoimmune rheumatic disease (e.g. RA, JIA, AS)	Synovitis hip
	Secondary OA of the hip
	Pyogenic arthritis of the hip
	Osteoporotic fracture
Maternal history of hip fracture; low body mass index; low bone mass; falls	Osteoporotic hip fracture
Multiple pregnancies	Osteitis pubis (± pelvic instability)
Footballers	Adductor tendonitis/apophysitis
	Osteitis pubis

- The adductor longus tendon can be palpated at its insertion at the pubic tubercle and distally along the upper medial thigh. The pubic tubercle is found by palpating slowly and lightly downwards from umbilicus over the bladder until bone is reached.
- Pain from **osteitis pubis or adductor apophysitis** is often significant, with abdominal rectus contraction (ask the patient to slowly lift their head and shoulders off the couch keeping your finger on the pubic tubercle).

Hip examination

The patient is supine. Tests generally help to discriminate articular and extra-articular disease, but not the causes of articular disease:

- Measure and determine actual or apparent leg length discrepancy: measure from the anterior superior iliac spine to the medial tibial malleolus; by flexing hips and knees, the site of shortening should become apparent.
- A fixed loss of extension is a sign of intra-articular hip disease. The patient flexes the hip and knee on one side until normal lumbar lordosis flattens out (confirmed by feeling pressure on your hand placed under their lumbar spine during the maneuver). If the other

hip flexes simultaneously, it suggests hip extension loss on that side (**Thomas' test**).

- Using the patella or tibial tubercle as pointers, test the rotational hip range in extension by rotating the straightened legs by holding the heels.
- Rotational movements are also tested by lifting the leg, flexed 90° at the knee, and swinging the foot out (internal rotation) or in (external rotation). Hip flexion can be tested in this position too (Plate 14). Patients without intra-articular pathology should have a pain-free range of movement.
- Rotational ranges in hip flexion and extension may differ between left and right in an individual. Also, variations in femoral neck anteversion contribute to variations in rotation range.
- To test hip abduction/adduction, fix the pelvis to avoid pelvic tilt by placing one hand firmly over the iliac crest (Plate 14). Occasionally, pain at the end of abduction or internal rotation occurs with a bony block (solid 'end-feel'). In an older patient this might suggest impingement of a marginal joint osteophyte.
- **Barlow's manoeuvre** checks for congenital dislocation of the hips in babies. Flex and adduct the hips exerting an axial force into the posterior 'acetabulum' to demonstrate posterior dislocation.
- Greater retroversion (allowing excessive hip external rotation) usually occurs in cases of slipped femoral epiphysis. External rotation is accentuated when the hip is flexed. The slip (usually inferoposterior) is thought to occur in association with a period of rapid growth.

Muscle activation tests

Specific muscle activation against resistance can be used to elicit pain, but results need to be interpreted cautiously in the context of known hip disease:

- Hip adduction against resistance (sliding their leg inwards towards the other against your hand) reproducing pain is a sensitive test for adductor longus tendonitis, but may be positive in osteitis pubis, hip joint lesions, and other soft tissue lesions in the adductor muscles.
- Test psoas by resisted hip flexion in slight internal rotation. Psoas bursitis or infection tracking along the psoas sheath is likely to give intense pain with minimal resistance.
- Hip abduction (sliding the leg outwards against your hand) may be particularly painful in cases of gluteus medius tears, but also in trochanteric bursitis or intra-articular pathology.

Palpate posterolateral structures

Ask the patient to lie on their side and palpate the posterolateral structures (Fig. 2.13):

- Tenderness over the greater trochanter is usually well-localized, although it may be anterior or posterolateral to the trochanter and refers a small way down the leg.
- The ischial tuberosity and its overlying bursa lie at the apex of the buttock.
- The soft tissues overlying the point where the sciatic nerve exits the pelvis is found midway between the ischial spine and the greater trochanter. There may be tenderness as a result of soft tissue lesions or trauma causing **sciatic nerve entrapment (piriformis syndrome)**, which can lead to foot drop.

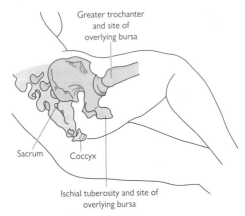

Fig. 2.13 Bony anatomy of the posterior hip and pelvis, showing the position in which lesions around the greater trochanter and ischial bursa can be palpated.

- A tender coccyx (**coccidynia**) can be palpated in this position. It can also be palpated (and the sacrococcygeal joint moved) from a bi-digital examination, though this requires the index finger to be placed inside the rectum, the thumb outside, the two digits then holding the joint.

Investigations

Radiographs

An AP radiograph of the pelvis is a good initial screening test in patients with pelvic, hip, or thigh pain. AP and lateral lumbar spine films may be warranted:

- The pelvis is a common site of involvement in myeloma, metastatic malignancy, and Paget's disease of bone (📖 Chapter 16, p 431).
- Established, but often not early, sacroiliitis can be ruled out. The main differential diagnoses of the causes of **sacroiliitis** are: AS, psoriatic or reactive arthritis, enteric arthropathy including Whipple's disease, brucellosis and other infections, hyperparathyroidism and osteitis condensans ilii (sclerosis of the SI joint on the lower iliac side; 📖 Chapter 8, p 281).
- Widening of the symphysis in children may be a sign of congenital disorders of development (e.g. epispadias, achondrogenesis, chondrodysplasias, hypophosphatasia), trauma and hyperparathyroidism (📖 Chapter 16, p 431).
- Widening of the symphysis pubis, osteitis pubis (bone resorption and sclerosis) and osteitis condensans ilii are signs associated with chronic pelvic pain in multiparous women.
- General osteopenia is a risk factor for general low bone mass measured by densitometry; however, it is not a sensitive or specific indicator of osteoporosis (i.e. may be osteomalacia or rickets).

- Regional osteoporosis confined to the femur is non-specific but may reflect hip synovitis, infection, or transient osteoporosis of the hip (rare).
- Early synovitis and infection may be demonstrated through subtle radiological signs such as joint space widening and change in soft tissue fat planes.
- A 'frog leg' (lateral) view of the hip shows the anterior and posterior femoral head more clearly than an AP view (useful in early osteonecrosis/Perthes', slipped epiphysis).
- The acetabulae are best visualized on 45° oblique views (acetabular fractures can be missed on a conventional AP view).
- 'Stork' views of the symphysis pubis (standing on one leg) are useful for confirming diastasis of the joint.

Diagnostic ultrasound

- US is a sensitive and simple way of confirming a hip joint effusion. Using US, fluid can be aspirated for culture and an assessment of the extent of synovial thickening can be made.
- Tendon damage in the groin area should be identifiable with US alone (guided steroid injection can then be done if necessary) but MRI may be needed either to characterize pathology further or rule out joint pathology.

Isotope bone scan

- Characteristic, though non-specific, patterns of bone scan abnormality are recognized in the hip/pelvic area. The following conditions can be recognized: sacroiliitis, bone malignancy, myeloma, Paget's disease, hip fracture, femoral head osteonecrosis (Plate 16), osteoid osteoma, OA and synovitis of the hip, osteitis pubis/adductor apophysitis (requires special seated 'ring' view), and bursitis/enthesitis at the greater trochanter.
- Scintigraphy is a useful investigation in children and adolescents as a screening investigation if other radiology tests are normal.

CT and MR

- CT/MR of the high lumbar region should be considered to confirm a nerve root lesion causing groin or thigh pain.
- Specific patterns of X-ray attenuation or signal change around the SI joints occur in sacroiliitis with CT/MR, although active and previous inflammation cannot easily be distinguished.
- A suspicion of bony malignancy from radiographs of the pelvis requires further characterization. CT is the technique of choice for characterizing bone lesions around the hip, such as femoral neck stress fracture, osteoid osteoma, or other bone tumours. CT may give more information about the lesion (and is valuable for 'guided biopsy'), but MR is useful in checking for pelvic visceral lesions.
- MR is the technique of choice if hip infection or osteonecrosis is suspected. In adults, patterns of signal change have been correlated with prognosis.
- During a single examination the pattern of hip synovitis (vascularity and thickness), cartilage loss, and subchondral bone erosion can be documented. This is particularly useful in children with JIA.

Laboratory investigations
- ESR and CRP may be normal in inflammatory SI joints, lumbar vertebral disc, and pelvic enthesis disorders.
- PMR is invariably associated with an acute phase response.
- Myeloma is unlikely if the ESR is normal.
- A high alkaline phosphatase is typically associated with an acute phase response, although in the elderly, it might suggest Paget's disease.
- ANA and RF are unlikely to help diagnostically.
- Major metabolic bone disease, such as osteomalacia and hyper-parathyroidism is usually excluded by a normal serum calcium and phosphate.

Treatment

Treatment of spinal and neuropathic pain is covered in the section on 'Low back pain and disorders in adults', (📖 Chapter 2, p 19):
- NSAIDs may be required for a number of the conditions described above, particularly OA, hip synovitis, and tendon inflammation.
- Physical therapy and rehabilitation play a vital and early part in management, maintaining mobility, preventing tissue contracture, and restrengthening/stabilizing the lower back, pelvis, and hip.
- Either physical therapists or podiatrists may help in accurately evaluating back and lower limb biomechanics. Asymmetry and muscular imbalance may be modifiable relatively simply with foot orthotics, for example.
- Steroid injections may be important in the following conditions:
  - meralgia paraesthetica;
  - osteitis pubis;
  - trochanteric bursitis/enthesitis;
  - ischial bursitis/enthesitis;
  - adductor tendonitis;
  - coccidynia;
  - hip synovitis (under imaging guidance);
  - sacroiliitis—in intractable pain and under X-ray or US guidance.
- Injection techniques are covered in 📖 Chapter 22, p 589.

Surgery
- When the hip has been damaged by an inflammatory arthritis or OA the principal surgical intervention is joint replacement. Osteotomy has been mainly superseded by more reliable replacement.
- Surgical synovectomy of the hip is a difficult procedure and opening the hip carries a risk of avascular necrosis. This procedure is very rarely done.
- Excision arthroplasty is only really necessary where infection or poor bone stock make reconstruction unwise. Power is often greatly reduced and even the previously fit young patient will not be able to ambulate without crutches.
- In children, in particular, it is important to assess spinal and knee disease, especially contractures, before embarking on hip surgery as the primary cause for flexion deformities or hip damage may be at these levels.

Knee pain

Anatomy of the knee

- The knee extends, flexes, and rotates.
- The main extensor quadriceps consists of four muscle segments—rectus femoris, vastus lateralis, medialis, and intermedius—which converge to form a tendon containing the patella that then inserts into the tibia. Rectus femoris arises from the pelvis and vastus muscles from the upper femur.
- The hamstring muscles (biceps femoris, semitendinosus, semi-membranosus) all arise from the ischial tuberosity and flex the knee. The biceps femoris inserts around the fibular head. The other two muscles insert into the tibia on the medial side and can externally rotate the femur.
- In the knee, the femoral condyles articulate within semicircular fibrocartilage menisci on the tibial condyles (Fig. 2.14). Only the peripheral 10–30% of the menisci is vascular and innervated and can potentially repair itself.
- As the knee approaches full extension, the femur internally rotates on the tibia (biceps femoris action) tightening each pair of ligaments relative to each other. This configuration confers maximum stability.
- As flexion is initiated, a small amount of femoral external rotation on the tibia occurs. This 'unlocking' is done by the popliteus—a muscle that arises from the posterior surface of the tibia below. It passes up obliquely across the back of the knee and inserts, via a cord-like tendon, into the lateral femoral condyle. The tendon partly lies within the knee joint capsule.
- Grooves on the femoral condyle articular surfaces allow tight congruity with the anterior horns of the menisci when the knee is extended. If full extension—and this optimal articulation configuration—is lost, then articular cartilage degeneration invariably follows. This is particularly important in inflammatory arthritis.
- The cruciate ligaments are the principal joint stabilizers. The anterior cruciate attaches above to the inside of the lateral femoral condyle and below to the tibia in front of the tibial spines though a slip attaches to the anterior horn of the lateral meniscus. Its main role is to control and contain the amount of knee rotation when the joint is flexed.
- The posterior cruciate attaches above to the inside of the medial femoral condyle. At the other end, it attaches in a (posterior) groove between tibial condyles. Its main role is to stabilize the joint by preventing forward displacement of the femur relative to the tibia when the knee is flexed.
- The cruciates are extra-articular and are covered by a layer of vascular synovium. Bleeding usually accompanies disruption.

The tibial or medial collateral ligament (MCL) has superficial and deep layers (Fig. 2.15). It stabilizes the knee against valgus stresses, mostly during flexion. The superficial MCL overlies, and moves relative to, the deep part and is separated from it by a bursa. The lower part of the superficial MCL is covered by the long adductors, gracilis, semitendinosus, and sartorius muscles, as they merge into the pes anserinus before inserting into the tibia. The MCL and pes anserinus are separated by the anserine bursa. Deeper MCL fibres attach to, and stabilize, the medial meniscus.

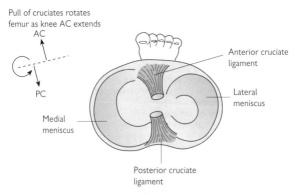

Pull of cruciates rotates femur as knee AC extends

AC

PC

Anterior cruciate ligament

Lateral meniscus

Medial meniscus

Posterior cruciate ligament

Fig. 2.14 Axial section of the right knee joint (looking down on the tibial plateau, where the foot is fixed on the floor). The femoral condyles articulate within the menisci. As the knee extends the cruciate ligaments tighten and pull the femoral condyles acting to internally rotate the femur through the last few degrees of extension. The knee therefore 'locks' and is stable when the leg is straight.

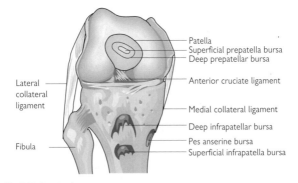

Patella
Superficial prepatella bursa
Deep prepatellar bursa

Lateral collateral ligament

Anterior cruciate ligament

Medial collateral ligament

Deep infrapatellar bursa

Pes anserine bursa

Fibula

Superficial infrapatella bursa

Fig. 2.15 Anterior knee structures.

- The fibular or lateral collateral ligament (LCL) joins the lateral femoral condyle to the fibular head and is separated from it by a bursa. It stabilizes the knee on its lateral side. It has no meniscal attachment. A small bursa separates it from the overlapping tendon insertion of biceps femoris.
- The patella is a seamed bone that articulates in the femoral condylar groove and makes quadriceps action more efficient. Patella articular facet configuration can vary; congenital bi/tripartite patellae are associated with anterior knee pain.
- The strongest force on the patella is from vastus lateralis (Fig. 2.15). Mechanical factors that increase the ratio of lateral to medial forces during patella tracking such as a wide pelvis, a more lateral origin of vastus lateralis, femoral neck anteversion, external tibial torsion, and a weak vastus medialis are risk factors for patella tracking problems and anterior knee pain.
- There are bursae between the quadriceps tendon and the femur (suprapatellar), the patellar tendon and tibial tubercle (deep infrapatellar), and overlying the patella (prepatellar) and patellar tendon insertion (superficial infrapatellar). The suprapatellar bursa communicates with the knee joint and large joint effusions invariably fill it.
- Posteriorly, bursae separate each of the heads of gastrocnemius (which arise from femoral condyles) from the joint capsule. The bursae communicate with the knee joint and can fill from joint effusions.

Taking a history

Ask about the site of pain

Try to establish whether pain is from articular, soft tissue, or anterior knee structures. Is it referred pain?

- Bursa, tendon, and most ligament lesions cause well-localized pain.
- Localized tibiofemoral joint line pain suggests meniscal pathology.
- Localized medial knee pain has a number of possible causes: MCL tear or chronic inflammation (calcification of MCL origin termed the Pellegrini–Stieda phenomenon), medial meniscus tear, meniscal cyst, **anserine tendonitis, bursitis, or enthesitis** (semimembranosus insertion).
- Enthesitis of structures at their insertion to the patella margins can result in considerable pain.
- Over-use in runners and cyclists can cause localized inflammation and pain of the iliotibial band (ITB) or its underlying bursa over the lateral femoral condyle (as the band moves across the bone as the knee flexes).
- Anterior pain in children, adolescents, and young adults invariably suggests an underlying mechanical abnormality. In older adults the most common cause is patellofemoral OA (Table 2.19).
- Anterior knee pain may be referred from the hip or L3 nerve root. Hip pain is an aching pain, root pain is sharp often with paraesthesias.
- Posterior knee pain associated with 'a lump' is often due to synovitis in the posterior knee compartment with popliteal cyst formation (**Baker's cyst**).

Ask about injury

Knee injuries are common; the most significant is anterior cruciate injury. Ask about injury and whether the knee feels unstable or 'gives way':

- Anterior cruciate injuries are invariably associated with a haemarthrosis, thus a painful effusion will have occurred immediately. Meniscus tears can cause immediate pain, but synovitis and swelling are delayed for about 6 h.
- Patients may volunteer that the knee 'keeps giving out on me'. This feeling may be the pivot shift phenomenon caused by reduced anterior cruciate stability against a valgus stress as the knee is flexing.
- Anterior cruciate and MCL injuries often co-exist (since they are attached). Ask about medial knee pain originally and subsequently.

Ask about knee locking

Knee locking is a mechanical effect of disruption of normal articulation by 'loose bodies':

- Suspect meniscus damage in the middle aged or if the patient plays a lot of sports. A meniscus tear is the most common cause of the knee locking. In adolescents, locking may be due to a tear in a discoid meniscus (>98% lateral). The morphologically abnormal discs are prone to degeneration.

Table 2.19 Causes of anterior knee pain

Commonly in adults	Patellofemoral OA (look for mechanical factors and generalized OA)
	Referred hip pain, e.g. hip OA
	Referred pain from L3 nerve root irritation
Specific to children and adolescents	Referred pain from the hip, e.g. slipped femoral epiphysis
	Bi-/tripartite patella
	Synovial plicae (synovial shelf clicking over femoral condyle on knee flexion)
	Recurrent patellar dislocation (tissue laxity, patella alta, trauma)
	Osteochondritis at patellar lower pole—over-use injury in jumping sports[*]
	Osteochondritis of tibial tubercle (Osgood–Schlatter's) (📖 Chapter 16, p 431)
	Non-specific ('chondromalacia patellae')
Causes at any age	Mechanical factors (patellar maltracking): wide pelvis, femoral anteversion, external tibial torsion; specific strengthening of lateral structures, e.g. iliotibial band syndrome; weakness or injury of vastus medialis or medial knee structures; tissue laxity, e.g. joint hypermobility syndrome
	Osteochondritis dissecans of patella (average age 18)
	Enthesitis at patellar margins (may be part of SpA)
	Bursitis (prepatellar, superficial/deep infrapatellar); gout (very rare in children unless inherited metabolic deficiency); autoimmune rheumatic disease; infection
	Tear/cyst of anterior meniscal horn
	Patellar fracture
	Fat pad syndrome (recurrent retropatellar tendon pain with swelling)

[*]Sinding–Larsen–Johansson disease.

- Chondral fragments (from osteochondritis dissecans lesions) can cause locking; the condition is most common in the 5–20-year age group (boys > girls).
- Synovial chondromatosis is a rare cause.
- Some patients with anterior knee pain describe the knee locking or giving way. This is due to reflex quadriceps inhibition rather than true instability.

Ask about the initial onset of pain
- Acute pain is usual with injuries of cruciates and vertical meniscal tears.
- Acute onset pain without trauma (but always with swelling) suggests **infection, crystal arthritis, or spontaneous haemarthrosis.**
- In the very elderly, traumatic lesions may be missed, since the presentation is not always striking, e.g. intra-articular fracture with haemarthrosis.
- An insidious onset of pain is usual in cleavage **tears of menisci** (horizontal tears), which occur typically in adults where the disc is degenerate, in adolescents with discoid menisci, and in early **osteochondritis dissecans**.

Ask about the pattern and type of pain
- Pain from synovitis is often associated with stiffness and is often worse after a period of immobility. Almost without exception knee synovitis can occur in all forms of arthritis.
- Pain from subchondral damage (e.g. OA) is almost always worse on weight- bearing, but this association is not specific.
- Pain on kneeling/squatting is characteristic of anterior knee pain.
- Burning pain may be neurogenic, e.g. L3 nerve root or reflex sympathetic dystrophy pain.

Past medical, family, occupational, and leisure history
- Knee synovitis and patellar enthesitis occur in adult and juvenile enthesitis-related arthritis. Ask about previous uveitis, low back pain, urethral discharge, sexually transmitted disease, dysentery, and psoriasis.
- Gout (📖 Chapter 7, p 269) is not uncommon around the knee. Ask about gout risk factors and whether the patient has ever had first MTP joint pain (i.e. podagra).
- There may be a family history of generalized OA (📖 Chapter 6, p 259), a hereditary disease of connective tissue, or hypermobility in young adults with OA.
- Prepatellar bursitis classically occurred in housemaids, hence the nickname '**housemaid's knee**'. Friction caused by repeated kneeling can cause it.
- Sports injuries are common. Anterior cruciate injury occurs characteristically in skiing. Meniscal injuries are common in soccer. Jumping events (e.g. high jump, basketball) can lead to patellar tendon apophysitis. Cycling is associated with anterior knee pain. MCL and meniscal injuries are common in skiing and weight-bearing activities where rotation and change of direction are frequent. Cycling and running are associated with ilio-tibial band (ITB)/bursa pain and inflammation.

Examination

From front and behind, observe the patient standing

- Look for mechanical abnormalities that might be associated with knee lesions: patella asymmetry, prominent tibial tubercles from previous **Osgood–Schlatter's** (anterior knee pain), flat feet, and hypermobility (patella dislocation, hyperextension of >10°).
- Check for mechanical abnormalities which might suggest specific pathology: **genu varum** (bowed leg, typical appearance with primarily medial compartment OA), obvious suprapatellar knee swelling (synovitis), psoriasis (associated synovitis or enthesitis), and **genu valgum** (knock-kneed). Marked genu varum occurs in the rare Blount's disease (developmental abnormality of the medial tibial physis typically in African-American boys).

Examination of the sitting patient

Ask the patient to sit on the examination table with legs hanging, knees bent. Patellar tracking and pain from medial meniscus damage can be assessed. An alternative approach is with the patient supine. Observe any muscle wasting. Palpate anterior, medial, and lateral structures:

- In patients with anterior knee pain, look for symmetric patellar alignment.
- Observe active knee extension. Patellar movement should be smooth, pain-free, and symmetric.
- Passively externally rotate each lower leg to its extreme. This is a reasonably sensitive test for conditions of the medial knee compartment (e.g. meniscus tear) and medial knee structures. Discomfort will be felt. If the MCL is totally deficient, an abnormally increased range of external rotation may occur.
- Quadriceps wasting (accentuated depression in muscle just above the patella) occurs with disuse after injuries and in chronic arthropathies.
- Sites of bursae, patellar tendon, and ligament insertions should be palpated in patients with localized pain (Fig. 2.16).
- Tibiofemoral joint line tenderness is likely to be due to either meniscus pathology or marginal osteophytes. Osteophytes give bony swelling.
- Anterior pain from patellofemoral joint disorders may be elicited by gentle pressure down on the patella. Mobilizing the patella sideways will give an impression of tissue laxity (possible underlying hypermobility).
- Factors that predispose to patellofemoral pain syndrome include: high or lateral patella, weak vastus medialis, excessive pronation, weak ankle dorsiflexors, tight hamstrings, reduced movement at the ankle, and a wide Q-angle. The Q-angle is formed between a line from the anterior superior iliac spine to the center of the patella, and a line extended upwards from the tibial tubercle through the center of the patella. The larger the angle the greater the lateral tensile pull on the patella (Fig. 2.17).
- Localized tenderness of the femoral condyle is often the only sign of osteochondritis dissecans in adolescents. The most common site is on the inside of the medial femoral condyle (75%).

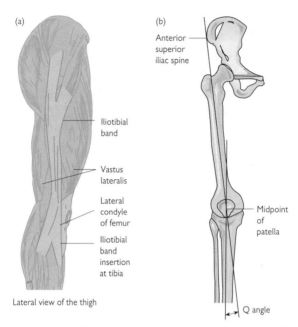

Fig. 2.16 (a) The iliotibial band. (b) The patella Q angle (normal values—men 10°, women 15°).

Examine for joint synovitis (synovial inflammation giving synovial thickening and/or tenderness) and an effusion

- The joint may be warm. Chronic synovitis does not always result in a warm joint, but infection, crystal arthritis, and haemarthrosis usually do.
- Gross synovitis can produce obvious effusions and/or synovial thickening most easily felt around the patellar edges.
- Effusions may be confirmed by the patellar tap test (Plate 17).
- Small effusions can be detected by eliciting the 'bulge sign'. Fluid in the medial compartment is swept firmly upward and laterally into the suprapatellar pouch. Firm pressure on the lateral side of the joint may then push fluid back into the medial compartment, producing a bulge.
- Thickened synovium can be detected by experienced examiners in the absence of a detectable effusion. It is not always tender.
- Posterior compartment synovial thickening and popliteal cysts can be felt by wrapping the fingers around under the knee when it is slightly flexed.
- In contrast to adults, popliteal cysts in children are not usually associated with intra-articular pathology. Investigation is not always necessary.

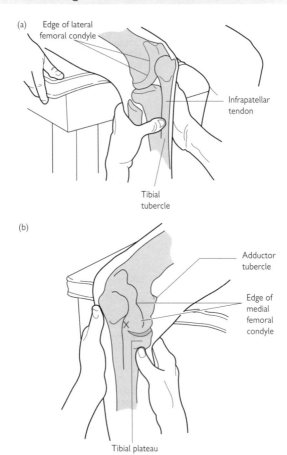

Fig. 2.17 Position of the knee for palpation of most of its structures. Palpating for enthesitis at the patellar tendon insertion. (a) Palpation over the insertion of semimembranosus and pes anserinus under the tibial plateau (b) The site of the majority of osteochondritis lesions in the knee is shown by the 'X'.

Test the knee for stability

- There are many tests for instability: instability may be straight or rotational and can be graded according to consensus criteria (consult orthopaedics texts).
- The **Lachmann test** (Fig. 2.18) is arguably the most sensitive test for eliciting anterior cruciate disruption: hold the knee flexed between 20–30°, grasped above and below the joint. Attempt to move the tibia

forwards and backwards on the femur. Ask about pain and feel for laxity or a 'clunk'.

- The anterior draw test is not as sensitive as the Lachmann test for detecting partial anterior cruciate tears, but is easier to do. The patient lies flat, hip flexed, the knee flexed at 90°, with the foot flat on the table. Fix the foot by gently sitting on it and pull the top of the lower leg forwards in the line of the thigh. Ask about pain and feel for laxity.
- The posterior draw test identifies posterior cruciate disruption: with the knee flexed to 90°, press the top of the lower leg backwards in the line of the thigh, ask about pain and feel for laxity.
- Test medial stability at 0° and 30° of flexion (MCL stabilizes maximally at 30°) by holding the upper leg still and applying a valgus force to the tibia. Laxity associated with widening of the tibiofemoral joint (with or without pain) is a positive test and suggests MCL deficiency.
- Lateral (LCL and ITB) stability is similarly tested, though using a varus force on the lower leg.
- MCL tears can accompany anterior cruciate injuries and deep lesions are associated with simultaneous tears of the medial meniscus. Such complex pathology can make specific examination manoeuvers difficult to interpret.

Test for meniscus damage

- **McMurray's test** (Fig. 2.19). Flex the knee, internally rotate the lower leg, then extend the joint. Repeat with the lower leg externally rotated. The fingers (over the joint line) may feel a 'clunk' as a femoral condyle passes over a torn meniscus. It is often positive (21–65% of cases) when surgery subsequently reveals no tear.
- Ask the patient to turn over. Lying initially on their side allows you to do **Ober's test** to detect lateral soft tissue injury. When prone, look and palpate for swelling in the popliteal fossa and proximal calf that may indicate a low lying popliteal cyst.
- Inflammation of the bursa underlying the iliotibial band (ITB) may result in tenderness over the lateral femoral condyle. The ITB may be tight. This is demonstrated using Ober's test. The patient lies on their side with the lower (non-affected) leg flexed at the hip. The upper (painful) knee is flexed to 90° and the thigh is extended and adducted. The test is positive if, when the examiner's hand is removed, the hip does not drop down (further stretching the ITB). Leg length inequality and foot over-pronation may be causative factors.
- Detecting specific structures in the posterior fossa is often difficult because of the lack of bony landmarks and overlapping soft tissue structures. Synovial cysts may form under pressure and are often hard and tender. Diffuse thickening suggests joint synovitis.

Investigations

Radiographs

AP and lateral weight-bearing radiographs are suitable screening views if the diagnosis is unclear after clinical assessment:

- Early synovitis may only be evident from the presence of an effusion, peri-articular osteopenia, or soft tissue swelling. Patterns of bone damage in chronic arthropathies may be recognized.

Anterior draw test

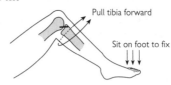

Pull tibia forward

Sit on foot to fix

Lachmann test

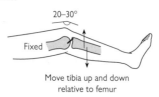

20–30°

Fixed

Move tibia up and down
relative to femur

Fig. 2.18 Dynamic tests of anterior cruciate function. Patients should be relaxed lying supine on a couch. Excessive laxity is the most important sign.

McMurray's test

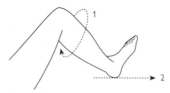

1

2

Action: Hold the knee and the heel.
Internally rotate the lower leg (1) then extend it (2)
Positive test: (Palpable) clunk at joint line

Fig. 2.19 Dynamic test designed to elicit signs of meniscus damage. 'Clunks', intra-articular pain, and coarse crepitus may indicate damage. The test is not specific and is open to misinterpretation.

- Signs of joint infection, which may not necessarily present acutely, are patchy bone osteolysis and irregular loss of bone cortex. Osteonecrosis is uncommon in the knee although it occurs in sickle cell anaemia.
- Loss of joint space, angulation deformity, osteophytes, subchondral bone sclerosis, and bone cysts are hallmark features of OA.
- In adults, linear or vague intra-articular calcification suggests chondrocalcinosis [associated with calcium pyrophosphate dihydrate (CPPD) arthritis]. Gross 'thumbprint' calcification is typical of synovial chondromatosis (mainly in children).

- In children check for an osteochondral fragment (e.g. osteochondritis dissecans), normal epiphyses, epiphyseal plates and metaphyses, normal patella shape, and osteochondritis at the tibial tubercle (Table 2.20).

Specialized radiographic views: tomographic views; 'skyline' (axial with knee bent) view; or lateral view taken with at least 30° of flexion

- Tomography is useful for clarifying non-peripheral osteochondral defects.
- Skyline views demonstrate anomalous patellar facet configuration and can reveal patellofemoral incongruity though multiple views may be needed. Subchondral patellar pathology is seen more clearly than on lateral views.
- Patella alta is most reliably seen on a lateral view with 30° flexion.

Further imaging

Further imaging depends on differential diagnosis and a discussion with your radiologist:

- Peri-articular soft tissue lesions can be characterized with MRI, although with superficial lesions adequate information needed for further management may be obtainable with ultrasound alone.
- Patterns of meniscus damage are recognized on MRI, give an indication of prognosis, and aid the surgeon's decision to proceed to arthroscopy.
- MRI is essential if there is likely to be a combination of lesions, e.g. anterior cruciate, MCL, and medial meniscus lesions.
- In children, both US and MR will confirm synovitis.
- MR is more sensitive than radiographs or US at identifying joint erosions in RA.
- The place of CT or MR in investigating radiographically detected bone tumours depends on the nature of the lesion.

Table 2.20 Interpretation of radiographic knee abnormalities in children

Radiographic abnormality	Possible conditions
Intra-articular calcific fragment	Osteochondritis dissecans, traumatic avulsion, synovial tumours, or chondromatosis (rare)
Epiphyseal defect/abnormality	JIA, sepsis, avulsion injury, bone dysplasias, rickets, haemophilia, hypothyroidism
Transverse radiolucent metaphyseal band or lysis	Leukaemia, lymphoma, neuroblastoma, metastases, infections (neonates),osteogenesis imperfecta, idiopathic juvenile osteoporosis, Cushing's disease
Joint space narrowing	JIA, sepsis, PVNS, haemophilia
Diffuse low bone density	Rickets, OI, osteoporosis, mucopolysaccharidosis
Periosteal reaction	Fracture, sepsis, infarction, tumours

Aspiration of joint and peri-articular fluid collections

- Early aspiration is essential if infection is suspected (Plate 18).
- The knee is a common site of monoarthritis (☐ Chapter 22, p 589). The principles behind management apply to all cases of single joint pathology.
- Send joint fluid for cell count, polarized light microscopy, and culture.

- In adults, the usual differential diagnosis of sepsis of knee structures is gout, so fluid should be examined by polarized light microscopy for urate crystals.
- Blood-stained fluid either suggests a traumatic tap or chondrocalcinosis. Frank blood suggests haemarthrosis, the major causes of which are cruciate tear, bleeding diathesis, intra-articular fracture, and pigmented villonodular synovitis (PVNS).
- Bursa fluid may be more successfully detected and aspirated using US guidance.

Laboratory investigations
These should be directed towards suspected underlying disease:
- FBC, acute phase reactants (ESR, CRP).
- Blood urea, electrolytes, creatinine, and urate.
- Blood calcium, phosphate, albumin, alkaline phosphatase, 25-OH vitamin D, and PTH to screen for metabolic bone disease.
- Autoantibodies: rheumatoid factor (RF), antinuclear (ANA), and extractable nuclear antibodies (ENAs) to characterize an autoimmune process where synovitis is chronic.
- Serum angiotensin converting enzyme (sACE) for sarcoidosis.
- IgM *Borrelia burgdorferi* serology for acute arthropathy in Lyme disease, streptococcal antibodies for reactive streptococcal arthritis.

Treatment
- In general, most soft tissue lesions will settle with rest and NSAIDs.
- Anterior knee pain may respond well to isometric exercises, adjustments to foot alignment, e.g. with sensible shoes, orthotics (support insoles), and hamstring stretching exercises.
- The acute swollen knee requires aspiration, rest for 24 h and gentle mobilization. If infection is considered, broad-spectrum antibiotics against staphylococcal and streptococcal agents should be started immediately while awaiting culture data. In infection, intra-articular antibiotics and steroids should be avoided. The patient should not bear weight on an acutely infected joint (Chapter 22, p 589).
- Acute and chronic inflammation can lead to joint destruction and instability. If RA is identified, early treatment may prevent long-term morbidity (Chapter 5, p 283).
- Physical therapy and splinting play an important role in maintaining function and preventing contractures, etc.

Address biomechanical factors
Input from a physical therapist may be helpful in cases of anterior knee pain. Success from McConnell (patellar) taping is more likely in non-patellofemoral OA-related anterior knee pain.
- Quadriceps strengthening exercises can be reviewed and reinforced by physical therapists in cases of knee OA.
- Knee pain, particularly anterior pain, may be linked to foot abnormalities (e.g. over-pronation), and hip alignment (Q-angle, above).
- Specific muscle strengthening exercises, foot orthotics, and knee braces should be considered.

Local steroid injection

Local steroid injections can be helpful in the following situations:

- Acute flare of non-infective inflammatory disease:
  - OA (especially where CPPD is present)—mild OA may also respond to hyaluronate injections;
  - autoimmune arthritis, e.g. RA, SpA;
  - intra-articular gout;
  - SpA
- Bursitis (may be gout):
  - pre- and infrapatella (superficial and deep) bursa (the latter may require US guidance);
  - anserine.
- Baker's cyst (note: the knee joint is injected at the site of the pathology assuming there is intra-articular communication between joint and cyst. Direct popliteal cyst injection should be under US guidance only to avoid damage to vascular and nerve tissues).
- Enthesopathy, e.g. semimembranosus insertion.
- Trauma, e.g. pain over medial collateral ligament insertion.
- Other soft-tissue: ITB syndrome.

The reader is referred to 📖 Chapter 22, p 589 for steroid injection techniques and to the relevant chapters for specific diseases.

Joint injection therapies

- In patients with large joint effusions, merely aspirating the effusion may provide some level of symptomatic relief.
- Knee OA may respond transiently to an injectible steroid, such as triamcinolone acetate. Saline irrigation and injections with hyaluronic acid preparations are also used, but response is variable.

Note: all intra-articular injection therapies are more effective when patient's knee is immobilized for 24 hours following the procedure.

Drugs

- NSAIDs will invariably be helpful in cases of inflammatory and septic arthritis.
- Colchicine 0.5 mg twice daily for 5 days is often useful in relieving pain from crystal arthritis in patients intolerant of NSAIDs.
- Paracetamol/acetaminophen may be as effective as NSAIDs for some patients.
- Glucosamine and chondroitin sulphate are controversial for the treatment of osteoarthritis. Although some studies demonstrate improved pain control and function, other studies clearly indicate that these are no better than placebo.

Surgery

- Arthroscopy is often used as a diagnostic tool in cases of undiagnosed monoarthritis and to confirm and trim cartilage tears. Synovium and synovial lesions (e.g. PVNS, synovial chondromatosis) can be biopsied or excised (synovectomy) and the joint can be irrigated.
- In appropriate cases joint replacement can be remarkably successful and is an important option to consider in OA and inflammatory arthritis, where pain is severe and present at rest, and when mobility is substantially restricted.
- Arthrodesis is rarely indicated.
- Unicondylar osteotomy can aid realignment of the tibiofemoral joint, e.g. in metabolic bone disease, such as Paget's disease.

Other

- In OA, capsaicin cream applied three or four times daily to painful superficial structures, e.g. patellar margins or marginal tibiofemoral joint pain, can ease symptoms. Response is cumulative and may not occur for 6–8 weeks.
- Topical lidocaine patches may also be useful for control of pain limited to one joint. Note lidocaine is often ineffective in all formulations in Joint Hypermobility Syndrome/Ehlers–Danlos syndrome hypermobility type (📖 Chapter 16, p 431).

Lower leg and foot disorders (adults)

Anatomy

Anatomy of bones and joints

- The leg absorbs six times the body weight during weight-bearing. Strong ligaments secure the ankle (formed by tibia above/medially and fibular malleolus laterally) and talocalcaneal (subtalar) joints and bones of the midfoot (Fig. 2.20).
- Anomalous ossicles in the foot are common. Some are associated with specific pathology. There are many potential sites, though the sesamoids in flexor hallucis brevis (FHB) are invariable.
- The foot is an optimal mechanical device to support body weight when walking or running over flat, inclined, and uneven types of terrain. The configuration of bones at synovial articulations allows dorsal flexion (foot pulled up), plantar flexion (to walk on toes), inversion (foot tips in), eversion (foot tips out), and small degrees of adduction and abduction. Midfoot movements allow pronation and supination.
- The normal ankle joint range is about 25° of dorsal flexion and 50° of plantar flexion from neutral (foot 90° to leg). The range of subtalar inversion–eversion is normally 10–15°.

Anatomy of the long muscles and tendons

- In the lower leg a strong fascia connects the tibia and fibula. Lower leg muscles primarily move the foot. They are separated into compartments by fascia and are prone to pressure effects.
- The foot dorsal flexors—tibialis anterior, extensor digitorum longus (EDL), extensor hallucis longus (EHL) and peroneus tertius—lie adjacent to the anteromedial side of the tibia. Their tendons pass in front of the ankle in synovial sheaths held down by strong retinaculae (Fig. 2.21). The tibialis anterior, the bulkiest flexor, inserts into the medial midfoot (medial cuneiform).
- In the posterior lower leg, the gastrocnemius (and plantaris), which arise from the femur, plantar flexes the foot by pulling the back of the calcaneum. The soleus, which arises in the lower leg, merges with them in the Achilles' tendon. This tendon has a deep and superficial bursa at its insertion site.
- Plantar flexion is assisted weakly by long muscles, which arise in the lower leg, pass behind the medial malleolus in synovial sheaths (Fig. 2.21), and insert into the sole. They mostly invert the foot. Tibialis posterior, the most bulky plantar flexor, inserts into the plantar surface of the navicular.
- The peroneus longus and brevis arise from the fibular side of the leg and pass around the lateral malleolus in a common synovial sheath held by a retinaculum. Longus passes into the sole and inserts into the medial cuneiform. Brevis inserts into the fifth metatarsal base. Both evert the foot.
- The tibial nerve and artery follow the course of the medial tendons under the flexor retinaculum (Fig. 2.21).

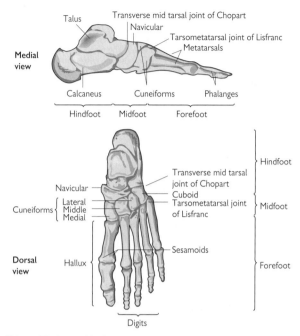

Fig. 2.20 The bones of the foot.

Anatomy of intrinsic foot structure

- Intrinsic foot structures have been greatly modified during evolution to combine provision of a flexible platform for support and a rigid lever for thrusting body weight forward when walking.
- In the sole of the foot, muscles are aligned longitudinally in four layers. The deepest layers include phalangeal interossei in the forefeet, tibialis posterior, peroneus longus, adductor hallucis, and FHB, which has two insertions into the proximal great toe phalanx, each containing a sesamoid.
- The superficial layers include flexor digitorum longus (FDL), which inserts into the lateral four distal phalanges, the phalangeal lumbricals, flexor digitorum brevis, and abductor hallucis. The latter two muscles arise from the plantar surface of the calcaneum deep to the plantar fascia.
- Flexor tendons merge with the deeper part of the plantar fascia, a swath of tissue that extends from os calcis to the metatarsal area.
- Longitudinal muscles, ligaments, and fascia contribute to stabilize the foot with a longitudinal arch—its apex at the talus, but also with some effect laterally. The foot arches transversely—its apex at medial cuneiform level.

Neuroanatomy
- The sciatic nerve splits into tibial and common peroneal nerves above the knee. The common peroneal is prone to pressure neuropathy as it runs superficially around the fibular head. The nerve then divides. A deep branch runs distally under the extensor retinaculum to the foot. It supplies tibialis anterior, EHL, and EDL. A superficial branch supplies the peroneal muscles and most of the skin over the dorsum of the foot.
- The tibial nerve runs in the posterior lower leg compartment supplying gastrocnemius and soleus. It then passes under the medial flexor retinaculum dividing into medial and lateral plantar nerves, which supply the intrinsic plantar muscles of the foot and skin of the sole.

Functional anatomy
- In a normal gait pattern, the foot is dorsiflexed and invertors/evertors stabilize the hindfoot for heel strike. As weight is transferred forward, the foot plantar flexes and pronates, the great toe extends (optimally between 65° and 75°), and push off occurs through the medial side of the forefoot.
- All metatarsals bear weight and can suffer weight-bearing injury.
- Ligamentous attachments around the hindfoot are strong. A fall on a pronated inverted foot without direct trauma can result in a fracture of the distal fibula. This is probably a consequence of the relative strength of the talofibular ligaments compared with bone.

Developmental factors
- Developmental characteristics often imply that different age groups are prone to a different spectrum of conditions.
- Due to ligamentous laxity, when babies begin to walk, the midfoot is flat to the floor. A longitudinal arch usually develops by 5 years.
- During growth, tendon insertions (apophyses) are often weaker than the tendons themselves. Traction strain on tendons can lead to apophysitis (osteochondritis). This is a common pattern of injury in the foot in active older children.

Conditions of the lower leg
- Patients with lower leg conditions may present with pain or deformity alone. In children, deformity may typically be due to spinal dysraphism (from birth), rickets (acquired age 1 year plus), or osteogenesis imperfecta (📖 Chapter 16, p 431).
- Pains in the calf may be due to local soft tissue or muscle conditions, but in adults are commonly due to referred lumbosacral pain. These pains are often described by patients as 'cramps'—suggesting a muscle problem at first. A detailed history may suggest nerve root pathology.
- Imbalance of muscles in the foot can lead to increased tension at tendon and fascial insertions in the calf and shin, resulting in '**shin splints**'. Shin splints usually present after activity and are relieved by rest. Conditions to consider include:
  - stress fractures of the tibia or fibula;
  - tibialis posterior fasciitis—often associated with a flat, pronated foot;
  - compartment syndrome (soft tissue and vascular swelling);

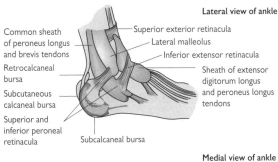

Lateral view of ankle

Common sheath of peroneus longus and brevis tendons

Retrocalcaneal bursa

Subcutaneous calcaneal bursa

Superior and inferior peroneal retinacula

Superior exterior retinacula

Lateral malleolus

Inferior extensor retinacula

Sheath of extensor digitorum longus and peroneus longus tendons

Subcalcaneal bursa

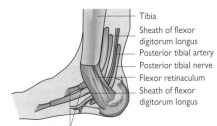

Medial view of ankle

Tibia

Sheath of flexor digitorum longus

Posterior tibial artery

Posterior tibial nerve

Flexor retinaculum

Sheath of flexor digitorum longus

Posterior tibial tendon end sheath

Fig. 2.21 Tendons, retinaculae, and bursae of the hindfoot.

- popliteal artery stenosis;
- referred nerve pain (spinal claudication);
- peripheral vascular disease (intermittent claudication).

Taking a history

Ask about site and quality of pain in the lower leg

- Localized anterior pain occurs in bony lesions of the anterior tibia, **e.g. stress fractures, periostitis**.
- Burning pain suggests a neurogenic cause. Diffuse burning pain may be caused by peripheral neuropathy, complex regional pain syndrome (☐ Chapter 18, p 489), or (rarely) erythromelalgia.
- Most commonly occurring in the elderly, bilateral leg pain with 'heaviness' or 'stiffness' limiting walking distance is typical of spinal stenosis. An alternative would be vascular claudication where often pain is more overt, and critical ischaemia can give night pain eased by hanging the legs over the side of the bed (gravity effects).
- Simultaneous knee problems may be relevant. Escape of synovial fluid from the knee into the soft tissues of the calf can present with acute pain and swelling and be misdiagnosed as a deep vein thrombosis

(pseudothrombophlebitis). Often a history of preceding joint effusion can be elicited.
- Low-lying synovial cysts connecting with the knee can cause calf pain (with or without swelling). This invariably occurs only with chronic synovitis.

Establish possible causes of hindfoot pain (Table 2.21)
- Establishing the cause of hindfoot pain from the history alone is difficult. There are important clues, mainly from patterns of injury or over-use.
- Posterior heel pain has a few causes. Often clinically indistinguishable from Achilles tendonitis or retrocalcaneal bursitis, enthesitis is usually associated with SpA (🕮 Chapter 8, p 281). An os trigonum may become damaged especially in soccer players and ballerinas (see below).
- The origin of plantar heel pain is varied. Mechanical plantar fasciitis is thought to occur more frequently in people who are on their feet for long periods of time, those who are obese, have thin heel fat pads, or poor footwear. Symptoms of arthritis and enthesopathy elsewhere, low back pain (sacroiliitis), eye inflammation (iritis), psoriasis, or previous gut or 'urethral' infection, might suggest SpA.
- Less common causes of plantar heel pain include fracture through a calcaneal spur and lateral plantar nerve entrapment between the fascia of abductor hallucis and quadratus plantae muscles (causing pain/paraesthesias on the lateral side of the sole).
- In the elderly and postmenopausal women, calcaneal stress fractures are a recognized feature of osteoporosis (🕮 Chapter 16, p 431) and can present with heel pain.
- Ankle and talocalcaneal synovitis, OA, ankle osteochondritis dissecans, and tendonitis around the hindfoot may be difficult to distinguish from the history alone. Synovitis or an effusion often accompanies OA of these joints.

Establish possible causes of midfoot and first MTP pain
- Gout (🕮 Chapter 7, p 269), OA (🕮 Chapter 6, p 259), enthesitis, and referred L5 nerve root pain are the most likely diagnoses of midfoot and first MTP pain.
- Gout should always be considered a possible cause of painful lesions in the foot in people at risk. Gout is not always intra-articular, intrabursal, or intratendonal. Local or diffuse soft tissue inflammation is common and often misdiagnosed as cellulitis. Swelling is usually marked.
- 1st toe is a common site for PsA; check X-ray for periosteal opposition.
- L5 pain is referred to the top (dorsum) and S1 pain to the sole of the foot.
- In older adults oa of midfoot joints is common. Mild synovitis can occur with it and may be caused by CPPD crystals (🕮 Chapter 7, p 269).

Establish possible causes of forefoot pain
- In those with forefoot pain, typically referred to as metatarsalgia, establish whether the condition is focal or due to arthropathy.

Table 2.21 Common conditions causing localized foot pain in children, adolescents, and adults

Site of pain	Common lesions
Ankle region	Ankle or talocalcaneal joint: synovitis (e.g. gout), OA. L4/L5 root pain
Posterior heel	Achilles tendonitis. Retrocalcaneal bursitis. Achilles enthesitis. Osteonecrosis of os trigonum
Medial side of heel	As for ankle region. Calcaneal fracture. Tibialis posterior tendonitis. Plantar fasciitis
Lateral side of heel	As for ankle region. Calcaneal fracture. Peroneal tendonitis. Fifth metatarsal base fracture[*]
Underneath heel	Plantar fasciitis. Calcaneal fracture. Infracalcaneal bursitis. Lateral plantar nerve entrapment
Top of foot	Midfoot joint synovitis (e.g. gout), OA. Navicular osteochondritis. Enthesitis. L5 root pain
Sole of foot	S1 root pain. Plantar fasciitis. Metatarsal stress fracture. Tibial/plantar nerve entrapment
Toes	MTP synovitis (e.g. RA, gout). MTP OA. Morton's metatarsalgia. Bursitis. Enthesitis/dactylitis

[*]Robert–Jones fracture from an inversion–pronation injury.

- Pain under the ball of the foot while walking is non-specific but might suggest any MTP joint abnormality, distal metatarsal stress fracture, Freiberg's disease, plantar nerve neuroma, or bursitis.
- Patients with RA often describe pain under the MTP joints and a feeling of 'walking on pebbles' (due to joint swelling and/or subluxation). Synovitis of the MTPS is a very common feature of early RA.
- Acute pain under the forefoot spreading into one or more (adjacent) toes and worse on walking suggests a plantar nerve neuroma (**Morton's metatarsalgia**) or intermetatarsal bursitis.
- Pain associated with paraesthesias or numbness under the forefoot might be due to S1 root irritation (common) or entrapment of the tibial nerve in the hindfoot (rare). Ask about back pain and other hindfoot problems.
- Non-traumatic toe pain associated with swelling of the entire toe suggests a dactylitis (associated with SpA). Although many toes may be affected, the dactylitis may be unilateral and affect just one toe.
- The development of hallux valgus is associated with tight footwear. The established deformity is associated with altered weight-bearing and a second toe (hammer) deformity. Big toe pain might be due to hallux rigidus. It is usually due to OA and important to recognize as it may prevent toe dorsiflexion sufficiently to lead to a compromised gait pattern.
- Pain specifically under the hallux may be due to damage of the sesamoids in the flexor hallucis brevis tendon and be misdiagnosed as a joint problem.

Ask for a description of the pain
- As in the hand, neurogenic pain is common and typical.
- Severe or unremitting pain when at rest suggests intrinsic bone pathology. Consider osteonecrosis, infection, fracture, and tumours, e.g. osteoid osteoma.
- Neurogenic pain may be sharp and well-defined (e.g. in acute L5 or S1 root pain), deep, achy, and less well-defined (e.g. chronic nerve root symptoms as in spinal or foraminal stenosis) or burning in quality. Paraesthesias and numbness may accompany both.
- If swelling accompanies neurogenic pain, consider a complex regional pain syndrome. There are numerous triggers, e.g. trauma, surgery. Patients may be unwilling to walk and apparent disability may appear profound.

Weakness
If true weakness is the major problem rather than pain, the diagnosis is usually between a spinal and peripheral nerve lesion (see Examination, below).

Examination
Observation
Observe the lower legs and feet from front and back, while the patient is standing. Note any swelling, deformities, or rashes:
- Lower leg deformities to note: tibia varum (or bow legs) in an older adult may be due to Paget's disease of the tibia. Muscle wasting might suggest disuse atrophy, old polio, or spinal stenosis (bilateral and subtle usually in older adults).
- **Oedema or soft tissue** swelling may be relevant to an underlying condition, e.g. ra. Although it may cause discomfort, oedema from cardiac failure, venous congestion, hypoproteinaemia, or lymphoedema is not painful unless there are ulcers or thrombophlebitis.
- Gout can cause swelling anywhere; gouty tenosynovitis can mimic the appearance of a cellulitis in the region of a joint.
- Calf swelling may be due to vein thrombosis or ruptured popliteal cyst.
- Common patterns of foot deformity are:
  - flat feet (pes planus);
  - high-arched feet (pes cavus) with high medial arch;
  - hallux valgus and rigidus;
  - over-riding, hammer, and claw toes.
- Skin conditions from venous abnormalities are common in the elderly. Other skin lesions which may be relevant include purpura, panniculitis—which is often subtle and over the shins—and pyoderma gangrenosum.

Ask the patient to walk in bare feet
Gait patterns should be noted:
- An antalgic ('limp and wince') gait is a non-specific indicator of pain.
- A wide-based gait (>10 cm wider than normal) suggests instability: joint instability, muscle weakness, or neurological lesions may be the cause.
- A foot that slaps down or a high stepping gait suggests tibialis anterior weakness (L4 nerve root or common peroneal nerve lesion).

- Significant weakness of gluteus medius and gluteus maximus in L5 and S1 root lesions, respectively, can result in lurching during gait. In the former, as weight is taken on the affected side, gluteus medius may be weak in controlling the small 2–3 cm lateral displacement in the weight-bearing hip that normally occurs. This can be compensated for if the body center of gravity is brought over the hip by lurching the upper body over the affected side. With gluteus maximus lesions (S1) extension of the hip, which helps mediate motion through the stance phase prior to toeing-off, may be weak. Thrusting the thorax forward with an arched back (forward lurch) compensates for the weakness and helps to maintain hip extension.
- A flat-footed gait with little or weak toe-off may suggest an S1 root lesion; however, 'flat-foot' (loss of the medial arch) with associated hind foot eversion and heel pain (plantar fasciitis) is extremely common. Often the arch weakness corrects when the patient is asked to walk.

Examine the lower leg

With the patient supine on the couch, examine the lower leg:

- After a ruptured popliteal (Baker's) cyst, calf tissues are often diffusely tender and swollen. Calf circumferences can be compared (e.g. 10 cm below tibial tubercle). There may also be mild skin erythema. Findings are not specific. Gout and infection (📖 Chapter 7, p 269 and 📖 Chapter 17, p 473) are the main alternatives if there is marked tenderness.
- Check for bruising, swelling, and tenderness around the fibula head in patients with foot drop (possible peroneal nerve palsy). Neurological examination may be done at this point.
- Localized anterior tibial tenderness is often found in patients with stress fractures or with pseudofractures (osteomalacia— 📖 Chapter 16, p 431).
- Tibial deformity in adults may be associated with diffuse bony tenderness and heat (arteriovenous shunting) in Paget's disease (📖 Chapter 16, p 431).

Examine the ankle and hindfoot

At the ankle and hindfoot, examine for joint and tendon synovitis, palpate specific structures and test passive hindfoot joint mobility:

- Synovitis of hindfoot joints is not always easily detected. With ankle joint synovitis, thickened tissue may be felt anteriorly in the ankle crease (where there may be a 'springy fullness') or laterally around the malleoli.
- Posterior tibial and peroneal tendonitis are associated with soft tissue swelling of the medial and lateral hindfoot, respectively. Synovial thickening from ankle and talocalcaneal joints may also be felt here and synovitis of structures may co-exist in RA or SpA. Pain from resisted movement of tendons may not be specific.
- Pathology of medial hindfoot structures may be associated with tibial nerve entrapment resulting in sensory symptoms on the sole of the foot. There may be a positive **Tinnel's sign**.
- Posterior heel pain may be due to Achilles' tendonitis, enthesitis and mechanical damage to the tendon, and retrocalcaneal bursitis. Deep tenderness may suggest an os trigonum lesion.
- The loss of passive hindfoot movements is not specific and can be associated with any cause of ankle or subtalar arthritis (20°–30° of

dorsiflexion and 45°–55° of plantar flexion is average for the ankle and a 10°–20° inversion–eversion range is average for the subtalar joint). Subtalar joint movement can be difficult to test accurately.

- The pain of **plantar fasciitis** may be elicited by firm palpation of the medial underside of the calcaneum. A negative test does not rule out pathology, as often the history is more sensitive. Full musculoskeletal examination is required to check for features of SpA, such as arthritis/enthesitis elsewhere and sacroiliitis.

Examine for midfoot lesions

Identifying specific midfoot lesions is difficult, though bony landmarks and discrete tender areas can be noted:

- Twisting the midfoot may elicit pain non-specifically. Common lesions include gout, OA, and synovitis associated with RA and SpA.
- Bony tenderness alone without soft tissue swelling does not rule out synovitis of an adjacent joint.
- The midfoot is a typical site for neuroarthropathy in diabetes.
- Bony lumps (exostoses) that may have formed at sites of pressure are common in the foot (e.g. medial or dorsal aspect of the first MTP joint, base or head of the fifth metatarsal, distal talus, or over the midfoot). In the elderly bony pain and skin sores may form at these sites.
- Both gout and infection result in swelling, skin erythema and localized tenderness. Gout of the first MTP joint occurs at any one time in 70% of patients with the condition. It can occur anywhere in the foot.

Examine the forefoot

Check for bony or other swelling, digit separation, and examine the sole of the foot. Squeezing the whole forefoot at the line of the MTP joints is a non-specific, but useful screening test for painful forefoot lesions:

- Tender swelling of the whole toe (dactylitis) occurs in SpA (📖 Chapter 8, p 281), sarcoidosis (📖 Chapter 18, p 489), and HIV infection (📖 Chapter 17, p 473). Swelling is soft not bony. Tender bony swelling suggests a bunion and is common on the dorsal aspect of the toes, and the first and fifth MTP joints.
- Forefoot splaying and interdigital separation suggests MTP synovitis or interdigital bursitis. MTP joints may be individually tender (simultaneously palpated with thumb below and finger above).
- Tenderness between metatarsal heads is typical in **Morton's metatarsalgia**. There may be a sensory deficit in the interdigital cleft. The differential diagnosis (in adolescents) may be osteochondritis of the second and third metatarsal head.
- Check for hallux rigidus—passive dorsiflexion should be at least 50°. Extending the big toe passively can reveal an ability to form a medial longitudinal arch in patients with flat feet (**Jack's test**).
- Discrete bony tenderness without swelling occurs with stress fractures.
- Uneven callus distribution under the forefoot may suggest an abnormally focused area of weight-bearing and an underlying mechanical abnormality.
- Rashes on the sole of the foot are uncommon but important to consider are: pompholyx, pustular psoriasis, and keratoderma blennorrhagica ('Reactive arthritis,' 📖 Chapter 8, p 281).

- Loss of sensation under the forefoot may be due to an S1 root lesion, peripheral neuropathy (e.g. diabetes), mononeuritis (e.g. vasculitis— 📖 Chapter 15, p 405), Sjögren's syndrome (📖 Chapter 12, p 353), undifferentiated (mixed) connective tissue disease), or, rarely, tibial nerve entrapment (examine hindfoot).

Neurological examination

Neurological examination is essential in cases where pain is neurogenic or there is weakness, numbness, or paraesthesias (Table 2.22).

Table 2.22 Patterns of common abnormal examination findings in lower lumbar nerve root lesions

Nerve root	Abnormal finding
L4	Weakness of ankle dorsiflexion (tibialis anterior)
	Patient finds walking on their heel difficult (strong ankle dorsiflexon needed)*
	Reduced knee reflex (L3 and L4)
L5	Weakness of big toe dorsiflexion (extensor hallucis longus)
	Weakness of foot eversion (peroneal muscles, also S1)
	Sensory deficit over dorsum of foot
	Reduced ankle reflex (L5 and S1)
S1	Weakness of ankle plantar flexion (gastrocnemius and soleus)
	Patient finds walking on, or repeatedly rising onto, tiptoe difficult*
	Sensory deficit over sole of foot
	Reduced ankle reflex

*Manoeuvres may be affected by pain, making interpretation difficult.

Investigations

Imaging of the lower leg

- Suspected tibial abnormalities such as stress fractures and pseudofractures in osteomalacia and Paget's disease have characteristic radiological appearances.
- Periosteal changes occur in trauma, psoriatic arthritis (above ankle), HPOA, and pachydermal periostitis.
- In athletes with exercise-related pain, a triple-phase isotope bone scan is part of the work-up for anterior shin pain.
- In suspected (but radiograph-negative) cases of bony disease, such as cortical stress fracture, periostitis, or cortical hyperostosis, an isotope bone scan may be useful to identify subtle pathology.

Imaging of the foot

Information available on radiographs of the hindfoot includes:

- Increased soft-tissue attenuation around the tendon insertion in cases of Achilles tendonitis or retrocalcaneal bursitis.

- Erosions or periostitis at the Achilles tendon insertion in enthesitis associated with SpA.
- Erosions in gout and RA-associated retrocalcaneal bursitis.
- Axial radiographs of the hindfoot are useful in showing talocalcaneal joint abnormalities, e.g. in RA.
- If radiographs are normal in patients with posterior heel pain, US can show patterns of tendon and bursal inflammation. MR can further characterize any discrete pattern of tendon injury.
- Osteonecrosis of an os trigonum or posterior talar process or tarsal navicular may be identified by radiographs. It is invariably located by bone scan and can be characterized further, usually with soft tissue swelling, by MRI.
- A **plantar spur** may denote recurrent plantar fasciitis.
- Plantar heel pain may be due to a fracture in a spur. Erosions just above the spur may be seen. The thickness of heel fat pad can be gauged from its X-ray attenuation (thin = risk for plantar fasciitis). A fat pad >23 mm thick in men and >21.5 mm thick in women is associated with acromegaly.
- **Calcaneal fractures** or an osteoid osteoma can be seen in some cases with radiographs alone. Isotope bone scan/CT are more sensitive.
- Patterns of joint, enthesis, and tendon inflammation can be documented using MR or isotope bone scan. This is useful information when characterizing an arthropathy.
- Bony abnormalities in the mid and forefoot are generally revealed by radiographs alone, though metatarsal stress fractures may be missed. MR can discriminate a plantar neuroma from interdigital bursitis and MTP joint synovitis. The former are probably best initially demonstrated by US.

Other investigations
- Neurophysiology (NCS) is a useful adjunct to clinical examination in diagnosis of lower limb neuropathies, and can help discriminate between peripheral (common peroneal or sciatic) or nerve root causes of foot drop, and also S1 root or tibial nerve entrapment causes of paraesthesias of the sole of the foot.
- Joint/bursa fluid aspiration is mandatory in suspected cases of sepsis and should be sent for culture (remember to consider gonococcus in young adults and TB in patients from endemic or inner-city areas). Fluid should be sent for polarized microscopy if a crystal-induced disease is suspected.
- Laboratory tests requested should reflect suspicion of specific infective, inflammatory, metabolic, or malignant pathology.

Treatment
Lower leg disorders
- Anterior shin pain should be treated according to cause. If there is also a problem of foot alignment then orthoses that support both the hind foot and mid arch may be very useful. Patients may volunteer that good walking shoes or 'trainers' ('sneakers') help (as is the case with plantar fasciitis).
- Exercise-induced lower leg pain has a number of causes and includes **shin splints and compartment syndrome**. The latter may require further investigation with pressure readings or exercise scintigraphy (^{99m}Tc-MIBI). In cases resistant to rest, analgesia, and modification of triggering factors, decompressive surgery may be required.

- Patients with **Paget's disease** of the tibia may require treatment with high-dose bisphosphonates and will need a biomechanical assessment.

Ankle and hindfoot disorders

- Tendonitis around the ankle should respond to treatment of its underlying cause. Chronic posterior tibial tendonitis left untreated will eventually accelerate the development of hindfoot valgus. Consider heel and arch support orthotics early.
- **Plantar fasciitis** may respond to a number of conservative measures:
  - Hind and mid-foot orthotics and/or supportive shoes
  - modification of weight-bearing activity
  - Achilles tendon stretching
  - hindfoot strapping
  - resting night splint (preventing ankle plantar flexion)
  - steroid injection around medial calcaneal tubercle
  - surgery

Forefoot disorders

- Localized forefoot pain, e.g. metatarsalgia, may respond to support pads and a change to a wider, more supportive, low-heel shoe. A podiatry/chiropody opinion should be sought as required.
- Forefoot stress fractures and metatarsal head osteochondritis require rest, supportive footwear and time to heal.
- Patients with chronic forefoot pain may benefit from a podiatric assessment. 'Stress offloading' foot orthoses for metatarsalgia and other biomechanical abnormalities (e.g. hallux rigidus) can be individually molded using thermoplastic materials.

Steroid injections

Steroid injections may be of value in the following:
- Ankle joint inflammation (e.g. RA, OA, gout) (Plate 19).
- Subtalar joint inflammation
- Tarsal tunnel syndrome
- **Achilles peritendonitis** (local steroid injections for Achilles' nodules should be avoided if possible as the risk of rupture is high. The same concern, though probably lesser risk, applies to Achilles' peritendonitis)
- Calcaneal apophysitis (**Sever's disease**—Achilles' tendon insertion)
- Retrocalcaneal bursitis
- Plantar fasciitis
- Gout/OA/enthesitis at first MTP joint

Surgery

- Minor surgical techniques can be curative in tarsal tunnel syndrome and in excising an interdigital (Morton's) neuroma. Consider excision of painful exostoses and troublesome rheumatoid nodules and amputation of deformed or over-riding toes.
- Major surgical procedures with good outcomes in appropriate patients include fusion of hindfoot joints and forefoot arthroplasty in chronic inflammatory arthritides. Osteotomy realignment of a hallux valgus deformity can be successful in the long term.

Child and adolescent foot disorders

For a review of classification criteria of autoimmune juvenile arthritides see 📖 Chapter 9, p 303.

Background

Lower limb and foot deformities of babies may be noticed first by parents. Diagnostic evaluation needs to focus on ruling out major congenital disease and exploring biomechanical factors.

- Neonatal deformities of the leg are uncommon.
- Talipes equinovarus (club foot) is an important deformity, which presents at birth. It is most commonly idiopathic and it is associated with wasting of the lower leg muscles. Causes to consider and rule out are spina bifida, spinal dysraphism, cerebral palsy, and arthrogryposis.
- With babies, persistence of certain sleeping postures is associated with patterns of angular and torsion deformity involving the whole leg. Postures include prone sleeping with knees tucked up under the chest, hips extended, or in a 'frog's-legs' position.
- In children able to walk, the most common conditions that present to pediatric orthopedic clinics are in-toeing and flat feet, though serious causes of flat feet usually affect only older children. Important points in evaluating an in-toeing deformity and flat feet are shown in Table 2.23. Some deformities in this group have been associated with persistence of sitting postures, e.g. cross-legged or 'reverse tailor' (floor sitting, knees bent and legs splayed out/back) positions.
- Achiness in the feet is the typical symptom in young children with torsional leg deformities of significance. If the biomechanical problem is sufficiently severe, shoes can wear out quickly.
- Regional musculoskeletal lesions in children <3 years of age are rare but most inflammatory arthritides can affect foot joints. Pain from an inflamed joint results in a miserable child and a refusal to walk.
- Periosteal pain (hyperostosis) in the tibia and other long bones occurs in Caffey's disease. There is usually symmetric limb enlargement in this rare condition, which usually occurs before the baby is 6 months old.

Taking a history

Ask about the site and quality of the pain

- Lower leg pain may be due to one of the causes of 'shin splints', a bone lesion, or algodystrophy.
- Localized anterior lower leg pain occurs in lesions of the anterior tibia e.g. stress fractures, periostitis, tibial tubercle osteochondritis, but deeper more diffuse anterior pain (often also medial) occurs in 'shin splints' (see below).
- Minimal or non-traumatic tibial fracture associated with fracture or bony deformity elsewhere raises the possibility of osteogenesis imperfecta.
- Localized or diffuse burning pain suggests a neurogenic cause. In children, disc prolapse is rare. Superficial burning pain may be due to peripheral neuropathy or algodystrophy.

Table 2.23 Common patterns of foot deformity in babies and infants

Deformity	Most common causes	Features
In-toeing	Metatarsus varus	Presents age 0–3 months or when starts to walk. Examination: forefoot varus only (heel is in neutral or valgus). Over 80% correct without surgery though predicting which will is difficult: 'wait and see until age 3' is appropriate
	Torsional lower limb deformity—medial tibial torsion and/or excessive femoral anteversion	Often related to regular prone knee–chest (foetal) sleeping position in babies and toddlers, and persistently sitting on the floor with legs forward internally rotated and knees bent out/backwards in children (Fig. 2.21)
	Cerebral palsy	Most often caused by excessive femoral anteversion
	Spinal dysraphism	Rare
Flat feet (pes planus)	Idiopathic or familial, hereditary connective tissue diseases, hindfoot disease: tarsal coalitions, arthritis, osteochondritis, infection etc.	Very common—often asymptomatic. Children often develop medial arch with time (passive big toe extension or standing on toes often reveals it). It is associated with conditions of general tissue laxity. If it occurs with pain and/or stiff flat feet look for peroneal muscle spasm and hindfoot pathology as the cause
Talipes equinovarus (club-foot)	Idiopathic, spina bifida, spinal dysraphism, tibial dysplasia, cerebral palsy, arthrogryposis	Incidence 1–2:1000 overall. Presents at birth. Idiopathic (aetiology unknown) is most common. Often a family history. Examination: calf wasting, hindfoot and forefoot in equinus (plantaris) and varus
Pes cavus	Idiopathic, peroneal muscular atrophy	High arch (medial and lateral sides), toe clawing. Associated with neurologic disease rarely e.g. Friedrich's ataxia

- Complex regional pain syndrome (📖 Chapter 18, p 489) typically gives burning pain, although it can occur with dull, aching pain or paroxysms. Pain often disturbs sleep. In children it is more common in the lower leg and foot than in the upper limb. Diffuse swelling and skin changes may be present. In many cases trauma is a triggering event but anything from simple sprains to arthroscopic knee surgery can trigger it; 25% are idiopathic.
- In children, algodystrophy (CRPS) may occur in the limb distal to an arthritic joint.
- Unremitting, sleep-disturbing pain that is worse on weight-bearing suggests bone or bone marrow pathology e.g. bone tumours, osteomyelitis, or periostitis (hypertrophic pulmonary osteoarthropathy, Gaucher's disease).

Ask about pain onset during sport

There are typical sports injuries of the lower leg that occur relatively often in active children and adolescents. Ask about pain onset during sport or recurrence during or after specific activities:

- Adolescents may refer to '**shin splints**'. Possible conditions include: tibial stress fracture, Osgood–Schlatter's disease, tibialis posterior fasciitis, compartment syndrome, popliteal artery stenosis, and mal-alignment of the hind- and midfoot.
- Tibial fascial inflammation and pain typically occurs as running begins, though patients can run through it, but it often returns severely after exercise and takes days to wear off. It is associated with hyperpronation of the foot (which increases stretch forces on the tendon).
- **Compartment syndrome** may be acute (due to muscle necrosis) or chronic. The chronic form occurs almost exclusively in endurance sports. Pain is absent at rest but builds as exercise progresses. It diminishes gradually—usually within a few hours. The pattern of pain and findings from perfusion scintigraphy suggest the cause of pain is ischaemic. Increased compartment pressures can be demonstrated by invasive monitoring.
- Pain from major vessel ischaemia occurs typically with walking. Muscle or a fibrous band in the popliteal fossa can compress the popliteal artery.
- Stress fractures occur in young athletes. In girls there may be an association with amenorrhea and generalized osteopenia.

Are there regional traumatic lesions?

In the foot, regional traumatic lesions are quite common, particularly in active children and athletes. Chronic arthritides should be considered:

- Apophysitides (**osteochondritides**) are quite common (Table 2.24). Most present with localized pain during exercise. There is tenderness and often swelling and pain on resisted movement of the appropriate tendon.
- Proximal midfoot pain may be caused by an accessory navicular, navicular osteochondritis (**Köhler's disease**), and tarsal coalitions (abnormal joins between bones leading to joint hypomobility, bilateral in 50% of cases). All lesions may be associated with a rigid flat foot (peroneal spastic flat foot) and will be more painful on weight-bearing.

Table 2.24 Localized painful foot disorders specific to school-age children and adolescents. Tumours are rare but osteoid osteoma should be considered

Site of pain	Disorder	Characteristics of disorder
Posterior heel	Calcaneal apophysitis (Sever's disease)	Traction osteochondritis. Both sexes age 8–10 years
Dorsal midfoot	Accessory navicular	Common finding in all children (50%). In 75% it fuses with main navicular. Majority not painful. Rarely it is associated with exercise-related pain
	Navicular osteochondritis (Köhler's disease).	Boys > girls. Presents with pain, limp and weight bearing on the outside of the foot
	Tarsal coalitions	Asymptomatic or with 'peroneal spastic' (rigid) flat foot (8–16 years)
Medial side of foot (may be diffuse)	Hypermobile flat foot	Children 1–5 years. May have generalized tissue laxity
Lateral side of foot	5th metatarsal base osteochondritis (Iselin's disease)	Children 10–12 years. Possibly due to tendon ossification and related to tight shoes
Dorsal and plantar distal midfoot	Stress fracture (rare)	Adolescents—2nd/3rd metatarsal
	Metatarsal head osteochondritis (Freiberg's disease)	Commonly 2nd metatarsal head. Affects active adolescent girls most frequently

- Joint synovitis (pain with immobility-related stiffness) is often difficult to detect clinically. Ankle synovitis is the easiest to be confident about. Soft or springy swelling with tenderness over the dorsal skin crease often suggests an effusion. Synovial thickening can be felt in florid cases circumferentially or just around the lower margins of the malleoli. In oligo-articular jia the ankle joint is sometimes painlessly swollen.
- Juvenile SpA/ERA is rare in children aged <8, and up until that age **oligo/polyarticular** JIA is a more likely cause of joint synovitis in the foot. Juvenile SpA/ERA may present with synovitis in a single lower limb joint, enthesitis at the Achilles tendon insertion or plantar fasciitis.
- **Dactylitis** ('sausage toe') raises the possibility of psoriatic arthritis or sarcoid. History usually discriminates the pattern of arthritis that helps in the differential diagnosis.
- The most common other arthritides to involve foot joints are viral and post-streptococcal arthritis and Lyme disease.
- Diffuse foot swelling occasionally occurs with synovitis in oligo/polyarticular JIA. The major differential is algodystrophy (CRPS).

Both pains are worse at night. Sensory symptoms are prominent and skin changes common in established algodystrophy.

- Forefoot pain in adolescents may be due to an interdigital neuroma (**Morton's metatarsalgia**) or osteochondritis of a metatarsal head (Freiberg's osteochondritis). Neuroma pain is often associated with dysaesthesia and numbness between the toes.
- Big toe pain from hallux rigidus (<50° passive dorsiflexion) is rare but can occur after injury and prevent running.
- Unlike in adults, gout occurs rarely in children and usually only in the context of renal failure, glucose 6-phosphatase deficiency (von Gierke's), malignancy, or X chromosome-linked disorders of uric acid metabolism.

Examination

Observe the lower legs from front and back while the patient is standing

- Lower leg muscle wasting occurs in hereditary sensorimotor neuropathy (bilateral) and typically accompanies spinal dysraphism. Diffuse muscle hypertrophy might suggest muscular dystrophy.
- Extremity swelling occurs in some forms of JIA (📖 Chapter 9, p 303), vasculitis (e.g. Henoch–Schönlein purpura (HSP)—📖 Chapter 15, p 405) and sepsis (📖 Chapter 17, p 473).
- Note the appearance and distribution of any rashes. Skin conditions from venous abnormalities are common. Other skin lesions which may be relevant include purpura (HSP) and panniculitis over the shins (erythema nodosum/sarcoidosis—📖 Chapter 18, p 489).

Observe the feet from front and back while the patient is standing

- Look for swelling and patterns of deformity. Patterns of deformity may require detailed orthopedic assessment. Check the gait.
- Look for localized oedema—an occasional sign of underlying jia but also present in nephrotic syndrome and in systemic vasculitides.
- Some torsional leg deformities are clinically significant. The most common pattern is with the hip internally rotated (usually excessive femoral anteversion), the tibia compensating in external rotation, and associated hindfoot valgus and forefoot varus.
- Torsional deformities will not spontaneously correct if they've not done so by the age of 7. There is speculation (based on the rationale of joint incongruity), but no proof, that torsional deformities in children are a risk for early OA.
- Flat feet are often asymptomatic and familial, and regress as the child grows (the medial arch becomes evident standing on tiptoe and with passive big toe dorsiflexion). Hindfoot pathology may be a cause.

Examine the sitting patient

With the patient sitting on the edge of the couch, check for tibial torsion.

Tibial torsion is measured as the angle between an imaginary line through the tibial tubercle in the sagittal plane and the perpendicular of an imaginary line through the malleoli (Fig. 2.22).

Examine the supine patient

With the patient supine on the couch, examine the lower leg:

- Check for bruising, swelling, and tenderness around the fibular head in patients with foot drop (peroneal nerve palsy).

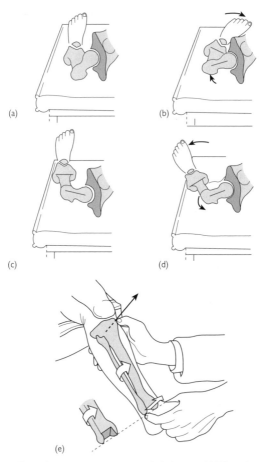

Fig. 2.22 Femoral anteversion, retroversion, and tibial torsion. (a) Where the femoral neck angulates excessively forward relative to an imaginary axis through the femoral condyles, the hip is anteverted. (b) Femoral neck anteversion can lead to a greater than usual range of hip internal rotation and a toe-in gait. (c) and (d) Retroversion, where the femoral neck angulates posteriorly relative to a femoral condyle axis, can cause a toe-out gait. (e) In-toeing can also be caused by excessive medial tibial torsion. Normally the ankle mortise faces 15° externally relative to a sagittal plane axis through the tibial tubercle (arrow) but in medial torsion it faces forward or internally.

- Localized anterior tibial tenderness is often found in patients with stress fractures.

Examine for swellings in the foot
- Bony lumps (exostoses) that may have formed at sites of pressure (e.g. posterior heel—'pump bump').
- Swelling, skin erythema and localized tenderness suggests infection, although synovitis, skin vasculitis, and panniculitis (e.g. erythema nodosum) should also be considered.

Examine the hindfoot
In the hindfoot, examine for joint and tendon synovitis, palpate specific structures, and test passive hindfoot joint mobility:
- Synovitis of hindfoot joints is not always easily detected. With ankle joint synovitis thickened tissue may be felt anteriorly in the ankle crease (where there may be a 'springy fullness') or laterally around the malleoli.
- The pain of plantar fasciitis may be elicited by firm palpation of the medial underside of the calcaneum. ERA should be ruled out.
- Posterior tibial and peroneal tendonitis are associated with soft tissue swelling of the medial and lateral hindfoot, respectively. Synovial thickening from ankle and talocalcaneal joints may also be felt there and synovitis of structures may co-exist in JIA or ERA. Resisting a tendon's movement aiming to elicit specific tendon pain may not be a specific test.
- Painful posterior heel structures are usually easily palpated, though pain may be due to a number of causes including Achilles' enthesitis, mechanical damage to the tendon, retrocalcaneal bursitis, and apophysitis.
- The loss of passive hindfoot movements is not specific. Often due to ankle synovitis, stiffness may also occur in other causes of joint pain (e.g. osteochondritis dissecans) and cases of peroneal spastic flat foot. The hindfeet of children are more mobile than those of adults.
- Peroneal 'spastic' (rigid) flat foot syndrome should be distinguished from flexible flat foot (when the medial longitudinal arch reappears when standing on the toes or with passive big toe dorsiflexion). Pain is centered on the dorsomedial side of the foot. The medial longitudinal arch is deficient. Associated peroneal muscle spasm may be painful. The age of presentation depends on the aetiology, the most common cause being tarsal coalition. It is always important to consider cerebral palsy and spinal dysraphism as well as local lesions: tumours (e.g. osteoid osteoma of calcaneum); navicular osteochondritis (Köhler's); local osteomyelitis or pyogenic arthritis; ankle or talocalcaneal joint synovitis (e.g. JIA). The diagnosis is of underlying cause but AP, lateral, oblique, and axial talocalcaneal radiographs, a three-phase isotope bone scan and hindfoot CT may all be useful in defining associated hindfoot lesions.

Examine the midfoot
- In the midfoot determine any sites of tenderness and stiffness: twisting the midfoot may elicit pain from lesions, though non-specifically.
- The major condition to rule out in teenagers is tarsal coalitions. These are fibrous, cartilaginous, or osseous joins between bones resulting in no or little mobility. The most commonly involved joints are the calcaneonavicular and the talocalcaneal. They may be tender.

Passive movement with inversion is usually painful and increases spasm in peroneal muscles.
- A tender navicular may also be due to osteochondritis.
- Synovitis associated with some forms of JIA can occur at any joint. Precise location is often difficult to identify clinically.

Examine the forefoot

Check for bony or other swelling, look for digit separation, examine the digits and the sole of the forefoot. Squeezing the whole forefoot at the line of MTPs is a useful but non-specific screening test for painful forefoot lesions:
- Dactylitis (psoriatic arthritis or sarcoidosis) swelling is soft, not bony.
- Forefoot splaying and interdigital separation suggests MTP synovitis. MTPS may be tender when palpated (simultaneously with thumb below and finger above).
- Tenderness between two metatarsal heads is typical in Morton's neuroma. The differential (in adolescents) may be osteochondritis of the second or third metatarsal head.
- Extending the big toe passively can reveal an ability to form a medial longitudinal arch in patients with flat feet (**Jack's test**).
- Discrete bony tenderness without swelling may occur with stress fractures.
- Loss of sensation under the forefoot is rare. Full back and neurologic leg examination may be necessary.

Investigations

Imaging of the lower leg
- Radiographs of the lower leg have characteristic patterns of abnormality in osteogenesis imperfecta, rickets, and some periosteal conditions, e.g. from stress fracture or periostitis, etc.
- Isotope bone scan is a sensitive investigation for radiograph-negative cases of suspected bone disease. It is also a useful initial investigation in adolescents with shin splints as it will rule out stress fractures and can show tibialis fasciitis.
- Treadmill or cycle ergometer exercise scintigraphy using ^{99m}Tc-MIBI can be useful in revealing compartmental perfusion defects in athletes with ischaemic-type pain during exercise (another cause of shin splints).

Imaging of the foot

Local lesions require investigation with radiographs, although in patients with inflammatory or bony lesions further imaging may be necessary:
- Routine AP and lateral hindfoot radiographs will reveal most cases of Sever's disease and osteochondritis dissecans of the ankle. Some cases of talocalcaneal coalition will require extra views and CT for diagnosis.
- In patients with a rigid flat foot additional oblique and axial view radiographs of the hindfoot help to show osteo-articular abnormalities if routine AP and lateral views do not. The gold-standard investigation is CT, which is used prior to, and to plan, surgery.
- Forefoot radiographs are a good screening test in those with forefoot pain. Though insensitive for detecting early synovitis, osteochondritides, hallux abnormalities, and the pattern of established arthritis can be identified.
- It is important to check a radiograph for first MTP osteochondritis dissecans in those with hallux rigidus.

- Isolated soft tissue swelling may be due to complex regional pain syndrome, underlying synovitis, or infection. Radiographs are mandatory. Scintigraphy may be non-specific in this setting, although the three-phase pattern of abnormality is characteristic in complex regional pain syndrome if synovitis can be ruled out.
- MRI of the whole foot or swollen area is the quickest way to an advanced differential diagnosis.
- Where swelling, pain, and tenderness co-exist infection must be ruled out using imaging. If it cannot and suspicion remains, tissue or fluid sampling should be undertaken. In most cases it is appropriate to do this under general anaesthesia. Complex regional pain syndrome should be excluded before any intervention.

Laboratory tests

Any possibility of joint synovitis (most likely to be ankle), enthesitis, tendonitis, or infection requires investigation with laboratory tests:

- ESR and CRP are likely to be raised in cases of autoimmune arthritis and infection and are more likely to be normal or only slightly increased in oligo-articular ERA compared with polyarticular and systemic JIA or infection.
- Normochromic anaemia (± mild microcytosis) is a non-specific sign of a systemic condition. FBC may be normal in oligo-articular JIA. Leukoctosis is typical with infection, with steroids and in systemic JIA.
- Moderately elevated titers of ANA may be present in 40–75% of patients with oligo-articular JIA and is a risk factor for associated uveitis. Even minimally symptomatic uveitis can threaten vision if not treated.
- Check for circulating rheumatoid factor (RF) in cases of synovitis. High titers are expected in (RF+) polyarticular JIA.

Treatment

Lower leg disorders

- Anterior shin pain should be treated according to cause.
- Treat foot alignment problems with appropriate orthotics.
- Avoid NSAIDs if possible.
- Review diagnosis if conservative treatment fails, e.g. is there an underlying stress fracture or periostitis? Consider obtaining an isotope bone scan.

Ankle and foot disorders

- The management of bony anomalies/deformities should be discussed with an orthopaedic surgeon and physical therapist early, to avoid missing an opportunity to prevent growth abnormalities.
- Be aware that soft-tissue steroid injection of a presumed local lesion may impair healing/growth at apophyses and may aggravate the symptoms of (missed) algodystrophy (CRPS).
- Consider intra-articular steroid injection of specific joints in oligo-articular JIA if joints can be clearly identified by isotope bone scan or MR. Injection under sedation (adolescents) or light general anaesthesia (toddlers/children) is appropriate.

Patterns of disease presentation: making a working diagnosis

Mono-articular pain in adults

When evaluating a patient with joint pain, it helps to know the number of joints involved:
- Mono-articular (one joint).
- Oligo-articular (2–5 joints).
- Polyarticular (>5 joints).

Each of these patterns is associated with its own differential diagnosis:
- The assessment of specific joints is discussed in detail in 🕮 Chapter 2, p 19.
- However, evaluation of a single, hot swollen joint—particularly, the knee, is a frequent occurrence.
- **Acute mono-arthritis** is commonly due to crystal arthropathies (particularly in the older patient) (🕮 Chapter 7, p 269), infection (particularly gonococcal in the younger patient; 🕮 Chapter 17, p 473 and 🕮 Chapter 24, p 609) or **haemarthrosis** [causes including trauma, bleeding disorder, vitamin C deficiency, synovial haemangioma, and **pigmented villonodular synovitis** (PVNS)] (🕮 Table 3.1).
- A fracture across the joint line may also cause an acute mono-arthritis. Stress fractures occur as the result of repetitive loading of bone, and can be found with occupational, recreational, or athletic activities. Stress fractures may be small and therefore can be missed on plain radiographs; MRI may be more sensitive and should be considered if the patient is at risk.
- **Non-gonococcal septic arthritis** is particularly important to consider in the elderly, who may not present with the signs and symptoms expected with infection. Non-gonococcal septic arthritis is a rheumatological emergency, and should be treated with intravenous antibiotics and joint aspiration. Although *S. aureus* is the most common culprit, in the elderly, it is prudent to consider atypical infections (e.g. Gram negative). Also remember that the presence of crystals does not completely exclude the possibility of a co-existing infection (🕮 Chapter 17, p 473 and 🕮 Chapter 24, p 609).

Oligo-articular pain in adults

Background

The assessment of an inflamed joint

- The clinical features of inflammation and pain at any given synovial joint and the differential diagnosis in the context of other possible regional musculoskeletal diagnoses are discussed in 📖 Chapter 2, p 19.
- **Synovitis** is the term given to inflammation of the synovial lining. This inflammation may be a consequence of a range of cellular processes, and is not specific for any one diagnosis. Joint effusions often accompany synovitis.
- Inflammation of peri-articular tissues may accompany synovitis. **Enthesitis** (inflammation at the tendon insertion into bone) or **tenosynovitis** (inflammation of the tendon itself) may be the most prominent feature.

History: general points

- Pain and stiffness are typical features of synovitis and enthesitis. Both are often worse in the morning, or after periods of immobility. The presence or absence of stiffness does not discriminate between different causes of synovitis.
- Pain is often severe in acute joint inflammation. In chronic situations, pain may be less severe (due to mechanisms that increase physical and psychological tolerance). There are no specific descriptors that discriminate pain from synovitis or enthesitis.
- Swelling, either due to synovial thickening or effusion, often accompanies synovitis. Enthesitis may be associated with peri-articular soft tissue swelling.
- A patient's report of swelling is not always reliable. Patients with carpal tunnel syndrome, for example, will frequently report that their hands are swollen, even when no swelling is visible.
- Reduced mobility in a joint affected by enthesitis/synovitis is almost universal regardless of its cause.

Examination: general points

- Swelling may be observed or detected by palpation. Its absence does not rule out synovitis or enthesitis. Synovial swelling needs to be discriminated from bony swelling, fat, and other connective tissue swellings (e.g. ganglia, nodules, etc.). Without imaging or attempting to aspirate joint fluid, it may be difficult to discriminate synovial thickening from effusion.
- Skin erythema (implying peri-articular inflammation) and warmth do not always accompany joint inflammation, but they are common with crystalline and septic arthritis. Erythema can also occur in reactive arthritis, rheumatic fever and with nascent Heberden's/Bouchard's nodes in osteoarthritis (OA; 📖 Chapter 6, p 259).
- Tenderness of thickened synovium is common, but is not always present. Severely tender swelling suggests joint infection, haemarthrosis, or an acute inflammatory reaction to crystals.
- Inflammation of entheses results in 'bony' tenderness at joint margins, and sites of tendon or ligament insertion.

Table 3.1 The most common causes of mono-articular and oligo-articular joint pain and typical patterns of presentation

Disease	Typical pattern
Gout (📖 Chapter 7, p 269)	Age >40 years. Initially presents as an acute mono-arthritis. Strong association with hyperuricaemia, renal impairment, and diuretics. Possible general symptoms mimicking sepsis. Possible family history. Acute phase reactants and serum WBC often high. Joint fluid urate crystals seen by polarized light microscopy (PLM). Joint erosions (radiographically typical) and tophi occur in chronic disease.
Spondyloarthritis (📖 Chapter 8, p 281)	Age <40 years, men more than women. Mostly oligo-articular lower limb joint enthesitis/synovitis. May occur with sacroiliitis, urethritis or cervicitis, uveitis, gut inflammation, psoriasis (scaly or pustular). Possible family history. ESR/CRP may be normal. More severe course if human leukocyte antigen (HLA) B27-positive.
CPPD arthritis (📖 Chapter 7, p 269)	Mean age 72 years. Oligo-articular, acute mono-articular (25%), and occasionally polyarticular patterns of synovitis.
Haemarthrosis	Obvious trauma does not always occur. Swelling usually considerable. Causes include trauma (e.g. cruciate rupture or intra-articular fracture), pigmented villonodular synovitis, bleeding diatheses, and chondrocalcinosis.
Osteoarthritis (📖 Chapter 6, p 259)	Soft tissue swelling is usually not as obvious as bony hypertrophy (osteophytes). Typical distribution (e.g. first carpometacarpal and knee joints).
Rheumatoid arthritis (📖 Chapter 5, p 283)	Can initially present with an oligo-arthritis that evolves into a symmetrical polyarthritis. Can rarely present as an acute mono-arthritis.
Septic arthritis (excluding *N. gonorrhoea*) (📖 Chapter 17, p 473)	Most common cause *Staphylococcus aureus*. Associated with chronic arthritis, joint prostheses, and reduced host immunity. Peak incidence in elderly. Systemic symptoms common and sometimes overt, but may not occur. Synovial fluid is Gram stain positive in 50% of cases and culture positive in 90% of cases.
Gonococcal arthritis (📖 Chapter 17, p 473)	Age 15–30 in urban populations and with inherited deficiency of complements C5 to C9. One form presents as an acute septic mono-arthritis. Organism detected by Gram stain of joint fluid in 25% and by culture in 50% in the second group.

- Decreased range of motion is almost always demonstrable in a joint affected by synovitis or enthesitis. The degree to which passive and active range of motion is reduced depends on a number of often interdependent factors (e.g. pain, size of effusion, peri-articular muscle weakness, or pain).

- Movement of a joint affected by synovitis or enthesitis will induce pain and stiffness, although neither is specific. Affected joints will demonstrate reduced range on active or passive range of motion exercises; moving the joint beyond that point will elicit pain.

Taking a history

Age, sex, and occupation

The age, sex, and occupation of the patient give non-specific, but important clues:

- Oligo-arthritis is uncommon in young adults. SpA, especially reactive arthritis, is likely to be the main cause; 75% of patients who develop reactive arthritis are less than 40 years old.
- Gout typically occurs in those more than 40 years old, and is the most common cause of inflammatory arthritis in men (self-reported in 1 in 74 men and 1 in 156 women).
- The mean age of patients with calcium pyrophosphate dihydrate (CPPD) arthritis is about 72 years (range 63–93 years).
- Areas endemic for tick infection (forestation) with *Borrelia* are at risk of **Lyme arthritis**.

Which joints are affected?

Some processes are more common in certain joints than others:

- Shoulder synovitis is typical in hydroxyapatite arthritis (**Milwaukee shoulder**/knee syndrome) and AL **amyloidosis** (📖 Chapter 18, p 489).
- Involvement of a shoulder or hip is extremely unusual in gout.
- CPPD arthritis (as pseudogout) occurs rarely in the small finger joints.
- The knee is the commonly involved in acute crystalline arthropathy and septic arthritis (both gonococcal and non-gonococcal).
- Large knee effusions are common with Lyme arthritis, but this is a non-specific finding. Large effusions can also be seen with septic and **psoriatic arthritis** (📖 Chapter 8, p 281).
- In theory, there are many causes of synovitis in a single first metatarsophalangeal (MTP) joint, but the majority of cases are due to gout; 50–70% of first attacks occur in this joint.

Preceding factors

Factors preceding swelling of a single joint or oligo-arthritis may be highly relevant. These include trauma and infection:

- Acute non-traumatic mono-articular synovitis is most commonly due to crystal-induced synovitis or synovitis associated with SpA.
- A preceding history of trauma typically suggests intra-articular fracture (with/without haemarthrosis), a meniscus tear (knee), or an intra-articular loose body, such as an osteochondral fragment (which may cause the patient to complain about a 'locking' knee).
- Twinges of joint pain often precede an acute attack of gout. Acute arthritis occurs in 25% of patients with CPPD arthritis.
- In hydroxyapatite arthritis, synovitis is usually mild-to-moderate, gradual in onset and typically worse at night.

- An acute mono-arthritis with fever in **Familial Mediterranean Fever** (FMF) (🕮 Chapter 18, p 489) is a mimic of septic arthritis. Such joint manifestations are present in up to 75% of cases.
- Septic arthritis should always be considered (and promptly ruled out) as a cause of acute joint swelling (🕮 Chapter 24, p 609).

Family and social history

There may be important clues from the family and social history:

- Both gout and SpA have a familial component. Between 6–18% of patients with gout also have a family history of gout. There may be a family history of SpA or uveitis in patients who have reactive, psoriatic, or enteropathic arthritis or ankylosing spondylitis (AS).
- Gout in young adults suggests an inherited abnormality (usually increased urate production from 5 phosphoribosyl-1-pyrophosphate synthetase activity, since the other enzyme deficiencies present in childhood).
- Excessive alcohol consumption is associated with gout. Alcohol can also contribute to lactic acidosis that inhibits urate breakdown.
- Consider Lyme disease if patients live, work, or visit endemic areas; outside of the United States, this includes Europe, Russia, China, and Japan. Peak incidence occurs during the summer.
- Brucellar arthritis is generally mono-articular and occurs primarily in areas where domesticated animals are infected and poor methods of animal husbandry, feeding habits, and hygiene standards co-exist.

Ask about other associated features

Associated extra-articular features include previous eye, gastrointestinal, cardiac, and genitourinary symptoms:

- Low-grade fever, malaise, and anorexia occur commonly in both septic arthritis and gout. Marked fever can occur in gout and only occurs in about a third of patients with septic arthritis.
- Ask about any current or previous features which might suggest SpA:
  - back or buttock pain (enthesitis or **sacroiliitis**);
  - swelling of a digit (**dactylitis**);
  - plantar heel pain (**plantar fasciitis**);
  - red eye with irritation (anterior **uveitis**);
  - **urethritis, balanitis, cervicitis** or acute diarrhoea (**reactive arthritis**);
  - psoriasis;
  - symptoms of inflammatory bowel disease.
- **Behçet's disease** (🕮 Chapter 18, p 489) can cause an oligo-arthritis. Other features include painful oral and genital ulcers, and uveitis.
- The involvement of more than one joint does not rule out septic arthritis. In up to 20% of cases, multiple joints can become infected.

Examination

General

- Always compare sides, to establish if the changes are symmetric or asymmetric.
- It is important to establish from the examination whether there is true synovial swelling. A history of swelling is not always reliable and

other, non-synovial, pathology can present with single or oligo-articular joint pain.

Examine the affected joints

Examine the affected joints for tenderness. Check passive range of motion for evidence of locking or instability:

- Acute processes such as crystal arthritis, infection and post-traumatic effusion often lead to painful swelling, marked tenderness of swollen soft-tissues, and painfully restricted active and passive movement of the joint. These features are usually less overt with chronic arthritis.
- Instability of an acutely inflamed joint or tests for cartilage damage in the knee may be difficult to demonstrate. Further examination will be necessary after drainage of joint fluid.
- Detection of enthesis tenderness around the affected joints or at other sites is a useful clue to the diagnosis of SpA.

Examine other musculoskeletal structures

- Examine the low back and typical sites of bony tenderness—sacroiliitis and enthesitis are common features of SpA.
- Tendonitis is not specific and can occur in gout, CPPD arthritis, SpA, and gonococcal infection.

Look for skin rashes and any inflammation

Oligo-arthritis may be part of a systemic inflammatory or infectious condition:

- Temperature and tachycardia can occur with some non-infectious causes of acute arthritis (e.g. crystal arthritis), although their presence in the context of oligo-articular joint swelling requires exclusion of joint infection.
- Gouty tophi may be seen in the pinnae and in other peripheral locations. They can be difficult to discriminate clinically from rheumatoid nodules. Polarized light microscopy of material obtained by needle aspiration will be diagnostic for tophi.
- The hallmark of **relapsing polychondritis** (📖 Chapter 18, p 489) is lobe-sparing, full thickness inflammation of the pinna.
- Mouth ulcers are common; however, crops or large painful tongue and buccal lesions associated with oligo-articular arthritis suggest Behçet's disease.
- A typical site for the osteitis (tender swelling of bone) of **SAPHO syndrome** (📖 Chapter 8, p 281) is around the sternum and clavicles.
- Skin erythema over a joint suggests crystal arthritis or infection.
- Associated skin rashes may include **erythema nodosum** (associated with ankle/knee synovitis in acute sarcoid), purpuric pustular rashes (Behçet's, gonococcal infection, and SAPHO syndrome), **erythema marginatum** (rheumatic fever) (📖 Chapter 4, p 193 and 📖 Chapter 18, p 489), or keratoderma blenhorragica (aggressive-looking rash of the sole of the foot in **Reiter's disease/Reactive arthritis**).
- Psoriasis may be associated with both synovitis and enthesitis.

Investigations

The presence of synovitis can be confirmed by obtaining US or MRI of the joints in question. At larger joints, both are sensitive for the detection of effusion and synovial thickening. Inflammation at peri-articular or capsular entheses can also be seen.

Joint aspiration

The most important investigation of a patient with mono-articular synovitis is joint aspiration and prompt examination of fluid. Fluid should be sent in sterile bottles for microscopy and culture:

- The appearance of synovial fluid is not specific; however, blood or bloodstaining suggests haemarthrosis from trauma (including the aspiration attempt), a haemorrhagic diathesis, haemangioma, PVNS, and synovioma.
- Turbidity (decreased clarity) of fluid relates to cellular, crystal, lipid, and fibrinous content. Synovial fluid in septic arthritis and acute crystal arthritis is frequently turbid due to the high number of neutrophils.
- Cell counts give some diagnostic guidance but are non-specific (Table 3.2). There is a high probability of infection or gout if the PMN differential is >90%.
- Joint fluid eosinophilia is not specific.
- **Polarized light microscopy** (PLM) of fluid can discriminate urate (3–20 μm in length, needle-shaped and negatively birefringent—blue and then yellow as the red plate compensator is rotated through 90°) and calcium-containing crystals such as calcium pyrophosphate (positively birefringent crystals, typically small and rectangular or rhomboid in shape).
- Lipid and cholesterol crystals are not uncommon in joint fluid samples, but their significance is unknown.
- Crystals appearing in synovium less commonly, but in typical settings include hydroxyapatite associated with Milwaukee shoulder (and knee) syndrome (alizarin red-S stain positive), calcium oxalate in end-stage renal failure on dialysis (may need scanning electron microscopy to confirm), cystine in cystinosis, and xanthine in xanthinosis.
- The presence of crystals in joint fluid does not exclude infection.
- The most common causes of non-gonococcal septic arthritis in Europe and North America are *Stapylococcus aureus* (40–50%), *Stapylococcus epidermidis* (10–15%), *Streptococcal* species (20%), and Gram-negative bacteria (15%).

Radiographs

Radiographs can confirm an effusion, show characteristic patterns of chondral and bone destruction (e.g. in infection or erosive gout) and can reveal intra-articular calcification associated with CPPD or hydroxapatite. arthritis.

- Septic arthritis causes patchy osteopenia and loss of bone cortex.
- 'Punched-out' erosions (within joints or around metaphyses), soft tissue swellings (tophi), and patchy calcification are hallmarks of chronic gout.

Table 3.2 Characteristics of joint fluid

Characteristic	Normal	Group I (non-inflammatory)	Group II (inflammatory)	Group III (septic)
Viscosity	Very high	High	Low	Variable
Colour	None	Straw	Straw or opalescent	Variable with organisms
Clarity	Clear	Clear	Translucent or opaque	Opaque
Leukocytes (cells/mm³)	200	200–2000	2000–50 000	>50 000
PMNs (%)	<25	25	Often >50	>75

- Intra-articular calcification may commonly be either chondrocalcinosis (fine linear or punctate fibrocartilage calcification) or larger loose bodies (often with prolific osteophytes)—both are associated with CPPD arthritis.
- Numerous regularly-shaped calcific masses in a joint may be due to **synovial chondromatosis** (most common in middle-aged men; 50% of cases affect the knee).
- The presence of erosions does not implicate RA. The arthritis may be due to an enthesitis associated with SpA.

Further imaging

Further imaging should be discussed with your radiologists:
- MRI confirmation of traumatized structures such as meniscus damage in the knee and labral damage in the shoulder should be sought if suspected.
- MRI can confirm synovitis, although appearances are usually non-specific. Characteristic MRI appearances of enthesitis and PVNS are recognized.

Laboratory investigations to consider
- FBC, acute phase response (ESR, CRP). Neutrophilia is not specific for infection and can occur in crystal arthritis.
- Blood urea, electrolytes, creatinine, and urate (e.g. hyperuricaemia and renal impairment associated with gout).
- Blood calcium, phosphate, albumin, alkaline phosphatase (±PTH), thyroid function tests and ferritin to screen for **hyperparathyroidism, thyroid disease, and haemochromatosis**, all of which can be associated with CPPD arthritis.
- Autoantibodies: rheumatoid factor and cyclic citrullinated peptide (CCP) may help identify early RA.
- IgM *Borellia burgdorferi* serology may help diagnose Lyme disease in patients at risk (e.g. acute arthropathy or migratory arthritis).
- Antibodies to the streptococcal antigens streptolysin O (ASOT) DNAase B, hyaluronidase, and streptozyme may be useful in patients who have had sore throat, migratory arthritis, or features of **rheumatic fever** (📖 Chapter 18, p 489).

Synovial biopsy

- If there is a haemarthrosis or suspicion of PVNS, MRI of the joint is wise before undertaking a biopsy to characterize the vascularity of a lesion.
- Consider a biopsy to evaluate a mono-arthritis of unclear aetiology. Biopsy may be helpful to diagnose **sarcoid** arthropathy (📖 Chapter 18, p 489), infectious arthritis, or crystalline arthropathy when the usual diagnostic tests are negative.
- Formalin fixation of samples is sufficient in most cases. Samples for polarized light microscopy are best fixed in alcohol (urate is dissolved by formalin). Snap freezing in nitrogen is essential if immuno-histochemistry is required.
- Arthroscopic biopsy will yield more tissue than needle biopsy and will allow joint irrigation.
- Congo red staining of synovium, ideally with polarized light microscopy, should be requested if AA, AL, or β_2-microglobulin **amyloid** is a possibility (📖 Chapter 18, p 489). This should be considered in patients with myeloma (AL) and long-term dialysis patients (β_2-microglobulin). AA amyloid is an uncommon, but recognized complication of RA, AS, Familial Mediterranean Fever, and Crohn's disease.

Oligo-articular and pauci-articular pain in children and adolescents

Background

Disease classification

Current practice is to use the 2001 (Edmonton, Canada) Juvenile Idiopathic Arthritis (JIA) classification developed by a working group under the auspices of The International League of Associations for Rheumatology (ILAR) (Table 3.4)

In addition several criteria exist for 'pauci-articular' disease and designed for the definition of the spondyloarthritis or 'late onset pauci-articular juvenile chronic arthritis' (LOPA). These include:

- *Juvenile*—age-specific criteria:
  - General classification for LOPA—Garmisch–Partenkirchen criteria
  - Specific disease subgroups: SEA syndrome (seronegative enthesopathy and arthritis); ERA (enthesitis related arthritis); atypical spondyloarthritis.
- No age specification, i.e. Adult and Child:
  - European Spondyloarthropathy Study Group (ESSG)
  - Amor classification (1995).

For more detail on juvenile spondylo-arthritides and JIA see 📖 Chapter 8, p 281 and 📖 Chapter 9, p 303 respectively.

Important issues pertinent to children and adolescents

- Compared to adults, it may be quite difficult to establish whether there is synovitis in a child's joint (see Table 3.3).
- An awareness of injuries and mechanical conditions that affect specific joints, notably at epiphyseal or apophyseal growth plates, is essential.
- In very young children, a history from both the child and the main care provider is important.
- It is important to note that mono-articular or oligo-articular synovitis:
  - may present with limb pain;
  - may not necessarily present with joint pain and stiffness;
  - may result in non-use, altered use, or irritability, any of which may be the main or only complaint.
- Systemic JIA [previously systemic onset juvenile rheumatoid arthritis (JRA; 📖 Chapter 5, p 233)] is defined as arthritis preceded by (or occurring with) daily recurring fever of more than 2 weeks' duration (documented for greater than 3 days) plus one or more of the following:
  - an evanescent, non-fixed, erythematous rash;
  - generalized lymphadenopathy; enlarged liver or spleen;
  - serositis.
- Persistent oligo-arthritis is defined by the involvement of no more than four joints throughout the disease course. Extended oligo-arthritis affects a cumulative total of five joints or more after the first 6 months of disease. Excluded from each group will be those with: a family history of psoriasis (first- or second-degree relative); a positive RF; HLA B27 (males >8 years old); or systemic arthritis.

Table 3.3 The major causes of mono-articular/oligo-articular joint synovitis or swelling in children

Condition	Distinguishing features
Septic arthritis	Systemically unwell child. With TB—pulmonary disease, lower limb, insidious onset, and rapid joint destruction
Trauma	Direct blow/forced hyperextension, haemorrhage into joint
Foreign body synovitis	History of injury
PVNS	Recurrent joint haemarthrosis
Thalassaemia	Episodic and migratory arthritis
Malignancy	Acute mono-articular joint swelling, associated with leukaemia and neuroblastoma
Viral arthritis	Associated with rash or immunization
Lyme disease	Exposure in endemic area, rash, positive serology
Post-streptococcal	Sore throat, migratory arthritis, signs of rheumatic fever
FMF	Ethnic grouping and familial aggregation, acute febrile episode with chest/abdominal pain
Behçet's disease	Rare. Orogenital ulceration and skin rashes
Oligo-articular JIA	Mono-articular in 60% of cases and involves two joints in 31% of cases. Diagnosis of exclusion, associated with asymptomatic uveitis
Enthesitis-related arthritis	Usually age 8 or over, boys > girls, iritis, most have enthesitis, HLA B27. Sacroiliac joint involvement, low back stiffness
Psoriatic arthritis*	Rash, nail pitting, or other changes
Sarcoid	Usually associated with rash and ocular symptoms
Vasculitis	Rash, high ESR/CRP
SLE	UV-sensitive skin rash, ANA

* In the new ILAR classifications, psoriatic arthritis is distinguished from enthesitis-related arthritis (see below).

- Enthesitis is a key-classifying criterion in the group of conditions previously classified as spondylarthropathy (SpA), now termed enthesitis-related arthritis (ERA).
- The definition of psoriatic arthritis will be broadened under the new ILAR classification (Table 3.4). The proposed classification criteria require arthritis beginning before 16 years of age and either typical psoriasis or at least three of the following:
  - dactylitis, nail pitting;
  - psoriasis-like rash;
  - family history of psoriasis (first- and second-degree relatives).

Enthesitis, iritis and HLA B27 are absent from this classification.

Table 3.4 2001 ILAR classification of arthritis in childhood (juvenile idiopathic arthritis)

ILAR classification of juvenile idiopathic arthritis (JIA)	Previous classification
Systemic arthritis*	Systemic onset JRA
Oligo-arthritis* which is either: persistent (always 4 joints or less) extended (after 6 months >4 four joints affected)	Oligo-articular JRA. Pauci-articular JRA
Polyarthritis (RF+)* 5 or more joints affected	Polyarticular JRA. Polyarticular JRA (RF+)
Polyarthritis (RF–)	Polyarticular JRA (RF–)
Psoriatic arthritis*	Psoriatic arthritis
Enthesitis-related arthritis (ERA)*	SpA

JCA = juvenile chronic arthritis; JRA = juvenile rheumatoid arthritis; RF = rheumatoid factor.
* See text for notes.

Taking a history

Epidemiology
Recall epidemiological features associated with different groups and ages:
- The peak incidence of oligo-articular **JIA** is between the ages of 1 and 3. It is relatively rare in onset after 12 years of age.
- **Enthesitis-related arthritis** (ERA) is more common in boys (ratio up to 10:1) and typically occurs after the age of 8.
- **Familial Mediterranean Fever** (FMF) can manifest in children as young as 1 year old. It occurs most frequently in Iraq, Turkey, Libya, Algeria, Morocco, and Tunisia, and in Sephardic Jews. Acute or chronic oligo-arthritis can occur.

Trauma
Mono-articular synovitis may be associated with trauma:
- Time to onset of joint swelling after trauma (<2 h) and intensity of pain (severe) may help discriminate whether a haemarthrosis is present. Intra-articular fracture should then be suspected.
- An absence of a history of trauma does not rule out the possibility of **osteochondritis dissecans** (only 10% are associated with trauma).
- Be aware that **non-accidental trauma** can present with traumatic joint swelling.

Infection/malignancy
Infection and malignancy must be ruled out in all cases of atraumatic mono-arthritis:
- An insidious onset does not rule out infection. This pattern is well recognized in TB. Joint destruction, however, may not be insidious.
- The most common neoplastic causes of mono-articular joint swelling in children are **leukaemia** and **neuroblastoma**.

Rare causes of symptoms

The rarer causes of mono-articular synovitis, joint swelling, or pain, and joint-specific causes of pain in a single joint should not be forgotten:

- Intra-articular **haemangiomas**, **osteoid osteomas**, synovial **chondromatosis** and **lipomatosis arborescens** can occur in most joints.
- Anterior knee pain (common in growing adolescents, especially girls).
- Isolated hip pain conditions such as **Perthes'**.
- Oligo-articular JIA of the hip is very rare.
- Osteochondritides/avulsion fractures, e.g. **Osgood–Schlatter's**.
- **Osteonecrosis** at typical sites, e.g. tarsal navicular, carpal lunate.

Preceding symptoms

Ask about preceding symptoms of infection and rashes. Consider viral (including vaccinations), streptococcal and enteric infections, and Lyme disease:

- Oligo-arthritis (or mono-arthritis) may be a reaction to an infection and may be short-lived usually lasting 3–6 weeks, but occasionally up to 8 weeks.
- A streptococcal sore throat can lead on to a migratory arthritis. The differential diagnosis would include **rheumatic fever** and **Lyme disease**.
- The most distinctive features of acute rheumatic fever should be sought in patients with oligo-arthritis, especially if it has been partially treated with aspirin or NSAIDs, which can mask its migratory nature; these include: carditis with prolonged PR interval, chorea, skin nodules, and erythema marginatum.
- *Salmonella, Shigella, Yersinia,* and *Campylobacter* enteric infections are associated with reactive arthritis.
- *Eschericia coli* and *Clostridium difficile* infections have the potential for triggering reactive arthritis.
- A facial rash occurs in rubella—coalescing erythema that clears as the limbs become affected; in most patients, however, a facial rash should make you think about parvovirus B19 infection (erythema infectiosum—**'slapped cheek' syndrome**).
- Pink or faintly red erythema on the trunk or limbs, but not the face is typical of the **erythema marginatum** of rheumatic fever. The outer rash margin is often distinct and continuous. Firm, non-tender skin nodules, which may have regressed, may also suggest rheumatic fever.
- Lyme disease causes **erythema chronicum migrans**, a spreading erythema from a tick bite. Because of heightened awareness, patients may present early, before the classic rash has a chance to evolve.
- Live attenuated rubella vaccines are associated, in up to 15% people, with subsequent arthralgias and myalgias. Arthritis may occur 2 weeks after the injection and clears in a week, but symptoms can remain for a year or so.

Family history

Ask about a history of illness in the family or a family history of enthesitis-related features:

- In children suspected of having septic arthritis due to TB, establishing a history of contact with sources may be important.
- Due to a link with HLA B27, there may be a history of similar musculoskeletal features in family members.

Examination

General principles of paediatric musculoskeletal examination
- Ensure that the child is comfortable in the environment and with the people present at the time of examination.
- Observe small children playing at first.
- Try to leave the painful area until last.
- Reassure the child that the examination will stop if it is painful.

Confirmation of synovitis/enthesitis in a joint
Review the features that help to confirm synovitis/enthesitis in a joint:
- It is important to establish from the examination whether there is true synovial swelling. Remember, a history of swelling is not always reliable and other, non-synovial, pathology can present with single or oligo-articular joint pain (e.g. enthesitis).
- Always compare both sides. Even subtle differences in range of motion may be important and denote synovial thickening.
- Doubt about synovial swelling can be addressed by obtaining US.

Additional musculoskeletal examination
Additional musculoskeletal examination must include a search for muscle atrophy, tenosynovitis, enthesitis, and spinal limitation:
- Adjacent muscle wasting may be a clue to the severity or chronicity of joint inflammation.
- **Tenosynovitis** is unusual in oligo-articular JIA, but can occur in sarcoid, occasionally in ERA, and in the polyarticular conditions.
- **Enthesitis** should discriminate between oligo-articular JIA and ERA. Commonly involved sites include Achilles, patellar tendon, and plantar fascia insertions.
- Clinical detection of spinal disease in patients who develop AS (◻ Chapter 8, p 281) or ERA is not always possible at the time of presentation of the first musculoskeletal manifestations of the disease, i.e. enthesitis, although spinal examination assessing localized pain and impaired mobility should be done.

Look for skin rashes and any inflammation
Oligo-arthritis may be part of a systemic inflammatory/infective condition. Look closely for skin rashes:
- Skin erythema overlying a joint suggests infection.
- Associated skin rashes may include **erythema nodosum** (◻ Chapter 18, p 489), the purpuric pustular rashes of **Henoch–Schönlein purpura** (HSP) (◻ Chapter 15, p 405) or **Behçet's** (◻ Chapter 18, p 489), **gonococcal infection** (◻ Chapter 17, p 473), **SAPHO syndrome** (◻ Chapter 8, p 281), erythema marginatum (rheumatic fever) and **psoriasis**.

Investigations

Although synovitis may be obvious clinically, its presence in any joint needs to be confirmed if there is doubt:
- The soft tissue appearances of joint radiographs are sufficient in confirming effusion and synovial thickening in many instances.
- US and MRI can identify effusion and synovial thickening.

Joint aspiration

Mono-articular synovitis and joint swelling requires joint aspiration and prompt examination of fluid. Fluid should be sent in sterile bottles for microscopy and culture. This procedure may be psychologically traumatic. Consider using sedation (at least) in older children and even a light general anaesthetic in younger ones:

• Synovial fluid appearances are not specific. Blood or bloodstaining suggests haemarthrosis from trauma (including the aspiration), **haemorrhagic diathesis, PVNS, synovioma, or haemangioma.**

• Turbidity (decreased clarity) of fluid relates to cellular, crystal, lipid, and fibrinous content; the joint fluid of **septic arthritis** (□ Chapter 24, p 609) and acute **crystal arthritis** (□ Chapter 7, p 269) is turbid due to the high number of neutrophils present.

• Crystals in synovial fluid in children are rare.

• The most common causes of non-gonococcal septic arthritis in Europe and North America are *Staphylococcus aureus* (40–50%), *Staphylococcus epidermidis* (10–15%), streptococcal species (20%), and Gram-negative bacteria (15%). Gonococcal infection should be considered a possibility in teenagers (□ Chapter 17, p 473).

Radiographs

Radiographs can confirm an effusion and show characteristic patterns of chondral epiphyseal and bone destruction (e.g. in infection or malignancy):

• In septic arthritis, osteopenia, and loss of bone cortex are classic signs (although their absence does not rule out septic arthritis). The main differential diagnosis is malignancy.

• If calcified, loose bodies due to osteochondritis dissecans may be visible.

• Erosions can occur in oligo-articular JIA or in ERA.

• Discriminating erosions from ossifying cartilagenous epiphyses in normal joints (which can appear irregular) is sometimes difficult. Bilateral views are sometimes helpful in this respect.

• Joint space narrowing is difficult to confirm from radiographs because of normal changes in epiphyseal cartilage thickness, operator error, and difficulty in weight bearing on painful joints.

• Joint destruction is a characteristic of polyarticular JIA.

Further imaging

Further imaging should be discussed with a radiologist. US and isotope bone scanning can confirm synovitis, and its pattern of joint involvement. CT and MRI are useful in discriminating against the causes of synovitis:

• US is a sensitive investigation for detection of synovitis.

• US and MRI can detect erosions earlier than radiographs.

• When malignancy and infection are suspected, isotope bone scan may help identify or rule out additional lesions.

• Because of its high sensitivity, bone scan can be useful in establishing whether significant bone/joint pathology is present in children with joint symptoms, but few clinical findings.

• In a normal joint, MRI differentiates all the major joint structures including epiphyses. Sedation may be needed in young children.

- MRI is an accurate and sensitive tool for identifying joint and epiphyseal damage at an early stage of a disease process. This may be invaluable, for example, if there is any doubt about the status of oligo-articular JIA or peripheral joint involvement in ERA, since early treatment can prevent permanent deformities and disability.

Laboratory tests

Laboratory tests should provide or exclude evidence of infection, give discriminatory diagnostic information, and exclude non-rheumatic diseases:

- A predominance of bands on FBC implies infection. Neutrophil predominance may be seen with a variety of inflammatory states, and is less specific for infection. Interestingly, mono-articular JIA can be associated with normal indices.
- A low platelet or white cell count but elevated acute phase indices may be suggestive of an underlying malignancy.
- Antibodies to streptolysin O (ASOT) may be helpful in patients who have had sore throat, migratory arthritis, or features of rheumatic fever. If there is persistent clinical suspicion despite a normal ASOT, antibodies to streptococcal DNAase B, hyaluronidase, and streptozyme may be of value.
- A single positive test for RF has little value. Repeatedly positive tests might suggest (RF+) JIA. ANAs are present in 40–75% of children with oligo-articular JIA. They are not disease-specific, but identify a subset within it at particular risk of (often asymptomatic) uveitis.
- Lyme serology may be helpful in a patient with an acute arthropathy or migratory arthritis.

Synovial biopsy

- If there is a haemarthrosis or suspicion of PVNS, MRI of the joint is wise before undertaking biopsy to characterize the vascularity of a lesion.
- Biopsy may be helpful to evaluate a persistent mono-arthritis of unclear aetiology; biopsy may help diagnose sarcoid arthropathy, malignancy, and chronic infectious arthritis due to atypical pathogens.
- Arthroscopic biopsy will yield more tissue than a needle biopsy. Direct viewing may add diagnostic information and allow joint irrigation.

Widespread pain in adults

Widespread (musculoskeletal) pain is a common reason for adults to seek medical advice (Table 3.5). Although some of these patients will have a polyarticular arthritis, many conditions are characterized by musculoskeletal symptoms, some of which may be diffuse or multicentric. In addition, the interpretation and reporting of symptoms varies considerably and can be a source of confusion.

The following section reviews important aspects of the history, examination, and investigations in the initial evaluation of patients who present with non-localized, multicentric pains.

Background

Initial impressions

- Think broadly about the possible diagnoses.
- Use what you know about the epidemiology of likely conditions. For example, a 25-year-old man with joint pains is more likely to have AS (📖 Chapter 8, p 281) than generalized OA (📖 Chapter 6, p 259), SLE (📖 Chapter 10, p 321) or PMR (📖 Chapter 15, p 405), although joint pains are characteristic of all of these diagnoses.

Age, sex, and racial background

What clues can be drawn from the age, sex, and racial background?

The degree to which these factors influence the likelihood of disease varies according to the prevalence of the disease in the local population. Review what you know about the epidemiology of the major diseases.

Previous diagnoses

Presenting features may be put in context early if you have knowledge of musculoskeletal associations of diagnoses that have already been made. For example:

- Synovitis in patients with (radiological) chondrocalcinosis.
- Arthropathy in patients with hyperparathyroidism and hypercalcaemia (📖 Chapter 16, p 431).
- Enthesitis/synovitis in patients with Crohn's disease or ulcerative colitis (📖 Chapter 8, p 281).
- Polyarticular synovitis and myalgia in patients with lymphoma.
- Crystal-induced or β_2-microglobulin deposition arthritis and osteodystrophy in chronic renal disease (📖 Chapter 16, p 431).

Taking a history

First, establish whether pains arise from joints or tendons/entheses, muscles, bone, or are neurologic (Table 3.5):

- Although the patient may report 'joint pains', take time to establish whether the pains are truly articular.
- Listen carefully to the description of the pains; try to determine if the patient has a single condition or a number of overlapping causes of pain.

Table 3.5 Broad categories of conditions that may present with widespread musculoskeletal pain

Common	Inflammatory polyarthritis (e.g. RA—📖 Chapter 5, p 233)
	Generalized (nodal) OA (📖 Chapter 6, p 259)
	Fibromyalgia/chronic pain syndromes (📖 Chapter 18, p 489)
	Non-specific myalgias and arthralgias* associated with infection (e.g. viruses) (📖 Chapter 17, p 473)
Less common	Myalgias, arthralgias* due to autoimmune connective tissue disease
	Myalgias, increased muscle inflammation (e.g. polymyositis) (📖 Chapter 14, p 385)
	Myalgias and arthralgias* associated with neoplasia (e.g. lymphoma)
	Skeletal metastases
	Polyostotic Paget's disease (📖 Chapter 16, p 431)
Rare	Metabolic bone diseases (e.g. osteomalacia, renal osteodystrophy; 📖 Chapter 16, p 431)
	Metabolic myopathies (e.g. hypokalaemia) (📖 Chapter 14, 385)
	Neurological disease (Parkinson's disease)

* In certain situations/conditions patients may complain of both muscle and joint pains. This is easily appreciated if you've ever had influenza!

Obtain a detailed history of the pain at different sites

- A good history should help narrow the differential diagnosis considerably. For example, a 70-year-old man referred with 'widespread joint pains mostly in his legs', could have multiple weight-bearing joint OA or lumbosacral nerve root claudication symptoms (📖 Chapter 2, p 19 and 📖 Chapter 20, p 525). A middle-aged woman with 'hand and neck pain' could have an arthropathy or radicular pain associated with cervical spondylosis (📖 Chapter 2, p 19).
- Widespread pain due to bone pathology could be due to skeletal metastasis. Bony pain is often unremitting, and changes little with changes in posture and movement.
- One pitfall is to assume that all pains arise from a single pathological process. For example, in an older patient, shoulder pain could be caused by PMR, OA, shoulder impingement syndrome, radicular pain, or a combination of all of these.

Joint pain at rest, after rest, or with joint use?

Establish whether pain arises from joints or tendons/enthuses.

- Pain occurring with inflammation is conventionally regarded as being associated with morning stiffness or stiffness after periods of rest. It tends to be prominent in conditions such as RA, SpA, PMR, and myositis. Inflammatory joint pain often improves during the day.
- Mild degrees of immobility-associated pain and stiffness occur in some other conditions, such as OA and fibromyalgia, although such forms of

stiffness generally last for less than 1 h. Stiffness may also be a feature of muscle spasm and soft-tissue oedema.
- Mechanical joint damage such as OA is also painful. Unlike inflammatory joint pain, mechanical joint pain is worsened by use, and improves with rest.

Ask, and document in detail, which joints are affected
- A symmetric polyarthritis affecting the small joints is typical for RA. RA can also present with carpal tunnel syndrome, tenosynovitis, tennis elbow, or an asymmetric pattern of joint involvement, and can be preceded by a palindromic pattern of joint pain (see below).
- Arthritis from parvovirus B19 infection may also be polyarticular and symmetric.
- Small joint pain in the hands occurs in nodal generalized OA. DIPs, PIPs, and thumb joints are usually affected. OA is also associated with pain in the spine, hips, and knees.
- The combination of sacroiliac (low back and buttock), pelvic, and lower limb joint/enthesis pain, typically in an asymmetric oligo-articular pattern, is suggestive of SpA. Typical sites of involvement include the anterior knee, posterior heel and inferior foot (plantar fascia).
- Enthesitis can affect the wrists and small joints of the hand and feet (e.g. plantar fascia origin and insertion at metatarsal heads) and may be difficult to distinguish from RA on clinical grounds alone.
- CPPD typically favours the large and medium-sized joints, but a picture of multiple joint involvement similar to that in RA is possible (including tenosynovitis).
- Widespread arthralgias/arthritis occurs in patients with leukaemia, lymphoma, myeloma, and certain infections.

Ask about the pattern of joint symptoms over time
- A short, striking history of marked, acute polyarticular symptoms often occurs with systemic infection (Table 3.6). Prominent malaise and fever should raise suspicion of infection.
- There may be a longer history than is first volunteered. Autoimmune rheumatic and connective tissue diseases may evolve over a period of time and often naturally relapse and remit; the first symptoms of disease may be dismissed by the patient as irrelevant.
- Conventionally, persistent inflammatory joint symptoms should be present for at least 6 weeks before RA is diagnosed.
- Migratory arthralgias occur in 10% of RA patients initially: a single joint becomes inflamed for a few days then improves and a different joint becomes affected for a few days and so on. A similar pattern can occur in post-streptococcal arthritis, Wegener's granulomatosis, sarcoidosis, Lyme disease, and Whipple's disease.
- Recurrent pains from various musculoskeletal lesions, which have occurred from injury or have developed insidiously, are typical in patients with underlying hypermobility [benign joint hyper-mobility syndrome or other heritable diseases of connective tissue such as Ehlers–Danlos syndrome (📖 Chapter 16, p 431)].
- The onset of enthesopathy may be insidious or acute.

Table 3.6 Common infections that can present with acute polyarthritis and a raised acute phase respons (also 📖 Chapter 17, p 473)

Infection	Common extra-articular clinical features	Key laboratory diagnostic tests in acute infection
Rheumatic fever (group A-haemolytic streptococci)	Acute infection 1–2 weeks earlier, fever, rash, carditis	Positive throat swab culture. High ASOT (in 80%).
Post-streptococcal	Acute infection 3–4 weeks earlier, tenosynovitis	As above
Parvovirus B19 (adults†)	Severe flu-like illness at onset, various rashes	Anti-B19 IgM
Rubella (also post-vaccine)	Fever, coryza, malaise, brief rash	Culture. Anti-rubella IgM
Hepatitis B	Fever, myalgia, malaise, urticaria, abnormal liver function	Bilirubin+, ALT+, AST+, anti-HBsAg, anti-HBcAg
Lyme disease (Borrelia burgdorferi)	Tick bites, fever, headache, myalgias, fatigue, nerve palsies	Anti-Bb IgM (ELISA + immunofluorescence)
Toxoplasma gondii	Myositis, paraesthesias	Anti-Toxo IgM

Even if serological tests have high sensitivity and specificity, the positive predictive value of the test is low if the clinical likelihood of the infection is low. Therefore, do not use serological tests indiscriminately.

ASOT = anti-streptolysin O titre.

†The presentation of parvovirus B19 illness may be quite different in children.

Is there widespread muscle pain?

If you think there is widespread muscle pain, remember to consider that:
- The myalgias may be fibromyalgia or enthesitis.
- Pain locating to muscle group areas may be ischemic or neurologic in origin, and not necessarily due to intrinsic muscle disease.
- The differential diagnosis of PM and dermatomyositis (DM) is broad, but many of these conditions are rare (Table 3.7 and 📖 Chapter 14, p 385).

Ask about the distribution and description of myalgias and weakness

- True weakness may denote either myopathy or a neurological condition. However, patients may report a feeling of weakness if muscles are painful, therefore, rely more on your examination before deciding muscles are weak.
- PMR (rare in patients less than 50 years old), myositis, and endocrine/metabolic myopathies typically present with proximal weakness.

- PMR does not lead to objective weakness; instead, patients experience proximal muscle pain and stiffness that is worse in the morning, and is frequently described by the patient as 'weakness'.
- Although rare, truncal muscle pain, and stiffness can be a presenting feature of Parkinson's disease.
- Cramp-like pains may be a presenting feature of any myopathy (e.g. hypokalaemic) or even motor neuron disease. However, some patients may interpret radicular (nerve root) pains as 'cramp-like'.
- Inflammatory and endocrine/metabolic myopathies are often not painful.
- Occasionally, some genetic muscle diseases (e.g. myophosphorylase, acid maltase deficiency), can present atypically late (in adults) with progressive weakness that may be mistaken for PM.

Ask about the pattern of muscle pains over time
- Severe, acute muscle pain occurs in a variety of conditions. The most common causes are viral, neoplastic, and drugs. Some toxic causes may result in rhabdomyolysis, myoglobinuria, and renal failure.
- Usually PM/DM is characterized by slowly evolving but progressive muscle pain and weakness (e.g. weeks to months).
- Low-grade episodic muscle pains may denote a previously undisclosed hereditary metabolic myopathy (📖 Chapter 14, p 385).
- Fibromyalgia (📖 Chapter 18, p 489) is chiefly a chronic pain syndrome and symptoms may have been present for a considerable time at presentation.

Are the pains ischaemic?
- Ischaemic muscle pain often occurs predictably in association with repeated activity and eases or resolves on rest ('claudication'). Consider this especially if pains are confined to a single limb or both legs.

Table 3.7 The major causes of myopathies and conditions associated with diffuse myalgia (also 📖 Chapter 14, p 385.)

Infectious myositis	Viruses (e.g. influenza, hepatitis B or C, coxsackie, HIV, HTLV-I)
	Bacteria [e.g. *Borrelia burgdorferi* (Lyme)]
	Other (e.g. malaria tooplasmosis)
Endocrine and metabolic	Hypo/hyperthyroidism, hypercortisolism, hyperparathyroidism
	Hypocalcaemic, hypokalaemic
Autoimmune diseases	Polymyositis, dermatomyositis, SLE, scleroderma, Sjögren's, RA, PMR
	Vasculitis (e.g. PAN, Wegener's granulomatosis, rheumatoid)
	Myasthenia gravis
	Eosinophilic fasciitis
Carcinomatous myopathy	
Idiopathic	Fibromyalgia (muscles should not be weak)
	Inclusion body myositis
	Sarcoid myositis
Drugs	Lipid-lowering drugs (e.g. fibrates, gemfibrozil, niacin)
	Anti-immune (e.g. colchicine, CyA, D-Pca*)
	Rhabdomyolysis (e.g. alcohol, opiates)
	Others (e.g. azathioprine (AZA) chloroquine*)
Muscular dystrophies	Limb girdle, fascioscapulohumeral
Congenital myopathies†	Mitochondrial myopathy
	Myophosphorylase deficiency Lipid storage diseases

*Drugs most likely to cause painful myopathy.
†Because of variable severity, some conditions may not present until adulthood.
Note: Guillain–Barré and motor neuron disease may be considered in the differential diagnosis of non-painful muscle weakness.

- The distribution of pains may give clues as to sites of underlying pathology, e.g. upper extremities are affected by subclavian artery stenosis and thoracic outlet syndrome; lower extremities are affected by atherosclerotic vascular disease or lumbar nerve root stenosis.
- Ischaemic pains in the context of a highly inflammatory state may suggest systemic vasculitis, such as polyarteritis nodosa.

Widespread pain may be due to bone pathology

- Bone pains are unremitting and disturb sleep. They could denote serious pathology—radiographic and laboratory investigations are important.

- The major diagnoses to consider include disseminated malignancy, multiple myeloma, metabolic bone disease (e.g. renal osteodystrophy, hyperparathyroidism, osteomalacia), and polyostotic Paget's disease.

Past medical history

Specific questions are often required because previous problems may not be regarded as relevant by the patient. For example:

- For those with joint pains a history of the following may be of help:
  - other autoimmune diseases (increased risk of RA, SLE, etc.);
  - Raynaud's phenomenon (association with scleroderma, RA, and SLE);
  - dry eyes (possible Sjögren's syndrome);
  - uveitis or acute 'red eye' (association with SpA);
  - recurrent injuries/joint dislocations (association with hypermobility);
  - genital, urine, or severe gut infection (link with SpA);
  - psoriasis (association with SpA);
  - diabetes (cheiro-arthropathy).
- For those in whom myalgias/myositis seems likely:
  - preceding viral illness (possible viral myositis);
  - foreign travel (tropical myositis);
  - other autoimmune disease (associated with PM/DM);
  - previous erythema nodosum (sarcoid);
  - drugs and substance abuse (see below).
- For all patients:
  - weight loss or anorexia (association with malignancy);
  - fevers or night sweats (association with infection);
  - sore throat (possible post-streptococcal condition);
  - persistent spinal pain (association with fibromyalgia);
  - rashes (association with Lyme disease, SLE, DM, vasculitis).
- For those with widespread bony pain:
  - history of rickets (association with osteomalacia);
  - chronic renal disease (will precede renal osteodystrophy and may predispose to crystalline arthritis and osteo-articular deposition of β_2-microglobulin).

Psychosocial and sexual history

- Preceding sexual activity and genital infection is important primarily because of an association of *Chlamydia trachomatis* infection with reactive arthritis and enthesitis/SpA (📖 Chapter 8, p 281).
- Reactive arthritis has an association with HIV. HIV is also associated with polymyositis, and is a risk factor for pyomyositis.
- There is an association of anxiety and depression with fibromyalgia (📖 Chapter 18, p 489).

Ask about travel

- Residence in, or travel to, rural areas populated by deer might be important in indicating a risk of exposure to *Borrelia burgdorferi* and contracting Lyme disease (the spirochete is carried by ticks that colonize deer, boar, and other animals and bite other mammals).
- *Plasmodium falciparum* (intertropical areas), trypanosoma (mainly South America), trichinella, and cystercercicae infections are associated with myalgias/myositis.

Family history

Ask about family with arthritis or autoimmune diseases:

- There is a hereditary component to large joint and generalized nodal OA, and hyperuricaemia/gout.
- The risk of developing any autoimmune condition is higher in families of patients with autoimmune diseases than generally.
- Hypermobility *per se* (not necessarily JHS) and FM show a strong heritability in twin studies.

Drug history

- The following drugs have been reported to cause a myopathy (those marked* are more likely to be painful): lithium, fibrates, statins, penicillin, colchicine, penicillamine*, sulfonamides, hydralazine, ciclosporin, phenytoin, cimetidine* (muscle cramps), zidovudine, carbimazole, and tamoxifen.
- The myositis that occurs with penicillamine is not dose- or cumulative dose-dependent. It can be life threatening.
- Drug-induced SLE, which is characterized commonly by arthralgias, aching, and malaise, and less commonly by polyarthritis, can occur with a number of drugs including hydralazine, procainamide, isoniazid, and minocycline. Quinidine, labetalol, captopril, phenytoin, methyldopa, and sulfasalazine may also cause similar symptoms.
- Mild myalgias and arthralgias may be caused by a number of commonly used drugs, e.g. proton pump inhibitors and quinolone antibiotics.
- Alcohol in excess and some illegal drugs are associated with severe toxic myopathy occasionally resulting in rhabdomyolysis (Table 3.7).

Ask about chest pain, dyspnoea, palpitations, cough, and hemoptysis

- Cardiac abnormalities are features of autoimmune rheumatic and connective tissue diseases, but are infrequent at initial presentation. Cardiac infection is associated with widespread aches and pains (e.g. rheumatic fever/post-streptococcal myalgias/arthralgias, infective endocarditis).
- Chronic effort-related dyspnoea due to interstitial lung disease occurs in many patients with autoimmune connective tissue and rheumatic diseases. Up to 40% of RA patients may have CT evidence of lung disease. In many sedentary patients, however, symptoms are not prominent. Dyspnoea may be present at presentation.
- Respiratory failure and aspiration pneumonia can occur as a result of a combination of truncal striated, diaphragmatic, and smooth muscle weakness in PM.
- There is an association between bronchiectasis and RA.
- The most common neoplasm in patients diagnosed with malignancy-associated myositis is of the lung.

Ask specifically about dysphagia, abdominal pain, and diarrhea

- Patients may not mention gastrointestinal symptoms if they have resolved. There are many links between bowel disease, and polyarthralgias or polyarthritis.
- Ask specifically about previous severe diarrhoeal or dysenteric illnesses; *Campylobacter, Yersinia, Shigella,* or *Salmonella*, may be relevant to diagnosing reactive arthritis/SpA.
- Gut smooth muscle may be affected in polymyositis and give rise to dysphagia and abdominal pain.

Examination

In patients with widespread pain a full medical examination is always necessary.

Skin and nails (📖 Chapter 4, p 193 and 📖 Chapter 18, p 489)
In all patients look carefully at the skin and nails:

- Nails may show prominent ridges or pits in psoriatic arthropathy (Plate 7), splinter haemorrhages in infective endocarditis, systemic vasculitis or antiphospholipid syndrome (APS), or peri-ungual erythema in scleroderma and the inflammatory myopathies.
- Look for skin rashes in conditions characterized by widespread pain. For example:
  - erythema migrans in Lyme disease;
  - erythema marginatum in rheumatic fever;
  - UV sensitive rash on face/arms in SLE;
  - violacious rash on knuckles/around eyes/base of neck in DM;
  - livedo reticularis in SLE and APS;
  - purpuric rash in vasculitis (e.g. HSP);
  - erythema nodosum in sarcoidosis.
- Lymphadenopathy may be present with either infection or inflammation and is non-specific. However, if prominent it may denote lymphoma.
- Signs of anaemia are a non-specific finding in many chronic systemic autoimmune diseases.
- Clubbing of the digits may be present in Crohn's disease and ulcerative colitis (associated with SpA) and bronchiectasis (associated with RA).
- Oedema can occur in both upper and lower extremities in a subset of patients presenting with inflammatory polyarthritis/tenosynovitis. The condition has been termed RS_3PE (remitting seronegative symmetric synovitis with pitting oedema). This condition is striking in that it occurs suddenly, often in patients between 60–80 years old and is very disabling. It may be associated with other conditions e.g. haematological, malignancy.

Examination of the joints
Important points to note when examining joints (detailed examination techniques that help discriminate synovitis from other pathology at specific joints are included in sections in 📖 Chapter 2, p 19).

- Each joint should be compared to the joint on the opposite extremity, first by observation, then palpation, then by its active and passive range of motion exercises.
- Useful examination tools include a tape measure to record swelling (circumferential) and a goniometer (protractor with arms) to measure the range of joint movement.

Patterns of abnormality

Note the specific cause of joint swelling and site of tenderness, distribution of affected sites, and hypermobility:

- In nodal generalized OA, osteophytes (bony swelling—may be tender) can be noted at DIPs (Heberden's nodes) and PIPs (Bouchard's nodes). Periosteal new bone at sites of chronic enthesitis may be palpable and tender.
- Nodules may occur in nodal OA, RA, polyarticular gout, ANCA-associated vasculitis (Churg–Strauss nodules), multicentric reticulohistiocytosis (Plate 6), or hyperlipidemia (xanthomata).
- Soft tissue swelling with tenderness and painful restriction of the joint on movement suggests an inflammatory arthritis. There is often adjacent muscle wasting. This is most easily appreciated in the interosseous muscles in patients with hand arthritis, or the quadriceps in patients with knee arthritis.
- The 'painful joints' may be inflamed tendons or entheses. Tender tendon insertions and peri-articular bone tenderness, often without any joint swelling, may denote enthesis inflammation associated with SpA.
- Tendonitis may be part of many autoimmune rheumatic or connective tissue diseases. Look specifically for thickening of the digital flexors and swelling of the dorsal extensor tendon sheath in the hand, and tenderness/swelling of both peroneal and posterior tibial tendons in the foot.
- Gross swelling with painful restriction of small joints is unusual in SLE. Often there is little to find on examination of joints.
- General joint hypermobility may lead to joint and other soft tissue lesions. An examination screen for hypermobility (🕮 Chapter 16, p 431) may be helpful (Table 3.8). Check also for associated features.

Table 3.8 Features of the benign joint hypermobility syndrome (JHS). ('Brighton' criteria – see also 🕮 p 470)

Examination screen (scored out of 9)	Ability to extend fifth finger >90°at MCPJ (score 1 + 1 for R + L)
	Ability to abduct thumb (with wrist flexion) to touch forearm (score 1 + 1)
	Extension of elbows >10°(1 + 1)
	Extension of knees >10°(1 + 1)
	Ability to place hands flat on floor when standing with knees extended (1)
Associated features	Prolonged arthralgias
	Skin striae, hyperextensibility, and abnormal scarring
	Recurrent joint dislocations
	Varicose veins
	Uterine/rectal prolapse
	Recurrent soft-tissue lesions
	Marfanoid habitus
	Eye signs: drooping eyelids, myopia, down-slanting eyes

Examination of patients with widespread myalgia

- Check for muscle tenderness and weakness. Document the distribution. Is there evidence of neurologic or vascular disease?
- The characteristic sites of tenderness in fibromyalgia should be confidently recognized (Fig. 3.1). Despite discomfort, the muscles should be strong.
- Examine the strength of both truncal and limb muscle groups (Fig. 3.2). In the presence of pain it may be difficult to demonstrate subtle degrees of muscle weakness.
- Patterns of muscle weakness are not disease specific; however, there are some characteristic patterns: symmetric proximal extremities in polymyositis and dermatomyositis; quadriceps and forearm/finger flexors in inclusion body myositis; limb muscles in mitochondrial myopathy. (Note: using specific apparatus physical therapists can help document isometric muscle strength in certain muscle groups.)
- Muscles in PMR are not intrinsically weak.
- Muscle wasting is not specific. If wasting is profound and rapid, consider neoplasia. Wasting will occur in most long-standing myopathies.
- Check for increased limb tone and rigidity—most evident by passive movement at a joint—consistent with extrapyramidal disease. There may be resting tremor in the hand, facial impassivity, and 'stiff' gait. Muscular tone in the limbs may also be increased in motor neuron disease (MND); however, if presenting with muscle pains, the patient with MND is more likely to have a lower motor neuron pattern of neuronal loss (progressive muscular atrophy) with muscular weakness/wasting, flaccidity, and fasciculations.
- The fatiguability of myasthaenia gravis can be identified by determining the length of time the patient can keep his arms extended in front of him, or maintain an upward gaze.
- Muscle pains or cramps owing to large-vessel ischemia are likely to be non-tender at rest and strong. Demonstrate absent pulses and bruits and substantiate findings with US Doppler examination.
- In suspected cases of polymyositis and dermatomyositis, carefully examine for cardiopulmonary abnormalities. Other associated signs in dermatomyositis include peri-ungual erythema/telangiectasia, erythematous violacious rash and skin calcinosis; include dysphonia and swallowing abnormalities in both polymyositis and dermatomyositis.
- Because of its associations (Table 3.7), patients with myositis should be carefully examined for the following signs: dry eyes/mouth [Sjögren's (📖 Chapter 12, p 353)], skin thickening/tenderness or discoloration [scleroderma (📖 Chapter 13, p 363)], skin rashes [SLE (📖 Chapter 10, p 321)], thyroid tenderness or enlargement [endocrine myopathy (📖 Chapter 4, p 193 and 📖 Chapter 14, p 385)].

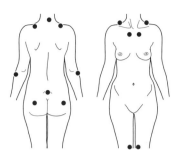

- Tenderness of skin overlaying trapezius
- Low cervical spine
- Midpoint of trapezius
- Supraspinatus
- Pectoralis, maximal lateral to the second costochondral junction
- Lateral epicondyle of the elbow
- Upper gluteal area
- Low lumbar spine
- Medial fat pad of the knee

Fig. 3.1 Typical sites of tenderness in fibromyalgia (📖 Chapter 18, p 489).

Investigations

General points

- ESR and CRP may be higher than normal in the setting of infection, malignancy, or active rheumatic disease. A slightly elevated ESR is a common finding in healthy elderly people.
- A positive ANA may occur in association with many autoimmune conditions, in other diseases (Table 3.9) and in some healthy people. It is, therefore, not diagnostic for SLE or any single condition; however, high-titer ANA may be significant and conversely, ANA-negative SLE is rare.
- Anti-CCP is more specific for RA than RF (📖 Chapter 5, p 233), which can be positive in a number of inflammatory conditions.
- Controversy exists about the diagnosis of FM. It is prudent to only make a diagnosis of FM when inflammatory disorders can be confidently excluded, bearing in mind that FM-like symptoms are often associated with inflammatory conditions.

Basic tests in patients with polyarthropathy

- Urinalysis (dipstick) may show proteinuria or haematuria. Both glomerular and tubular damage are possible. Glomerulonephritis (in SLE, vasculitis, or endocarditis, for example) is usually associated with significant proteinuria and haematuria simultaneously. These patients will need urgent evaluation by a nephrologist.
- ESR and CRP are non-specific and may be normal in the early stages of these conditions. If very high then consider infection or malignancy. There is often no evidence of an acute phase response in patients with enthesitis (even though pain and bony tenderness may be widespread). A mild anaemia and thrombocytosis may accompany inflammation.
- Throat swab, ASOT, anti-DNAaseB antibodies may be useful to identify a post-streptococcal condition.
- Other simple blood tests which should be considered in the appropriate setting:
  - random blood sugar (diabetes);
  - TFTs/thyroid antibodies (hyper/hypothyroidism);
  - prostatic specific antigen (malignancy).

Table 3.9 Examples of the prevalence of antinuclear antibodies (ANA) in some diseases using Hep2 cells as substrate

Population group		Prevalence of ANA
Normal population		8%
SLE		95%
Other autoimmune rheumatic diseases	Systemic sclerosis	90%
	Sjögren's syndrome	80%
	Rheumatoid arthritis	60%
	Polymyositis	40%
	Polyarteritis nodosa	18%
Other diseases	Chronic active hepatitis	100%
	Drug-induced lupus	100%
	Myasthenia gravis	50%
	Waldenstrom's macrogobulinaemia	20%
	Diabetes	25%

- Joint fluid aspiration and culture is mandatory for patients in whom sepsis is a possibility. Fluid should be examined by polarized light microscopy in suspected cases of crystal-induced synovitis.
- In patients who are ANA-positive, testing serum for extractable nuclear antigens (ENAs) may be useful for characterizing the type of autoimmune process. Ro, La, Sm, and RNP positivity are each found in a slightly different spectrum of disorders.

(a) **Functional**

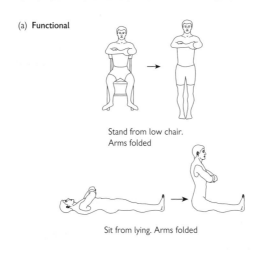

Stand from low chair.
Arms folded

Sit from lying. Arms folded

(b) **Specific resisted**

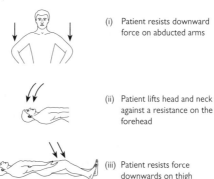

(i) Patient resists downward force on abducted arms

(ii) Patient lifts head and neck against a resistance on the forehead

(iii) Patient resists force downwards on thigh

Fig. 3.2 Screening examination for proximal myopathy. (a) Functional movements requiring truncal and proximal lower limb muscle strength. (b) Resisted movement testing of deltoid (i), longitudinal flexors of the neck (ii), and iliopsoas/quadriceps (iii) strength.

- In many patients presenting with a short history of widespread joint pains, radiographs will be normal. An early sign of joint inflammation is peri-articular osteopenia, but this is not specific for any particular disorder. Recognized types of erosions and their distribution can be noted by experienced radiologists in specific conditions (e.g. RA, psoriatic arthritis, gout).

- Referral to a sexual health clinic for further detailed investigations if there is a suggestion of recent or recurrent genital infection may help to strengthen the evidence for a diagnosis of reactive arthritis.

Basic laboratory tests in patients with widespread muscle pain/weakness
- Dipstick urinalysis: to screen for haematuria or myoglobinuria.
- FBC and measures of acute-phase response.
- An endocrine and metabolic screen: urea/electrolytes, creatinine, free thyroxine and TSH, blood calcium, phosphate and 25-hydroxyvitamin D, LFTs.
- Elevated CK or aldolase occurs in most cases of PM. ALT, AST, and LDH are non-specific markers of muscle damage. Note that specific muscle isoenzymes of CK and LDH exist and the normal range of all enzymes may vary in different populations. Muscle enzymes may be elevated after non-inflammatory causes of muscle damage, e.g. exercise/trauma.
- Check for ANA and, if positive, screen for ENAs. Antibodies to certain (cytoplasmic) tRNA synthetases (e.g. Jo-1) are myositis-specific.
- All of the above tests may reasonably be done in cases where you think muscle pains are due to FM, but want to rule out other pathology.
- Think of checking for urinary myoglobin in cases where acute widespread muscle pain may be associated with myolysis—causes include excessive alcohol or ingestion of certain drugs (cocaine, amphetamines, ecstasy, heroin), exercise, or trauma. Such patients may be at risk of renal failure.
- Polymyositis can be a presenting feature of HIV. In HIV-positive patients, infections causing muscle disease include TB and microsporidia.
- Viral myositis may be clinically indistinguishable from PM. Serology may yield diagnostic clues.

Electrophysiology and imaging in patients with muscle conditions
- Electromyographic abnormalities occur in two-thirds of patients with muscle inflammation. More information is likely if studied in the acute rather than the chronic phase of the illness. In the acute phase, denervation and muscle degeneration give rise to fibrillation potentials in 74% of polymyositis and 33% of dermatomyositis patients (☐ Chapter 14, p 385). Other features include: low-amplitude short-duration motor unit and polyphasic potentials.
- Electromyography is poor at discriminating on-going muscle inflammation in myositis from steroid-induced myopathy.
- There are characteristic MR patterns of abnormality in polymyositis and dermatomyositis. MR can be used to identify potential muscle biopsy sites to avoid false-negative results associated with patchy muscle inflammation.

Muscle biopsy
- Muscle biopsy should be considered in all patients evaluated for polymyositis or dermatomyositis.
- In polymyositis, inflammatory infiltrates predominate in the endomysial area around muscle fibers without perifascicular atrophy. In dermatomyositis, inflammation is more prominent in the perimysial

area and around small blood vessels and there is typically perifascicular atrophy.
- Routine tests do not reliably distinguish polymyositis from cases of viral myositis. Some of the glycogen storage diseases will become apparent from light microscopy of biopsy material.

Investigations for malignancy

Investigations in adults with widespread bony pain should aim to rule out malignancy, particularly myeloma and malignancies from breast, renal and prostate cancers:

- Investigations may include: mammography, urine cytology, PSA, renal US, serum and urinary protein electrophoresis.
- Hypercalcaemia may accompany these conditions; check blood calcium, phosphate and albumin (also PTH).
- PTH should also be checked in suspected cases of osteomalacia (raised due to calcium/vitamin D deficiency) together with 25-hydroxyvitamin D levels (low or low/normal), alkaline phosphatase (high/normal), and 24-h urinary calcium (low).
- Radiographs of affected sites are important. Include a chest radiograph (CXR).
- Isotope bone scan can identify sites of neoplasia, Paget's disease, polyostotic osteoporosis, or osteomalacia (Plate 15). Although characteristic patterns exist, it is generally not specific for any condition.
- Bone biopsy (maintained undecalcified by placing sample in 70% alcohol) of affected sites will be diagnostic in some, but not all, cases of osteomalacia, osteoporosis, renal osteodystrophy, malignancy, and Paget's disease (Chapter 16, p 431) as good samples are hard to obtain. The best samples are obtained from a transiliac biopsy. Bone marrow can be aspirated for examination at the same time.

Widespread pain in children and adolescents

Background

Disease classification

The classification of JIA and the differential diagnosis has been discussed earlier in this chapter (Table 3.4).

As with adults it is important to consider the breadth of differential diagnosis including myopathies (Tables 3.10 and 3.11).

Conditions such as FM and JHS manifest in similar ways to that seen in adults.

Table 3.10 The differential diagnosis of JIA

Infection (multiple sites in immunodeficiency)	*Staphylococcus* septic arthritis
	Haemophilus influenzae septic arthritis
Reactive to an infectious agent	Parvovirus B19, hepatitis, rubella, rubella vaccination
	Post-streptococcal, rheumatic fever
Autoimmune connective tissue disorders	SLE
	MCTD, overlap syndromes
	Poly/dermatomyositis
Systemic vasculitis syndromes	Kawasaki disease (young child, high fever, desquamating extremity rash)
	Polyarteritis nodosa
	Wegener's granulomatosis
	HSP, Behçet's disease, familial Mediterranean fever
Sarcoid arthritis (polyarthritis, rash, uveitis)	
Haematological disorders	Sickle cell disease
	Constitutional bleeding disorders
	Acute leukaemia (bone and joint pain)
Other causes	Chronic recurrent multifocal osteomyelitis
	Diabetic cheiro-arthropathy

Taking a history

Are the pains due to myalgias or myositis?

- Acute viral myositis is distinguished from chronic myositis by its localization to calf muscles, severe pain, and its resolution within 4 weeks.
- Chronic muscle weakness suggests an autoimmune connective tissue disease, such as juvenile dermatomyositis. Myalgias and muscle cramps occur in hypothyroidism, uraemia, and electrolyte imbalance.

- Myalgias are common in paediatric SLE, but myopathy occurs rarely (10%).
- Episodic cramping or muscle pain related to exercise in early childhood might reflect muscular dystrophy, congenital myopathy, myotonic disorders, or genetic defects in glycogen or glucose metabolism.
- A pain syndrome (e.g. fibromyalgia, FM) is a diagnosis of exclusion. Enthesitis should be carefully excluded.

Is there bone pain?

Do the pains represent bone pain—persistent, deep-seated pains that change little with posture or movement?

- Night-time pain is typical of bony involvement in malignancy or osteomyelitis. Acute lymphoblastic leukaemia, lymphoma, and neuroblastoma are the most common malignant lesions.
- Achy 'bony' pain around joints may be due to enthesitis. Patients with ERA/SpA can present with enthesitis alone.
- Migratory bone pains are typical in multifocal osteomyelitis.

Is the child with arthritis systemically unwell?

- Malignancy should be ruled out and vasculitis and autoimmune connective tissue diseases considered in all children with persistent polyarthritis or widespread pains who have systemic symptoms.
- Fever is non-specific but essential to making a diagnosis of systemic JIA (Fig. 3.3), which is associated with spiking fevers, chills, and sweats. Anorexia and weight loss are common. Vasculitis (📖 Chapter 15, p 405) and FMF (📖 Chapter 18, p 489) should be considered in appropriate patients.
- There may be several years between the onset of systemic features and the arthritis of systemic JIA.
- Low-grade fever can often be present in patients JIA.
- Serositis is typical in systemic JIA but also occurs in SLE.
- In children <1 year, fever and arthralgias raise the possibility of chronic infantile neurological cutaneous and articular (CINCA) syndrome (📖 Chapter 9, p 303) and hyperimmunoglobulin D syndrome.

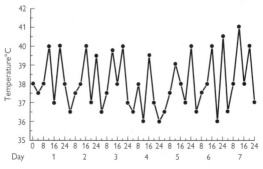

Fig. 3.3 Double-daily fever spikes with rapid return to below 37°C in systemic JIA.

Table 3.11 Classification of childhood disorders characterized by myalgias and muscle weakness

Muscular dystrophies	X-linked, e.g. Duchenne
	Autosomal dominant, e.g. fascioscapulohumeral
	Autosomal recessive, e.g. limb girdle
Congenital myopathies	e.g. myopathic arthrogryposis
Myotonic dystrophy	
Metabolic disorders	Glycogen storage disease, e.g. acid maltase/phosphorylase/phosphofructokinase deficiency
	Familial periodic paralyses
	Due to endocrinopathies, e.g. Addison's disease, Cushing's disease
Inflammatory diseases	Post-infectious, e.g. viruses—influenza B, coxsackie B, echo, polio
	Autoimmune, e.g. RA, dermatomyositis, SLE
Genetic abnormalities	Osteogenesis imperfecta
	Ehlers–Danlos syndrome
	Mucopolysaccharidoses
Trauma	Physical, e.g. rhabdomyolysis
	Toxic, e.g. snakebite
	Drugs, e.g. steroids, hydroxychloroquine, diuretics
Neurogenic atrophies	Spinal muscular and anterior horn cell dysfunction
	Peripheral nerve, e.g. peroneal muscular atrophy
	Neuromuscular, e.g. congenital myasthenia

- A catastrophic illness can occur in children with systemic JIA. It is termed macrophage-activation or haematophagocytic syndrome, and is characterized by cytopenias, hepatic dysfunction, encephalopathy, and disseminated intravascular coagulation with bleeding.
- A history of recurrent infections and arthritis may suggest immunodeficiency. The most common is X-linked humoral deficiency.

Is there a rash?
Does the child have a rash or did one precede the onset of pains?
- Rashes raise the possibility of preceding infection: EBV, rubella, and adenovirus are common and are associated with myalgias, arthralgias, and fever.
- The rash of systemic JIA is a salmon-pink macular rash. Lesions may either persist or come and go and may exhibit Köebner phenomenon—the exaggeration of the rash at sites of trauma.
- UV skin sensitivity may indicate SLE or dermatomyositis.

- Check for a vasculitic rash (e.g. HSP, cutaneous PAN). Systemic vasculitis can be associated with recurrent fevers and joint pains.

Are there ophthalmic symptoms?

Eye symptoms are an important indicator of underlying autoimmunity in the context of persistent joint or muscle pains:

- Uveitis is associated with most forms of JIA (particularly in association with ANA), but also may indicate an ERA/SpA (uveitis = pain/discomfort, blurring of vision, photophobia and a 'red eye').
- Impairment of visual fields suggests a retinal abnormality—a typical manifestation in juvenile dermatomyositis (due to occlusive vasculopathy).

Examination

Full medical examination

A full medical examination is essential:

- Pharyngeal erythema is non-specific and swabs should be cultured for streptococci. Sterile pharyngitis is a known feature of systemic JIA.
- Lymphadenopathy is common, but non-specific.
- For skin examination in detail see 📖 Chapter 4, p 193. UV sensitivity occurs in DM and SLE; healing psoriasis may mimic Gottron's lesions; calcinosis and pretibial hypopigmentation are signs of DM.
- The cardiovascular examination is important. Pericarditis is common in systemic and other forms of JIA, but is infrequently detected clinically. Myocarditis and heart failure also occur (rarely) in systemic JIA. Persistent tachycardia without anaemia/fever raises the possibility of myocarditis. Cardiac conduction defects are common in juvenile DM.
- A variety of cardiac conditions occur in (RF+) JIA including aortic valve insufficiency. The latter also occurs in ERA/SpA (8–30%).
- Respiratory examination may be abnormal if the arthralgias/arthritis are associated with respiratory tract infection; however, fixed crackles may indicate fibrosis [e.g. (RF+) JIA, PM] and a simultaneous reduction in expansion, breath sounds, and vocal fremitus suggests pleural effusion [e.g. (RF+) JIA].
- Bedside eye examination may be unrevealing even in those with ophthalmic symptoms. Thrombosis of dilated blood vessels at the margin of the upper lid is characteristic of dermatomyositis and polymyositis. Dry eyes are a common complaint, and may be the result of medication side effects; dry eyes are also found in association with a number of rheumatic diseases.
- As with all chronic conditions of childhood, growth and maturation (skeletal, endocrine/pubertal, and psychological) assessments should be considered at regular intervals.

Musculoskeletal examination—general principles

- Synovitis of a joint is characterized by soft-tissue swelling, effusion, and a reduced range of joint movement.
- Enthesitis may not be accompanied by an effusion; it can appear alone at bony insertions of ligaments/tendons with joint stiffness, but without swelling.
- Tendonitis can be difficult to distinguish from synovitis. Its diagnosis requires a precise knowledge of anatomy. The inflamed tendon may be more painful on active range of motion exercises.

- If the condition is chronic, an assessment of limb growth should be done, e.g. measuring leg length discrepancy (Plate 20).

Musculoskeletal examination—patterns of joint, tendon, and enthesis involvement

A full examination should be undertaken:

- Ligament/tendon insertion tenderness, not necessarily associated with swelling, may denote enthesitis. Enthesitis, which is probably more common (or at least more commonly recognized in lower limbs) raises the possibility of ERA/SpA.
- Within 2 years of the onset of symptoms, most cases of systemic JIA would be called oligo-articular because few joints are affected at first. Almost any joint can be involved, including those in the cervical spine. Hip joint involvement is almost always symmetric.
- There is no consistent pattern of joint or tendon involvement that distinguishes polyarticular (RF+) JIA from the majority of conditions associated with, or characterized by, polyarticular (RF–) JIA.
- Subsets of polyarticular (RF–) arthritis have been suggested on the basis of features such as 'painful' or 'dry' synovitis, stiffness, and other laboratory and genetic indices.
- Muscle tenderness is not specific. If confined to the calves, consider viral myositis. Weakness can accompany metabolic and endocrine myopathies and is not specific for inflammatory myopathy.
- Muscle weakness at rest may be present in children with severe forms of inherited metabolic muscle diseases. Often weakness only becomes apparent after exercise in these conditions (Table 3.12).

Laboratory investigations

- Laboratory abnormalities are non-specific in polyarticular (RF–) JIA.
- Because RF may appear in association with infections, ILAR criteria propose that significant titers of RF should be demonstrated on two occasions at least 3 months apart to make a diagnosis of polyarticular (RF+) JIA.
- A range of laboratory investigations is suggested when considering a diagnosis of systemic JIA (Table 3.13).
- Lymphopaenia is a hallmark of DM and SLE, and is not a feature of inflammatory arthritis.
- Neutrophilia and thrombocytosis are invariably present and can be marked in systemic JIA, whereas leucopaenia and thrombocytopenia are uncommon.
- Urinalysis is important in all children with widespread pains and may detect blood or haemoglobinuria in some muscle diseases (actually is myoglobin). Protein and blood may be a sign of underlying kidney inflammation in connective tissue diseases.
- Conventional acute phase markers can be normal in polymyositis (PM)/ dermatomyositis (DM). A sensitive indicator (though non-specific) of active disease is von Willebrand factor.
- A raised creatine phosphokinase (CK), alanine transaminase (ALT)/ aspartate transaminase (AST), or aldolase is a sensitive, but not specific sign of autoimmune myositis.

Table 3.12 Characteristics of rare inherited causes of muscle pain and/or weakness

Condition	Musculoskeletal features	Other features
Malignant hyperthermia (muscle sensitivity to severe physical or metabolic stress)	Acute rigidity and subsequent rhabdomyolysis	Acute—fever. Hyperkalaemia
McArdle's disease (myophosphorylase deficiency)	Painful (temporary) muscle contractures triggered by exercise	Autosomal recessive. Genotypic and phenotypic heterogeneity
Tauri's disease (phosphofructokinase deficiency)	Similar to McArdle's	Haemolytic anaemia (reticulocytosis)
Von Gierke's disease (glucose 6 phosphatase deficiency)	Skeletal myopathy	Hepatomegaly. Growth retardation. Hypoglycaemia. Lactic acidosis
Pompe's disease (acid maltase deficiency)	Severe skeletal muscle weakness and cardiomyopathy	Death in first year
Cori–Forbes disease (debrancher enzyme deficiency)	Variation from severe childhood myopathic to symptomless adult forms	
Mitochondrial myopathies	Severely limited exercise capacity	Dyspnoea. Lactic acidosis

Imaging investigations: radiographs
- A positive ANA is found in association with many autoimmune connective tissue diseases and some JIA subsets. ANA (speckled) is positive in 60–70% of children with polymyositis and dermatomyositis.
- Additional initial investigations in those suspected of having myopathic pains include bone biochemistry and thyroid function tests (TFTs).
- Seek specialist paediatric radiologist opinion.
- Proper X-ray beam coning, high-speed intensifying screens, gonadal shielding, and digital radiography all reduce radiation dose.
- Soft tissue swelling and joint-space widening are important, but non-specific, signs of early arthritis in young children.
- The most easily recognized sign of early polyarthritis in an older child will be peri-articular osteopenia.
- At joints also look for joint space narrowing, erosions, growth abnormalities, subluxation, and ankylosis. All occur at multiple joints in systemic JIA and polyarticular JIA.

- In children with abnormalities in stature or skeletal morphology look for diffuse, but subtle changes in bone quality and epiphyses.
- Destruction of bone cortex at sites of pain in patients with myalgias, arthralgias, or polyarthritis may suggest malignancy.

Imaging investigations: US, skeletal MR, and bone scan

- The role of US is expanding. It is non-invasive, non-ionizing, can be done at the bedside, and is generally accepted well by children.
- With US, cartilagenous forms of bones can be visualized. This is especially advantageous in the hip, where femoral head position and abnormal movement can be seen in young children.
- US is very useful for identifying effusions, notably in the hip, and for discriminating effusion from synovial thickening.
- Bone scan provides critical information in musculoskeletal pain when radiographs can be unrevealing. Although of less use when joints are involved, bone scan should be considered when pain originates in bone or infection is a possibility.
- CT is a reliable way of documenting sacroiliac disease in children suspected of having ERA / SpA.
- MR has become the imaging modality of choice, especially when the diagnosis of JIA is not straightforward. It is more sensitive than radiographs for detecting soft-tissue and most bone lesions.
- MR is more sensitive than radiographs for detecting changes in joints associated with chronic arthritis. MR should provide diagnostic information if there is doubt about the presence of arthritis in a joint after clinical examination and radiographs.
- The discrimination of synovitis and enthesitis by MR may have implications for the diagnosis of ERA (SpA) compared with JIA.

Investigations of muscle pains

- EMG patterns of abnormality occur in muscular dystrophy, myasthenia gravis, and autoimmune myositis, but each is not specific.
- Evidence of an inflammatory myopathy on EMG is not specific to juvenile dermatomyositis and may be due to a myositis-component of another autoimmune connective tissue disease.
- MR can confirm myositis and reveal potential sites of biopsy in what can be a patchy process.

Table 3.13 Useful tests in investigating suspected systemic JIA

In all patients:	Full blood count (FBC), ESR, CRP
	Renal and liver biochemistry, serum albumin
	Serum immunoglobulins
	Clotting screen
	Blood cultures
	Electrocardiogram (ECG), CXR, abdominal/pelvic US
	ANA
	Bone marrow aspiration and biopsy
	Ocular slit-lamp examination
	Joint aspirate (single joint)
	Radiographs of selected affected joints
In selected patients:	Muscle enzymes (CK, ALT/AST, and aldolase)
	RF
	Isotope bone/gallium scan
	Upper GI series/small bowel follow-through
	Tissue biopsies
	Viral serology—parvovirus, adenovirus, others
	Echocardiogram
	ASO/antihyaluronidase antibodies
	Urinary homovanillic/vanillylmandelic acid
	Serum IgD

The spectrum of non-musculoskeletal disorders in rheumatic disease

Skin disorders and rheumatic disease

The importance of examining the skin

- The skin is the most accessible organ to examine.
- Pattern recognition of skin symptoms and lesions is valuable in aiding diagnosis (e.g. acute or chronic **sarcoid**) and prognosis of rheumatic diseases (e.g. nodules and vasculitis in **RA**).
- Musculoskeletal abnormalities may be mirrored by skin abnormalities (e.g. **joint hypermobility** and skin laxity with bruising, scarring, and striae).
- Some **anti-rheumatic drugs** produce highly specific and potentially serious cutaneous reactions that require prompt diagnosis and management.
- A number of rarer conditions associated with musculoskeletal symptoms can manifest primarily with skin pathology (🕮 Chapter 18, p 489).

Regional abnormalities

The scalp

Scalp symptoms and lesions may be subtle:

- Scalp tenderness and the description of scalp 'lumps' (due to atypical aneurysms) are recognized in giant cell arteritis.
- C2 root/occipital neuropathy (e.g. in RA) or shingles may be associated with dysaesthesia over the scalp and occipital neuralgia.
- Alopecia may be localized (areata) or diffuse [e.g. in systemic lupus erythematosus (**SLE**) or iron deficiency]. Scarring alopecia is typical of discoid lupus.
- Scalp **psoriasis** may be patchy and discrete.

Face and ears

Face and ears are in sun-exposed areas. Consider ultraviolet (UV) skin sensitivity.

- A variety of patterns of SLE-associated, UV-sensitive rashes may occur. The rash is often diffuse. Shaded areas (e.g. nasolabial folds) may not be affected (🕮 Chapter 10, p 321).
- As in SLE, **rosacea** can present with an erythematous facial rash. Distinction is sometimes difficult without biopsy.
- Peri-orbital oedema occurs in dermatomyositis, angioedema (which may be a presenting feature of SLE), and in nephrotic syndrome.
- Heliotrope rash refers to violaceous oedema/erythema of the eyelids in **dermatomyositis** (🕮 Chapter 14, p 385).
- The cutaneous infiltration of chronic sarcoid (**lupus pernio**) (🕮 Chapter 18, p 489) across the nose and cheeks may be overt (papular) but also may be quite subtle (Plate 21).
- Saddle nose deformity/nasal cartilage destruction has a number of causes: **Wegener's granulomatosis** (WG) (🕮 Chapter 15, p 405), **relapsing polychondritis** (🕮 Chapter 18, p 489), hereditary connective tissue disease (e.g. **Stickler's syndrome** 🕮 Chapter 16, p 431), and lethal midline granuloma. Nasal septal perforation can also occur in the setting of cocaine use.
- Oral aphthous ulcers are common. Oral ulceration may follow disease activity (e.g. in SLE). Ulcers in **reactive arthritis** are typically painless. Oral aphthous ulcers are frequently idiopathic, and not associated with systemic disease.

- Large punched-out and numerous tongue and buccal ulcers that scar are a hallmark of **Behçet's** disease (📖 Chapter 18, p 489). They may remain for several weeks.
- Strawberry erythema of the tongue and lips should not be missed in children. It may denote self-limiting streptococcal infections but may also herald the desquamating palmar (and sole) rash of **Kawasaki disease** (📖 Chapter 14, p 385).
- Lacy white streaks on the buccal mucosa suggest **lichen planus**.
- The pinna is a common site for gouty tophi and discoid lupus. Relapsing polychondritis typically causes softening and distortion of cartilage.
- Lipid skin deposits around the eye occur in hyperlipidemia and **multicentric reticulohistiocytosis**.

Hands and nails

Hands and nails should be examined closely:

- A photosensitive eruption spares the finger webs and palms.
- Erythema on the back of the fingers may help distinguish dermatomyositis from SLE.
- In patients with **Raynaud's phenomenon** (RP), finger ulceration, finger pulp atrophy (with smooth tapering of the finger tips), induration, and tethering of the skin indicate scleroderma (📖 Chapter 13, p 363). Unlike normal skin, the skin of scleroderma does not form fine wrinkles when pinched.
- **Onycholysis**, nail-**pitting**, salmon patches, and subungual hyperkeratosis are typical of psoriasis (📖 Chapter 8, p 281).
- Subungual **splinter haemorrhages** may be associated with trauma, infective endocarditis, systemic vasculitis, or thromboangiitis obliterans.
- Nailfold capillaries can be examined with an ophthalmoscope at 40 diopters after applying a drop of oil (or surgical lubricant) to the cuticle. Enlarged (dilated) capillary loops and capillary 'dropout' suggests an underlying autoimmune connective tissue disease, particularly scleroderma.
- Nailfold vasculopathy is non-specific, and can occur in association with systemic vasculitis, dermatomyositis, and infective endocarditis.

Types of eruption

Macular rashes

Macular rashes are flat (non-palpable) areas of altered skin colour. Papules are lumps <1 cm in diameter:

- Maculopapular rashes are typical of viral infections.
- A short-lived, pinkish, maculopapular eruption occurs on the trunk and limbs in **Still's disease** (📖 Chapter 5, p 233). It is often prominent in the late afternoon, and coincides with temperature spikes. If scratched, the rash may blanch ('Köebner phenomenon').
- Erythema that enlarges to form erythematous patches with pale centres suggests **rheumatic fever** ('erythema marginatum').
- A 'bulls-eye' erythematous lesion around a tick bite may be the erythema migrans of **Lyme disease**.
- Maculopapular eruptions can occur from NSAIDs, gold, penicillamine, sulfasalazine, azathioprine hypersensitivity, and leflunomide (📖 Chapter 21, p 545).

Pustules and blisters

Blisters may be vesicles (<0.5 cm diameter) or bullae (>0.5 cm diameter):
- The most common pustular rash is due to folliculitis.
- Pustules confined to the hands and feet suggest reactive arthritis, although local forms of psoriasis may be indistinguishable. Psoriasis can also occur as 'raindrop' erythematous lesions, also known as guttate lesions.
- Generalized pustular rashes can occur in **vasculitis**, the **neutrophilic dermatoses**, intestinal bypass syndromes, **Behçet's disease**, and gonococcal bacteraemia.
- Bullous eruptions may be due to SLE and drug reactions, **pemphigus**, and **pemphigoid**.

Plaques

Plaques are slightly raised, circumscribed areas of skin, often disc shaped:
- Plaques are the hallmark of psoriasis. Skin may be scaly and flake off easily. Lesions are often red.
- **Psoriatic plaques** can occur anywhere on the skin, but typical sites are over the extensor surfaces of the joints, in the intergluteal cleft, and the umbilicus.
- Scaling may be a feature of discoid lupus; scaling tends to occur at the periphery of the lesion.

Vascular lesions

Bleeding into the skin that does not blanch is called purpura. It may sometimes be palpable. **Telangiectasia's** are dilated small vascular lesions that blanch on pressure:
- Non-palpable purpura may be due to thrombocytopenia, platelet dysfunction, trauma (± capillary/skin fragility, e.g. chronic steroid use), haemophilia, anticoagulation, and hereditary connective tissue diseases [e.g. Ehlers-Danlos syndrome (📖 Chapter 16, p 431)].
- Palpable purpura suggests vasculitis, including drug-induced (📖 Chapter 15, p 405).
- Widespread telangiectasia occurs in **limited cutaneous scleroderma** (📖 Chapter 13, p 363), hereditary haemorrhagic telangiectasia, and dermatomyositis.

Ulcers and ulcerating rashes

Ulcers are defined as a loss or defect of dermis and epidermis produced by sloughing of necrotic tissue:
- Cutaneous ulceration may have more than one cause in autoimmune diseases. For example, vasculitis, venous stasis in an immobile patient, and ulceration over nodules or pressure points may all contribute to the same set of lesions. Trauma may be an important cause of cutaneous ulcers in a patient who is already predisposed towards forming these lesions.
- An indurated, expanding, plum-coloured plaque or acneiform pustule that then ulcerates suggests **pyoderma gangrenosum** (📖 Chapter 18, p 489). The ulcer has irregular, bluish margins.
- Neurotropic ulcers are a classic sequelae of diabetes, but they can also occur in association with mononeuritis multiplex (from vasculitis) and other rheumatic diseases.
- Severe widespread ulceration developing rapidly in a child may suggest dermatomyositis.

- Vasculitic ulcers in the context of **livedo reticularis** and antibodies to phospholipids (e.g. cardiolipin) may denote **antiphospholipid syndrome** (APS) (📖 Chapter 11, p 343).

Textural abnormalities

Abnormalities of the texture of the skin may be difficult to discern. Atrophy and thinning, laxity, thickening, and induration may all be associated with disease:

- Generalized skin atrophy and thinning is an age-related process, but this can be accelerated by chronic steroid use; hereditary diseases of connective tissue should also be considered.
- Skin laxity can best be demonstrated over elbow and knee extensor surfaces. Generalized laxity of connective tissue may result in varicose veins and internal organ prolapse.
- True acral and digital puffiness in a patient with Raynaud's is suggestive of scleroderma. Skin thickening has a variety of causes (see below). Scleroderma and scleroderma-like skin may be localized, limited, or diffuse—this distinction is important (Table 4.1).

Diagnostic issues in patients with skin thickening

- **Raynaud's phenomenon** (RP) invariably precedes the onset of systemic sclerosis (scleroderma), but is not a characteristic of morphea or linear scleroderma.
- In patients with RP, abnormal nailfold capillaries on capillaroscopy may indicate the presence of scleroderma or 'pre-scleroderma' (Plate 8).
- The specificities of autoantibodies are often predictive of the scleroderma subtype. In patients with RP, ANA has predictive value for identifying patients who may progress to scleroderma; anti-centromere antibody can predict progression to limited cutaneous scleroderma; anti-topoisomerase I (SCL-70) and anti-RNA polymerase antibodies are linked with progression to **diffuse cutaneous scleroderma**.
- Patients with diffuse cutaneous scleroderma have a preponderance of visceral organ involvement in the first 5 years of disease; screening investigations are usually useful, and should include pulmonary function tests, an echocardiogram, and a high-resolution CT of the chest to screen for pulmonary hypertension and pulmonary fibrosis.
- **Eosinophilic fasciitis** (📖 Chapter 13, p 363) may occur as a paraneoplastic syndrome, and is associated with haematological malignancies.
- Linear scleroderma in children can produce lifelong deformities because limbs to develop correct length and bulk.
- Scleroderma-like syndromes may occur secondarily to exposure to some industrial chemicals: vinyl chloride, chlorinated organic solvents, and silicon and epoxy resins.

Table 4.1 Pattern recognition in patients with skin thickening

Classification	Skin features
Morphea may be localized (guttate) or generalized	Early small skin areas affected (itchy). Progression to hidebound skin, typically on trunk (areola spared) and legs. Lesions become waxy and hypo/hyper-pigmented guttate (small <10 mm) Papules usually on neck and anterior chest
Linear scleroderma	Linear band-like pattern often in dermatomal distribution. Atrophy of muscles is common. Fixed joint deformities and growth abnormalities can occur
'Coup de sabre'	Linear scleroderma on the face/scalp can be depressed; ivory in appearance. Hemi-atrophy can occur
Systemic sclerosis (early)	Early morning 'puffiness' in hands and feet, facial 'tightness'. Non-pitting oedema of intact dermal and epidermal appendages. High degree of suspicion needed
Systemic sclerosis (classic)	Firm, taut, hidebound skin proximal to MCP joints. Skin may be coarse, pigmented, and dry. Epidermal thinning, loss of hair, and sweating can occur. Telangiectasia and skin calcinosis become obvious. Skin creases disappear. Such change proximal to elbows or knees in the limbs or below the clavicles (in those with face and neck involvement) classifies disease as diffuse as opposed to limited systemic sclerosis
Systemic sclerosis (late)	2–15 years after onset of classical phase, skin softens, but pigmentation changes remain. Skin becomes atrophic and can ulcerate
Eosinophilic fasciitis	*Phases:* early—pitting oedema; progressive—*peau d'orange*; late—induration ('woody feel') with venous guttering when limb elevated. Arms and legs most commonly affected, but fingers mainly spared. Synovitis and low-grade myositis may occur. Eosinophilia is usually striking, but not always present
Lipodermato-sclerosis	Fibrotic induration of lower legs associated with venous stasis ('champagne-bottle legs')
Diabetes	Waxy thickening of extremities. Insidious progression. Joints of the hands become stiff, the tendons can thicken. Skin changes proximal to wrist and on the face very unlikely, but stiffening of elbow and shoulder joints not uncommon
Dependent lymphoedema	Feet/ankles/lower legs. Often pitting. Chronic presence may give hyperkeratosis. Main causes: R- or L-sided heart failure, renal failure, nephrotic syndrome, and low-protein states

Skin vasculitis in adults

Background

There are a variety of ways in which systemic vasculitis may present, including fever of unknown origin, organ infarction, gastrointestinal bleeding, and high acute phase reactants in a generally unwell patient. However, a vasculitic skin rash is one of the most common presenting features of systemic vasculitis, and can be an important diagnostic clue (📖 Chapter 15, p 405).

When to consider a diagnosis of vasculitis

- Primary systemic vasculitis is rare. Overall, the annual incidence is about 40 per million.
- Cutaneous vasculitis, however, is not rare; it can follow viral or bacterial illness, can be triggered by drugs, and is associated with malignancy. Biopsy generally demonstrates degranulation of neutrophils ('leucocytoclasis') and evidence of vessel destruction. The list of causes is long (Table 4.2); however, in about 50% of cases no cause may be found.
- Cutaneous vasculitis may also occur in association with another autoimmune disease not normally characterized by vasculitis, such as **SLE, RA, and Sjögren's syndrome**.

Important considerations

The following important points of clinical assessment should be followed in patients with possible vasculitic rashes:

- Determine whether the patient has been taking a new drug. Many antibiotics, including penicillins, sulfonamindes, and cephalosporins, commonly cause cutaneous vasculitis.
- Evaluate the patient for evidence of chronic infection; Hepatitis B, Hepatitis C, and HIV all are worth considering. Endocarditis should also be considered (e.g. the elderly, or patients who use intravenous drugs).
- Look for evidence of a primary autoimmune disorder that may be associated with cutaneous vasculitis. Inflammatory bowel disease, for example, can occasionally cause a leucocytoclastic vasculitis in addition to oral ulcerations and pyoderma gangrenosum. Because SLE is common, it may be worthwhile to check ANA and serum complements as well.
- Look for evidence of cryoglobulinaemic vasculitis. Serum cryoglobulins tests are often mishandled, leading to false-negative results, primarily because the sample needs to be kept warm (usually by simply holding in the closed palm of the hand) and should be taken straight to the laboratory.
- Rheumatoid factor is detected in 80% of patients with **mixed essential cryoglobulinaemia**, and may be a better screening test.
- Age-appropriate screening for malignancy should be performed. Serum and urine electrophoresis with immunofixation may be of value.
- Urinalysis may demonstrate 'active sediment'; evidence of **haematuria, proteinuria**, or red blood cell casts may be the first clue that a patient has a systemic vasculitis.

Systemic vasculitis

- Untreated primary systemic vasculitis is generally characterized by inflammation; many patients will complain of B-type symptoms, including fevers, weight loss, and night sweats. Patients with idiopathic cutaneous vasculitis, on the other hand, often feel quite well
- The extra-cutaneous signs and symptoms may provide clues to the correct diagnosis:
  - *Henoch–Schönlein purpura (HSP):* colicky abdominal pain
  - *Churg–Strauss syndrome:* adult-onset asthma, eosinophilia
  - *Wegener's granulomatosis:* chronic sinusitis, pneumonitis
  - *Microscopic polyangiitis:* haemoptysis, red blood cell casts
- **Mononeuritis multiplex,** which presents as a 'wrist drop' or 'foot drop', is suggestive of systemic vasculitis in a non-diabetic patient.

Table 4.2 Precipitants and associations of hypersensitivity (allergic) small vessel vasculitis

Drugs	Sulfonamides and penicillins, for example—there are many
Infections	Hepatitis B, hepatitis C, HIV
	β-haemolytic streptococcus
Foreign protein	E.g. serum sickness
Autoimmune disease	Rheumatoid arthritis
	Sjögren's syndrome (anti-Ro positive)
	Systemic lupus
Inflammatory diseases	Sarcoid
	Crohn's disease, ulcerative colitis
	Chronic active hepatitis
Malignancy	Myelo- and lymphoproliferative disorders
	Solid tumours
Cryoglobulinaemia	

Investigations

Skin biopsy

- Discuss the case with the histopathologist.
- Punch biopsy is simple, and may be sufficient to yield a diagnosis. Elliptical biopsy provides more tissue, and may increase yield.
- Use a needle to lift the skin sample—this avoids forceps-induced damage.
- Biopsy should extend to the subcutaneous fat, which generally includes the arterioles and venules affected by primary systemic vasculitis. Idiopathic leucocytoclastic vasculitis affects the capillaries but generally spares the arterioles and venules.

- Biopsy should be sent for routine histology and for direct immunofluorescence, which may yield important clues regarding the underlying cause:
  - *IgA:* HSP;
  - *IgM, C3:* cryoglobulinaemic vasculitis;
  - IgG, IgM, IgA, C3: SLE;
  - minimal immunoreactant staining: ANCA-associated vasculitis.
- Samples for immunofluorescence should be snap frozen in liquid N_2 or dry ice or transported immediately to the laboratory. Immunofluorescence cannot be performed on samples that have been treated with formalin.

See Table 4.3 for a list of laboratory investigations to be carried out in patients with suspected vasculitis.

Table 4.3 Laboratory investigations in patients with suspected vasculitis

Haematology	FBC, ESR
Biochemistry	Electrolytes, urea, creatinine
	Liver function enzymes, serum ACE
	CRP
	Serum and urine protein electrophoresis
	Urine microscopy for red cell casts
Microbiology	Blood cultures
	Hepatitis B and C serology. Consider HIV
	Streptococcal antibodies
Immunology	Immunoglobulins, cryoglobulins, complement
	ANA, ENAs, rheumatoid factor
	ANCA

Skin vasculitis in children and adolescents

Epidemiology

- Classification of childhood vasculitis is difficult. A system that has clinical utility is shown in Table 4.4.
- Statistically, the most common form of vasculitis is **HSP**, followed by **hypersensitivity angiitis**.
- **Kawasaki disease** (KD) affects primarily children under 5 years old.
- **Wegener's granulomatosis** is rare. As in adults, it may be characterized by a limited localized form involving the respiratory tract. Subglottic stenosis, nasal septum disease, and respiratory infections may all have occurred.
- Testicular pain is a rare, although fairly specific feature for **polyarteritis nodosa**. This can also occur with Wegener's granulomatosis.
- Abdominal pain is not specific. Gut bleeding can occur in HSP and **juvenile dermatomyositis** especially.
- Vasculitis can occur in association with **Familial Mediterranean Fever**.
- All of the systemic vasculitides may be associated with features such as fatigue, fever, gastrointestinal symptoms, lymphadenopathy, myalgias, and arthralgias.
- Drugs or infection are often identified as a precipitant of a cutaneous leucocytoclastic vasculitis. Infectious triggers have also been implicated for cutaneous polyarteritis nodosa and KD.

Examination

Characteristic examination features of the rash

- Erythematous rash with swelling progressing to desquamation of palms and soles of the feet is typical of KD.
- Lower limb and buttock palpable purpura is typical of, but not specific for, HSP and hypersensitivity angiitis.
- Skin nodules are not specific but are common in cutaneous polyarteritis and frequently occur in hypersensitivity vasculitis. A nodular, painful rash on the medial sides of the feet is frequent in cutaneous polyarteritis.
- Extensive necrotic and ulcerative rash with notable muscle pains suggests dermatomyositis. Peri-ungual erythema and both eyelid and nail bed **telangiectasia** are typical.
- **Livedo reticularis** is a feature of cutaneous polyarteritis nodosa (often with painful skin nodules), but also occurs with SLE and the antiphospholipid syndrome (📖 Chapter 10, p 321 and 📖 Chapter 11, p 343, respectively).

Other typical or specific examination features

- Bilateral conjunctival injection, lip/oral/buccal inflammation, and acute non-purulent cervical lymphadenopathy are typical features of KD.
- The incidence of cardiovascular manifestations is 35% in KD. Murmurs, gallop rhythm, and coronary artery aneurysms (30%) can occur.

- Pulselessness may suggest a large vessel vasculitis.
- Severe oral aphthous ulceration raises the possibility of **Behçet's disease** syndrome. It is rare, but does occur in children.

Table 4.4 A classification of childhood vasculitis

Polyarteritis	Macroscopic
	Microscopic
Kawasaki disease (mucocutaneous lymph node syndrome)	
Granulomatous vasculitis	Wegener's granulomatosis
	Churg–Strauss vasculitis
Leucocytoclastic vasculitis	Henoch–Schönlein purpura
	Hypersensitivity angiitis
Cutaneous polyarteritis	
Vasculitis and autoimmune connective tissue disease	SLE
	JIA
	Mixed connective tissue disease
	Dermatomyositis
	Scleroderma
Large vessel vasculitis	Giant cell arteritis
	Takayasu's disease
Miscellaneous vasculitides	

Investigations

- Leucocytosis, thrombocytosis, anaemia, and an acute phase response are typical in all forms of systemic vasculitis and are not specific.
- ECG and echocardiography are essential in suspected KD.
- Glomerulonephritis is not specific and should be ruled out in all cases (urinalysis, urine microscopy, spot urine protein/creatinine ratio). In patients with an active sediment, kidney biopsy can be valuable to confirm the diagnosis.
- ANCA is not specific, but C-ANCA with antibodies to proteinase-3 in appropriate patients is highly suspicious for Wegener's granulomatosis.
- Biopsy of the skin rash is a key investigation in all patients.
- Impaired renal function with nephrotic range proteinuria is an indication for renal biopsy in patients with suspected HSP.
- Investigate of suspected polyarteritis nodosa might include mesenteric and renal angiography looking for aneurysmal changes.

Cardiac manifestations

Subclinical cardiac involvement is found in many of the rheumatic diseases, and it is not uncommon for a cardiac abnormality to be discovered incidentally. As our ability to treat the underlying rheumatic diseases improves, our ability to identify and to treat the cardiac complications of these diseases becomes increasingly important.

Pericardium

- **Pericardial effusion** is not uncommon, and has been reported in association with a large number of rheumatic diseases, including scleroderma, Sjögren's, polymyositis, mixed connective tissue disease, the spondyloarthropathies, and the systemic vasculitides.
- In the majority of cases, these effusions are discovered incidentally. These effusions are often small, clinically asymptomatic, and require no specific therapy.
- Pericardial effusions can also occur in the setting of non-rheumatic illness. When a patient with a known rheumatic disease presents with a symptomatic effusion, it is important to consider other possible explanations, such as infection (e.g. TB, viral), malignancy, and other unrelated conditions (uraemia, hypothyroidism).
- Pericardial effusions are a common manifestation of SLE, largely due to immune complex deposition into the pericardium. These effusions can be serous, serosanguinous, or haemorrhagic. Analysis of the pericardial fluid generally demonstrates evidence of complement, immune complexes, and leucocytes, consistent with an active inflammatory state.
- Although pericardial effusions are common with SLE, they are generally trivial. **Cardiac tamponade** is found in less than 1% of patients with SLE. Since the effusion tends to reflect the overall disease state, generally treatment of the underlying disease is adequate to resolve the effusion. Rarely, therapeutic pericardiocentesis may be required.
- Pericardial effusions are found in up to 30% of patients with RA, although only a small number of these patients will present with pericarditis or evidence of tamponade. Pericardial effusions are more common in RF-positive patients with a history of rheumatoid nodules. Chronic pericardial effusions can become superinfected, and in rare cases lead to a constrictive pericarditis.
- For both groups of patients, the presence of a symptomatic pericardial effusion is associated with increased mortality. In one study of patients with SLE who presented with cardiac tamponade, the 5-year survival was only 46%.

Myocardium

- **Myocarditis** is a relatively uncommon manifestation of rheumatic disease. Myocarditis can be found among patients with active SLE and RA, although it generally does not lead to clinically significant dysfunction.
- Cardiomyopathy among patients with RA and SLE is more likely to be due to premature coronary artery disease, followed by the development of ischaemic heart disease.
- Although uncommon, the possibility of hydroxychloroquine-induced cardiomyopathy should be considered in a patient who develops congestive heart failure in the absence of coronary artery disease. This diagnosis can be confirmed with myocardial biopsy, and often responds to drug cessation.
- The Churg–Strauss syndrome can lead to an acute eosinophilic myocarditis that can be life-threatening if not treated promptly.
- One-third of patients with Wegener's granulomatosis may have cardiac dysfunction as a consequence of the underlying vasculitis. The majority of these patients will have wall motion abnormalities on echocardiography, but valvulitis and ventricular **aneurysm** have also been reported. The majority of these lesions will be asymptomatic, but the 5-year survival rate for patients with cardiac lesions attributable to Wegener's granulomatosis is 57%.

Valvular disease

- **Aortic regurgitation** is an important potential consequence of aortitis, which can occur with any of the large-vessel vasculitides (including Takayasu's arteritis, giant cell arteritis, and Behçet's disease). In these cases, aortitis leads to aneurysm formation, which creates valvular incompetence.
- Aortic regurgitation can also occur as a consequence of AS. Unlike the vasculitides, AS cause's inflammation at the aortic root, this leads to dense scarring of the aortic valves. Although the mechanism is unique to this disease, it should be monitored and treated like any form of aortic insufficiency.
- Mitral regurgitation and **mitral valve prolapse** (MVP) are common manifestations of SLE, particularly among patients who have antiphospholipid antibodies. MVP may also be a feature of Joint Hypermobility Syndrome/Ehlers–Danlos Syndrome.
- A more serious valvulitis can occur in association with SLE. In the process of healing, the valves become scarred and calcified, a process that can eventually lead to clinically significant valvular disease.
- **Libman–Sacks endocarditis** is a classic manifestation of SLE. In this disease, vegetations form from immune complexes, mononuclear cells, and fibrin, which attach to the valves. Although not infectious, these vegetations can embolize
- Haemodynamically insignificant valve lesions have also been reported in association with RA, mixed connective tissue disease (MCTD), scleroderma, and Sjögren's.

Coronary artery disease

- Surprisingly, the primary vasculitides rarely lead to coronary artery inflammation, although coronary artery vasculitis has been reported in association with polyarteritis nodosa and the ANCA-associated vasculitides.
- The antiphospholipid syndrome is associated with a substantial increased risk of myocardial infarction, even in the absence of true coronary artery disease.
- Both RA and SLE are strongly associated with **coronary artery disease**. This may be the result of systemic inflammation or a response to chronic immunosuppression. Regardless, patients with these diagnoses should undergo early cardiac evaluation to address modifiable risk factors for coronary artery disease.
- Accelerated atherosclerosis may be an important consequence of glucocorticoid exposure. Even chronic low dose prednisone may place some patients at increased risk of cardiovascular disease.

Conduction abnormalities

- Clinically insignificant **dysrhythmias** and conduction defects are common among patients with inflammatory myopathies (dermatomyositis, polymyositis) and scleroderma.
- Clinically significant abnormalities (including heart block) can be seen in patients with spondyloarthropathies as a result of the same scaring process that leads to the valvular abnormalities noted above.

Pulmonary manifestations

Pleura

- An exudative (see below) **pleural effusion** is found in up to 50% of patients with SLE. These effusions can be unilateral or bilateral, and frequently are found in association with a pericardial effusion.
- Pleural disease is also a common manifestation of RA, which is associated with both pleural effusions and pleural thickening. These effusions are generally asymptomatic, and are found in the setting of active disease.
- Asymptomatic pleural effusions can also be found in 10–30% of patients with ANCA-associated vasculitis.
- Pleural effusions are classified as transudates, typically arising as a consequence of left ventricular, renal and hepatic failure, and SLE (📖 Chapter 10, p 321), or exudates, usually due to infection, malignancy or pulmonary embolism.
- By the 'Light' criteria (with a 75–80% sensitivity) a transudate is defined as:
  - Clear;
  - specific gravity <1.012;
  - fluid protein <2 g/dL;
  - fluid:serum protein ratio <0.5;
  - fluid:serum LDH ratio <2/3rd;
  - cholesterol <45 g/dL.
- In the same criteria an exudate is defined as:
  - Cloudy;
  - specific gravity >1.020;
  - fluid protein >2.9 g/dL;
  - fluid:serum protein ratio > 0.5;
  - fluid:serum LDH >2/3rd;
  - cholesterol >45g/dL.
- If an exudate is identified fluid should be examined for:
  - *amylase:* in oesophageal rupture, pancreatitis
  - *glucose:* decreased in infection, malignancy and RA
  - *pH:* low in empyema
  - Gram stain
  - Polymerase chain reaction (PCR) for tuberculosis.

Pulmonary nodules/masses

- Both Wegener's granulomatosis and sarcoidosis are often diagnosed incidentally, after the discovery of lung masses. Sarcoidosis is associated with **hilar lymphadenopathy**, while Wegener's granulomatosis generally presents with multiple peripheral **pulmonary nodules** that can be mistaken for lung cancer.
- In a patient with a known rheumatic disease who presents with a lung mass, it is always important to consider the possibility of malignancy. Lung cancer risk is increased among patients with RA and scleroderma, and many rheumatic diseases are associated with an increased risk of lymphoma.
- Wegener's granulomatosis (and less commonly, AS and RA) can lead to **cavitating apical lesions** that can be mistaken for TB.

Interstitial lung disease

- **Pulmonary fibrosis** (with a predilection for the lung bases and periphery) is a common feature of both scleroderma and the inflammatory myopathies.
- Pulmonary fibrosis is found in 20–65% of patients with scleroderma. Radiographically, the lesions take on the appearance of ground glass infiltrates that gradually lead to honeycombing and fibrosis.
- Pulmonary fibrosis may be the initial manifestation of an inflammatory myopathy, and pulmonary symptoms may precede clinical evidence of muscle involvement.
- RA is also associated with an interstitial lung disease, although this has become increasingly rare. It may be a side effect of MTX.
- Apical fibrosis can be found in 1% of patients with ankylosing spondylitis. Apical fibrosis is also an uncommon feature of rheumatoid lung.
- Pulmonary fibrosis can also occur as the long-term sequelae of pulmonary capillaritis, which may occur in patients with Wegener's granulomatosis and microscopic polyangiitis.

Vasculature

- **Haemoptysis** can be the result of pulmonary capillaritis, which can be found in association with the so-called 'pulmonary renal syndromes': SLE, ANCA-associated vasculitis (predominantly microscopic polyangiitis), and anti-glomerular basement membrane (GBM) syndrome.
- Cryoglobulinaemic vasculitis can also cause pulmonary capillaritis, although this is not one of its more common manifestations.
- **Pulmonary artery hypertension** (PAH) is most commonly associated with limited cutaneous scleroderma. Isolated PAH can also be seen with diffuse cutaneous scleroderma, although it generally appears as a consequence of pulmonary fibrosis.
- Scleroderma causes PAH by narrowing of the small arteries and arterioles that gradually leads to obliteration of the pulmonary vascular bed.
- RA, SLE, inflammatory myopathy, mixed connective tissue disease, and Sjögren's syndrome can also be associated with PAH, but it is considered an uncommon feature of these diseases.

Airways

- RA can lead to **laryngeal obstruction** when it affects the cricoarytenoid joints. Such patients will present with hoarseness or odynophagia.
- Subglottic stenosis is a common feature of Wegener's granulomatosis, which can lead to significant **stridor**.
- Uncontrolled relapsing polychondritis can cause tracheomalacia, which is a significant cause of morbidity and mortality for this disease.

Renal manifestations

Evaluation of renal failure: overview

- The kidneys are a key component to the evaluation and management of the rheumatic diseases. Many conditions affect the kidneys directly, and a careful examination may yield important clues to the correct diagnosis. For other patients, the kidneys must be considered because many treatments have renal toxicity or are renal cleared.
- In terms of time course, renal failure is frequently divided into 'acute renal failure' and 'chronic renal failure.' The GFR value classifies renal function as stage 1 to 5: normal (>90), mild (60–89), moderate (30–59), severe (15–29), and severe failure (<15) in units of mL/min/1.73m^2.
- Acute renal failure (ARF) is often divided by the source of the injury. Acute renal failure due to renal hypoperfusion is called 'pre-renal'; acute renal failure due to urinary tract obstruction is called 'post-renal'.
- Intrinsic renal failure (i.e. renal failure due to direct involvement of the renal parenchyma) should be evaluated with a careful examination of the urine. The presence of red blood cells and protein, or red blood cell casts (i.e. 'active sediment') implies **glomerulonephritis**, which can occur with vasculitis and SLE.

Pre-renal azotaemia

- Hypovolaemia is an important cause of pre-renal ARF. Dehydration and anaemia can both lead to pre-renal azotaemia.
- Renal hypoperfusion can also be caused by diminished blood flow to the kidneys. Diseases involving the renal artery (such as renal artery stenosis, polyarteritis nodosa affecting the renal artery, or renal artery thrombosis) may cause pre-renal azotaemia. If long-standing, this leads to intrinsic renal failure.
- Conditions associated with low cardiac output (including shock, congestive heart failure, myocarditis, tamponade, and pulmonary arterial hypertension) may all predispose the patient to pre-renal ARF.
- **Hyperviscosity**, which is seen with type I (monoclonal) cryoglobulinaemia, is a rare cause of pre-renal azotaemia.
- All of these conditions may be exacerbated by drugs that decrease renal perfusion, including NSAIDs and ACE-inhibitors.
- With pre-renal azotaemia, the fractional excretion of sodium [FENa = (UNa × PCr)/(PNa × UCr)] is less than 1.0; this test is not reliable in patients treated with diuretics.

Post-renal azotaemia

- Nephrolithiasis is not a common cause of post-renal azotemia, but should be considered in a patient with gout. 5–10% of renal calculi in the United States are caused by uric acid; this is particularly common among patients with gout who have been treated with uricosuric agents (e.g. probenecid).

- Sarcoidosis can cause hypercalcaemia and hypercalcuria, which in turn can lead to nephrolithiasis and nephrocalcinosis, both of which can rarely cause post-renal azotaemia.
- Methotrexate and trimethoprim/sulphamethoxazole can cause crystalluria and renal obstruction.
- Ultrasound is a useful modality to evaluate both for the presence of obstruction leading to hydronephrosis and renal calculi.

Intrinsic renal failure—'active sediment'

- The **nephritic syndromes** are an important cause of rapidly progressive renal failure among patients with rheumatic diseases, particularly vasculitis and SLE.
- The presence of haematuria, proteinuria, and red blood cell casts strongly suggests the presence of glomerulonephritis.
- A renal biopsy is crucial to determining the underlying diagnosis and the severity/chronicity of the disease.
- Nephritic syndromes can be divided into 'focal proliferative' and 'diffuse proliferative' based on histology.
- Causes of focal proliferative glomerulonephritis include SLE, Henoch–Schönlein purpura (HSP), and other forms of small vessel vasculitis.
- Diffuse proliferative glomerulonephritis is caused by cryoglobulinaemia, SLE, anti-glomerular basement membrane (GBM) disease (**Goodpasture's syndrome**), and small-vessel vasculitis (including Wegener's granulomatosis, microscopic polyangiitis, and renal-limited vasculitis).
- Direct immunofluorescence can also provide valuable information regarding the correct diagnosis. SLE biopsy demonstrates multiple immunoreactants ('full house' staining pattern). IgA deposition implies Henoch-Schönlein purpura. Cryoglobulinaemic vasculitis leads to IgG and C3 deposition. Sparse or absent immunoreactants on biopsy is sometimes called 'pauci-immune', and implies an ANCA-associated vasculitis.

Intrinsic renal failure—'bland sediment'

- A bland sediment refers to a urine sample that is acellular; transparent hyaline casts may be seen. Remember that bland sediment is also seen in pre-renal and post-renal azotaemia.
- **Acute tubular necrosis** (ATN) or acute kidney injury (AKI) is used to describe causes of acute, intrinsic renal failure associated with a urine sediment that has muddy brown casts and tubular epithelial cells.
- Nephrotoxic tubular injury from drugs is a common cause of ATN in patients with rheumatic disease.
- Prolonged pre-renal azotaemia can lead to permanent kidney damage; therefore, diseases of the renal artery [including polyarteritis nodosa and renal artery thrombosis from antiphospholipid antibody syndrome (APS)] should be considered.
- **Interstitial nephritis** is most commonly seen as a drug reaction (e.g. gold, penicillamine)
- Interstitial nephritis can also be seen as a manifestation of several rheumatic diseases, including Sjögren's, SLE, sarcoidosis, and the Churg–Strauss syndrome.

- NSAIDs cause renal vasoconstriction and interstitial nephritis, both of which can eventually lead to a chronic analgesic nephropathy.
- Unlike the other forms of ANCA-associated vasculitis, the mechanism of renal failure among patients with the Churg–Strauss syndrome is an interstitial nephritis; glomerulonephritis is relatively rare with this diagnosis.
- The most common causes of secondary renal **amyloidosis** (📖 Chapter 18, p 489) are RA and Familial Mediterranean Fever. Glomerular deposits of amyloid lead to proteinuria (which can be nephrotic range) and progressive renal failure.

Scleroderma renal crisis

- Scleroderma renal crisis is a rheumatologic emergency characterized by acute renal failure and malignant hypertension (📖 Chapter 24, p 609).
- Patients with diffuse cutaneous scleroderma are at greatest risk; scleroderma renal crisis generally occurs within the first 4 years after diagnosis, but it can occur at any time. Patients who are treated with corticosteroids may be at the highest risk.
- Urinalysis generally demonstrates a bland sediment. Kidney biopsy demonstrates evidence of a thrombotic micro-angiopathy that histologically cannot be distinguished from malignant hypertensive nephrosclerosis, haemolytic-uraemic syndrome, SLE, or APS.
- The cornerstone of therapy is gradually escalating doses of ACE-inhibitors, followed by angiotensin II receptor blockers (ARB) and calcium channel blockers if adequate blood pressure control is not achieved.

Renal tubular acidosis

- **Renal tubular acidosis** (RTA) causes a non-anion gap metabolic acidosis caused by a failure of the renal tubules to maintain acid-base status (📖 Chapter 16, p 431).
- Type I RTA, caused by an inability to excrete acid, is found with Sjögren's syndrome and SLE.
- Type IV RTA is most commonly caused by hyporeninaemic hypoaldosteronism, can occur as a result of treatment with non-steroidal anti-inflammatory drugs (NSAIDs), ACE-inhibitors, and ARBs. This is commonly associated with hyperkalaemia.

Endocrine manifestations

Well-characterized musculoskeletal conditions occur in many endocrine disorders. Some are specific for certain disorders; others are non-specific, but occur with greater frequency among patients with endocrine disease. Musculoskeletal manifestations occur either as a result of metabolic disturbances or are influenced by a common link through their autoimmune pathophysiology.

Diabetes

- **Dupuytren's contracture**, **trigger finger**, **carpal tunnel syndrome**, diffuse idiopathic skeletal hyperostosis (DISH), and **adhesive capsulitis** all occur with greater frequency among patients with diabetes.
- Some form of tissue or joint hypomobility/stiffness is common among patients with diabetes (Table 4.5); in some cases, this can appear similar to scleroderma. These scleroderma-like skin changes are more prevalent among patients with type I diabetes.

Table 4.5 Patterns of joint and tissue hypomobility or stiffness in diabetes by reported series. Tissue changes are thought to occur from excessive hydration (a consequence of an excessive local production of sugar alcohols)

Patient series	Major abnormalities	Associations
Diabetics overall	In about 30–40% mainly in long-standing disease: slow decrease in hand mobility; waxy skin thickening ('scleroderma-like')	Occasional lung fibrosis. Microvascular diabetic complications
Adults	55–76% prevalence of joint hypomobility in type 1/type 2 diabetes, respectively	Not associated with diabetic complications
Mature onset diabetes (mean 61 years)	Stiffening of connective tissue (assessed in hands)	Diabetic nephropathy
Children with type 1 diabetes	31% have limited joint mobility	None with glycaemic control, retinopathy, or proteinuria
Juvenile and young adult onset (age 1–24 years) diabetes	34% had skin thickening. Changes rarely proximal to MCPs and never proximal to wrists. Joint contractures in >50%, often third or fourth fingers	No flexor tendon rubs (as seen in scleroderma)

- Hand weakness may be due to **diabetic neuropathy** and may be mistaken for carpal tunnel syndrome. Neurophysiology tests help discriminate between these two diagnoses.
- Calcification of soft tissues around the shoulder occurs in approximately 20% of diabetics, and is associated with variable symptoms and disability.
- **Diabetic amyotrophy** is uncommon. It presents acutely with pain, weakness, and wasting of the proximal lower limb muscles. It may be unilateral. Differential diagnosis includes myositis (📖 Chapter 14, p 385) and polymyalgia rheumatica (📖 Chapter 15, p 405). It is associated with uncontrolled hyperglycaemia. The aetiology is unknown, but it is probably a neuromyopathy.
- Though rare (1:500 diabetics), neuropathic arthritis can occur in advanced disease. Most patients are aged 40–60 years and have poor glycaemic control. Tarsal and metatarsal joints are most frequently affected (60%). The usual presentation is of swelling of the foot with no or little pain. Trauma may have occurred. Early radiographic changes can resemble OA (📖 Chapter 6, p 259).
- Asymptomatic **osteolysis** can occur at the distal metatarsals and proximal phalanges with relative joint sparing. The aetiology is unknown.
- **Osteomyelitis** is not uncommon and needs to be discriminated from cellulitis and neuropathic arthritis (Charcot's joint). A triple-phase bone scan should be helpful. Osteomyelitis is usually disclosed by prominent blood flow in the dynamic (first) phase and increased uptake of tracer by soft tissue and bone in later stages. Cellulitis is associated with minimal uptake of tracer in bone in the delayed (third) phase. Neuropathic joints display minimal first-phase abnormalities but prominent tracer uptake in the third phase.
- Diabetic muscle infarction can present as a painful muscle mass and is a result of arterial narrowing. Often mistaken for thrombophlebitis, myositis or vasculitis, this is a late complication of diabetes. Biopsy may be needed to confirm this diagnosis.
- Diabetes may be associated with a **'metabolic syndrome'** — hypertension, DM, hyperuricaemia, obesity.

Hypothyroidism

- Over 25% of patients with hypothyroidism have an arthropathy. Because this arthropathy can lead to an erosive arthritis, it can be mistaken for RA (📖 Chapter 5, p 233).
- Thyroid disease may also be autoimmune and the serum ANA positive, again often mistaken for assuming the presence of a primary rheumatic condition.
- This arthropathy commonly involves the knees and hands; in children, the hips are most likely to be affected. It is characterized by pain, stiffness, effusions, and synovial thickening due to glycosaminoglycan deposition. Calcium pyrophosphate deposition may contribute to this arthropathy (📖 Chapter 7, p 269).
- Radiographically-defined **chondrocalcinosis** is only marginally increased compared with controls (17% vs 10%). About 1/10 patients with pseudogout are hypothyroid.

- **Carpal tunnel syndrome** is common (7%). Up to 10% of patients with carpal tunnel syndrome may have hypothyroidism.
- **Hyperuricaemia** is common, but gout attacks are rare. However, screening for hypothyroidism in patients with gout is recommended. Treated hypothyroidism then requires review of the need for uric acid-lowering therapy.
- Musculoskeletal symptoms are common, and may improve with treatment of hypothyroidism.
- Consequences of hypothyroidism in children included retarded bone age, short stature, and **epiphyseal dysgenesis** with premature epiphyseal plate closure and increased probability of slipped femoral epiphyses.
- Myopathy is relatively common. About 1 in 20 cases of acquired myopathy are due to hypothyroidism. The presentation can mimic **polymyositis** with elevation of muscle enzymes, but muscle biopsy typically shows no inflammatory cell infiltrate. Improvement with thyroxine replacement is sometimes complicated by muscle cramps, but these should resolve in a few weeks.
- The combination of weakness, muscular stiffness, and an increase in muscle mass in an adult with myxoedema is termed **Hoffman's syndrome**. Muscle mass increase is sometimes striking and can take many months to resolve on treatment. The same condition occurs in children (**Kocher–Debre–Semelaigne syndrome**).
- Lymphocytic thyroiditis (Hashimoto's) is an autoimmune condition characterized by hypothyroidism and autoantibodies to thyroglobulin and thyroid microsomes. These antibodies are found in 40% of patients with primary **Sjögren's syndrome**, but only about 10% are or have been overtly hypothyroid.

Thyrotoxicosis

- Hyperthyroidism can cause a **proximal myopathy** (70%), shoulder peri-arthritis (7%), acropachy (thickening of extremities), and **osteoporosis** (◻ Chapter 16, p 431).
- Acropachy is rare (<2% of patients with thyrotoxicosis) and most often occurs in treated patients who are hypo/euthyroid. It consists of clubbing, painful soft tissue swelling of hands and feet, and periosteal new bone on the radial aspect of the second and third metacarpals. Clinically, this occurs most frequently in patients who have the opthalmopathy or dermopathy associated with autoimmune thyroid disease.
- Graves' disease is frequently associated with **fatigue** and muscular weakness. It is associated with autoimmune rheumatic and connective tissue diseases.

Hyperparathyroidism (◻ Chapter 16, p 431)

The following points refer to both primary and secondary disease:
- Musculoskeletal symptoms are the initial manifestation in up to 16% of patients with primary hyperparathyroidism.
- Hyperparathyroidism, chondrocalcinosis, and pseudogout frequently coexist. Pseudogout (CPPD) can be triggered by parathyroidectomy.
- A polyarthropathy can occur that can mimic RA. Unlike RA, synovial proliferation is absent. Radiographically, erosions have a predilection

for the ulna side of distal upper limb joints, the joint space is preserved, pericapsular calcification is often present, and reactive bone formation may be observed.

- An erosive polyarthritis favoring the large joints can occur with renal osteodystrophy in patients with chronic renal failure on dialysis. It does not appear to be related to CPPD.
- Hyperparathyroidism is associated with a specific shoulder arthropathy characterized by intra/peri-articular erosions of the humeral head. This may be sub-clinical.
- Subjective muscle weakness and fatigability are common complaints. Typically, muscle enzymes are normal and biopsy shows type II fibre atrophy; the features of an inflammatory myopathy are generally absent.
- The hallmark of radiographic changes is bone resorption: subperiosteal (typically on the radial side of second and third phalanges), intracortical, subchondral, trabecular, subligamentous, and localized (**Brown's tumours**) resorption patterns are seen. Bone **sclerosis**, **periostitis**, and **chondrocalcinosis** also occur.
- Fragility fracture is common and often precedes a diagnosis of primary hyperparathyroidism. Although significant and fast accretion of bone occurs after surgery, bone mass often remains low long term.

Acromegaly

- Over-stimulation of bone and connective tissue cells from excessive growth hormone can result in several features: bursal and cartilage hyperplasia, synovial and bony proliferation, an OA-like picture, backache, and hypermobility.
- Joint complaints usually manifest about 10 years after the onset of clinical acromegaly. Knees are frequently affected.
- Joint symptoms are not typical of an inflammatory arthritis—morning stiffness is not prominent and joint swelling is present in <50% of patients.
- **Carpal tunnel syndrome** affects >50% of patients and is frequently bilateral.
- Back and neck pain and radicular symptoms from nerve root compression or spinal stenosis are not uncommon and are related to axial bony proliferation (📖 Chapter 2, p 19 and 📖 Chapter 20, p 525).
- A painless proximal myopathy occurs infrequently.
- Radiographs characteristically show widened joint spaces (e.g. >2.5 mm in adult MCPs) and a thickened heel pad (>23 mm in men and >21.5 mm in women).
- Diagnosis relies on demonstration of a failure of growth hormone to be suppressed by a glucose tolerance test, but a lateral skull radiograph is a good screening test as 90% have enlargement of the pituitary fossa.

Gut and hepatobiliary manifestations

- Musculoskeletal features frequently occur in patients with gut or hepatobiliary disease (Table 4.6).
- Data on the frequency of rheumatological features are largely based on studies of hospital patients with clinically overt gut or biliary disease. This may lead to an underestimate of the frequency of association.
- Well established associations include:
  - toxic effects of medications (☐ Chapter 21, p 545);
  - functional gastro-intestinal disorders (e.g. in Fibromyalgia and Joint Hypermobility Syndrome);
  - **sacroiliitis**, arthritis, and enthesitis in patients with inflammatory bowel disease;
  - inflammatory arthritis in **coeliac disease** and **viral hepatitis**;
  - degenerative arthritis in **haemochromatosis** and Wilson's disease;
  - dysmotility (scleroderma).
- The frequency of enthesitis in patients with inflammatory bowel disease may be underestimated. Enthesitis may be detected at the medial/lateral humeral epicondyles, Achilles' tendon insertion, calcaneal plantar fascia origin and insertion, and the patellar tendon origin and its insertion at the tibial tubercle.
- Radiology studies in patients with inflammatory bowel disease suggest that sacroiliitis is under-recognized by clinicians.

Severity of rheumatologic manifestations

- Optimal surveillance strategies for the musculoskeletal manifestations of gut or biliary disease are not known in many instances.
- Life-threatening vasculitis may occur from chronic viral infection. Hepatitis B is associated with polyarteritis nodosa, and hepatitis C may lead to cryoglobulinaemic vasculitis.
- In most patients who develop joint inflammation or enthesitis after bacterial dysentery, the condition is self-limiting. Chronicity and severity may be linked to HLA B27. Progressive spondylitis is rare.

Gut and hepatobiliary conditions in patients with rheumatic diseases

(Tables 4.7 and 4.8)

- The most common problem among patients with RA is dyspepsia associated with gastroduodenal erosions or ulcers due to NSAIDs. Peptic lesions may be clinically silent and may present with dropping haemoglobin levels or an acute bleed.
- RA may be the most common cause of AA amyloidosis. Biopsies of the upper gastrointestinal tract will demonstrate amyloid deposits in 13% of patients. There are numerous gastrointestinal manifestations of amyloidosis, including **gastrointestinal haemorrhage, malabsorption, obstruction,** and **hepatosplenomegaly**.

Scleroderma has numerous gastrointestinal manifestations including refractory gastro-oesophageal reflux disease, gastric antral vascular ectasia ('watermelon stomach'), **oesophageal dysmotility**, bacterial over-growth syndrome, and faecal incontinence. The reflux associated

Table 4.6 Associations between gastrointestinal and rheumatic disorders

Gastrointestinal disorder	Rheumatic manifestation	Association
Enteric infection	Reactive arthritis: self-limiting in most	Arthritis in 2% who get Shigella, Salmonella, Yersinia, Campylobacter C. difficile overall but in 20% of infected who are HLA B27+
Crohn's disease	Arthritis 20%. AS 10%. Sacroiliitis in 26%	60% of spondylarthropathy patients have histological evidence of bowel inflammation. See also below
Ulcerative colitis	Arthritis 20%. AS 7%. Sacroiliitis 15%	See also above. Severity of gut and joint inflammation varies in its association but SI joint/spine inflammation does not
Whipple's disease	Migratory arthritis in >60%	T. whippelii identified in small bowel. Diarrhoea occurs in >75% ultimately
Intestinal by-pass surgery (blind loop syndrome)	Polyarticular symptoms 50% in scleroderma	Intestinal bacterial overgrowth in small bowel? Associated with joint symptoms
Coeliac disease	Arthritis is rare	?Increased intestinal permeability
Viral enteritis	Rare (<0.5%)	Most common: coxsackie or echo
Hepatitis A	Arthralgia 15%. Vasculitis rare	Causal association
Hepatitis B	Arthralgia 10–25%. PAN	Aetiological
Hepatitis C	Sialadenitis in >50%. Vasculitis (cryoglobulinaemic)	?Aetiological in Sjögren's. Hepatitis C identified in 27–96% of patients with cryoglobulinaemia
Primary biliary cirrhosis	Polyarthritis 19%. Scleroderma 18%. Sjögren's 50%	Autoimmune 'overlap'. Features may be subclinical
Chronic active hepatitis	Polyarthralgia or arthritis in 25–50%	Autoimmunity
Haemochromatosis	OA 50%	Iron storage disease
Wilson's disease	OA in 50% adults. Chondrocalcinosis	Copper storage disease

with scleroderma often requires treatment with high dose proton pump inhibitors. 'Watermelon stomach' can lead to significant acute and chronic haemorrhage. The bloating and abdominal distension caused by bacterial overgrowth may respond to cyclic courses of antibiotics.

Table 4.7 Gut and hepatobiliary manifestations in rheumatological diseases (I: General)

Disease	Abnormalities	Presentation with
Rheumatoid arthritis (📖 Chapter 5, p 233)	TMJ arthritis. Oesophageal dysmotility	Impaired mastication Dysphagia, reflux
	GI vasculitis (0.1%)	Ulcers, pain, infarction
	Portal hypertension	Splenomegaly (Felty's)
	Liver involvement (Felty's)	Enzyme abnormalities
	Hepatosplenomegaly	Palpable viscera
Systemic lupus (📖 Chapter 10, p 321)	Oesophageal dysmotility	Dysphagia, reflux
	GI vasculitis	Ulcers, pain, perforation
	Protein-losing enteropathy	Hypoalbuminaemia
	Peritonitis	Ascites (10%), serositis
	Hepatosplenomegaly (30%)	Palpable viscera
Scleroderma (📖 Chapter 13, p 363)	Oesophageal dysmotility	Heartburn/dysphagia
	Delayed gastric emptying	Aggravated reflux
	Intestinal dysmotility and fibrosis (80%)	Malabsorption, pseudo-obstruction (<1%)
	Pseudo and wide mouth diverticulae	Haemorrhage, stasis, bacterial overgrowth
Polymyositis and dermatomyositis (📖 Chapter 14, p 385)	Muscle weakness	Aspiration, dysphagia
	Disordered motility	Dysphagia, constipation
	Vasculitis (rare)	Ulcers, perforation
MCTD	Hypomotility	Dysphagia, reflux, pseudo-obstruction

Table 4.7 *(Cont'd)*

Disease	Abnormalities	Presentation with
Sjögren's syndrome (📖 Chapter 12)	Membrane dessication	Xerostomia, dysphagia
	Oesophageal webs (10%)	Dysphagia (>60%)
	Gastric infiltrates/atrophy	Masses, dyspepsia
	Pancreatitis	Pain, amylasaemia
	Hepatic dysfunction	Hepatomegaly ($\cong$ 25%)
	Hepatic cirrhosis	Primary biliary cirrhosis
Spondyloarthritis (📖 Chapter 8)	Ileocolonic inflammation	May be asymptomatic
Adult onset Still's	Hepatitis, peritonitis, hepatosplenomegaly	Pain or abnormal enzymes ($\cong$75%)
Systemic JIA (📖 Chapter 9, p 303)	Serositis	Abdominal pain
	Hepatomegaly	Abnormal enzymes
Marfan, JHS Ehlers–Danlos (📖 Chapter 16, p 431)	Defective collagen	Hypomotility, Malabsorption, visceral rupture/laxity
		Functional GI disorders

Table 4.8 Gut and hepatobiliary manifestations in rheumatic diseases [II: Vasculitis (📖 Chapter 15, p 405)]

Disease	Frequency of GI vasculitis and features
Polyarteritis nodosa	80% (mesenteric). Buccal ulcers, cholecystitis (15%), bowel infarction, perforation, appendicitis, pancreatitis, strictures, chronic wasting syndrome
Henoch–Schönlein Purpura	44–68%. Abdominal pain, melena, haematemesis, ulcers, intussusception, cholecystitis, infarction, perforation, appendicitis
Churg–Strauss Syndrome	~40%. Haemorrhage, ulceration, infarction, perforation
Behçet's disease	Buccal and intestinal ulcers, haemorrhage, perforation, pyloric stenosis, rectal ulcers
Systemic lupus erythematosus	2%. Buccal ulcers, ileocolitis, gastritis, ulceration, perforation, intussusception, volvulus (1%), pneumatosis
Kawasaki disease	Abdominal pain, intestinal obstruction, non-infective diarrhoea
Wegener's granulomatosis	<5%. Cholecystitis, appendicitis, ileocolitis, infarction
Juvenile dermatomyositis	Well recognized. Perforation, pneumatosis
MCTD	Rare. Ulceration, perforation, pancreatitis
RA and JIA	0.1%. Buccal ulcers, abdominal pain, peptic ulcers, acalculus cholecystitis, gut infarction, and perforation
Polymyositis and dermatomyositis	Very rare. Mucosal ulcers, perforation and pneumatosis
Cryoglobulinaemia	Rare. Ischaemia and infarction

- In SLE, serious gut and hepatobiliary manifestations are relatively uncommon (5%), but nausea, anorexia, vomiting, and diarrhoea are quite frequent.
- Mesenteric vasculitis is classically caused by polyarteritis nodosa, but can be seen with a variety of rheumatic illnesses, including Takayasu's arteritis, ANCA-associated vasculitis, and (rarely) with SLE. Although mesenteric angina is the symptom most strongly associated with mesenteric vasculitis, the earliest sign of intestinal ischaemia is diarrhoea.
- Henoch–Schönlein purpura is an IgA-mediated small vessel vasculitis that presents with colicky abdominal pain and purpura. Although generally mild and self-limited in children, it can occasionally cause intussusception and bowel necrosis.

Gut and hepatobiliary side-effects from drugs used in treating rheumatic and bone diseases (📖 Chapter 21, p 545)

Such side-effects are common:

- NSAIDs are a common cause of gastrointestinal distress. COX-2 inhibitors were developed to decrease the risk of **peptic ulcer disease**; most have been withdrawn from the market due to concerns regarding increased risk of cardiovascular events and those remaining may be no more effective than taking a conventional NSAID with a proton pump inhibitor.
- Glucocorticoids are also associated with **gastritis**, peptic ulcer disease, and **gastrointestinal haemorrhage**. Although the absolute increase in events is small, the combination of steroids and NSAIDs results in a synergistic increase in the risk of gastrointestinal sequelae.
- MTX may cause **stomatitis**, which may respond to supplemental folate. Nausea, emesis, and altered taste may also occur, which may respond to dose reduction. MTX can cause a **transaminitis**; it is therefore recommended that patients treated with methotrexate abstain from alcohol.
- Sulfasalazine gut and hepatobiliary side-effects are common and may occur in up to 20% of patients. The most frequent are mostly mild: indigestion, nausea, vomiting, anorexia, and abdominal pain. Gut ulceration, bloody diarrhoea, and serious liver problems are rare. In about 65% of side-effects occur in the first 3 months of treatment.
- Azathioprine (AZA) can cause nausea (15%), vomiting (10%), and abdominal pain (8%). **Diarrhoea** is rare (5%). Liver enzyme abnormalities are often mild and may remit on lowering the dose. The GI side effects can occur in patients with normal levels of thiopurine methyltransferase.
- Penicillamine causes altered taste (25% within the first 3–6 months), nausea or vomiting (18%), and stomatitis/mouth ulcers (5%). Hepatotoxicity and haemorrhagic **colitis** are rare.
- Chloroquine and hydroxychloroquine, used in mild SLE particularly, can cause non-specific GI intolerance (10%). The onset is often insidious.
- Ciclosporin causes **gingival hyperplasia**, nausea, diarrhoea, and elevation in hepatic enzymes.
- Effects of cyclophosphamide on the gut are frequent and include nausea, vomiting, diarrhoea, and stomatitis. Serious hepatotoxicity is rare.
- Chlorambucil has a low incidence of GI side-effects.
- Leflunomide can cause nausea (8–13%), diarrhoea (up to 25%), and abnormal liver enzymes. In studies to date, most rises in transaminases have been mild (<two-fold) and are reversible on drug withdrawal.
- Oral bisphosphonates (such as alendronate and risedronate) and strontium ranelate can cause nausea, dyspepsia, and diarrhoea. Oesophageal ulceration has occasionally been noted with alendronate, although it is thought this occurs only in people who do not follow the instructions for taking them. Myalgias and arthralgias can also occur with bisphosphonates.
- Calcitonin either given as subcutaneous injection or as nasal spray can give abdominal pains and diarrhoea.

Malignancy

Rheumatic features may be clues to the existence of cancer; these may be caused directly (through tissue invasion) or indirectly (as a paraneoplastic phenomenon).

Primary and secondary neoplastic diseases of bone and joints

- Synovial tumour's are rare. Sarcoma (synovioma) is more common in men than women and unusual in those over 60. It usually occurs in the legs (70%) and can occur around tendon sheaths and bursa. At diagnosis, pulmonary metastases are common.
- Para-articular involvement by bone tumors may give a monoarticular effusion. Invasion of synovium may occur and malignant cells can be detected in joint fluid. Breast, bronchogenic carcinoma, GI tumours, and melanoma can all metastasize to joints.
- Lymphomas and leukaemias may simulate various conditions and cause synovitis in a single or in multiple joints.
- Arthritis complicating the presentation of myeloma or an acute leukemia is most likely to be polyarticular and asymmetric.
- In adults, arthritis complicating leukemia is rare (5% of cases).
- Leukaemia is the most common cause of neoplastic skeletal symptoms in childhood and adolescence (15% of leukaemia cases).
- Neuroblastomas are the most frequent cause of a solid tumour metastasizing to the skeleton in children.

Clues that may lead to a suspicion of malignancy directly causing musculoskeletal symptoms

- Constitutional symptoms.
- The co-existence of bone pain from metastases (Plate 15; also consider metabolic bone diseases, sarcoid, and enthesitis-related conditions).
- Haemorrhagic joint fluid [also consider trauma, pigmented villonodular synovitis (PVNS), chondrocalcinosis].
- Radiographs that show adjacent bone destruction, perhaps with loss of cortex (also consider infection).
- Radiographic calcification in soft-tissue mass (consider synovioma).

Paraneoplastic myopathies

- Myopathy may be due to carcinomatous neuromyopathy.
- **Polymyositis, dermatomyositis, Eaton–Lambert myasthenic syndrome (ELMS)** and **hypophosphataemic (oncogenic) osteomalacia** are all found in association with malignancy (Table 4.9).
- Carcinomatous neuromyopathy is a condition characterized by symmetric muscle weakness and wasting. Can pre-date malignancy.

Non-myopathic paraneoplastic syndromes

- The non-myopathic paraneoplastic syndromes are rare:
- **Hypertrophic pulmonary osteoarthropathy** (HPOA) consists of clubbing, periostitis of tubular bones, and an arthropathy (may range from arthralgias to diffuse polyarthritis). Suspicion of this should prompt a request for an isotope bone scan, which typically shows

Table 4.9 Myopathy and links with malignancy

Condition	Typical pattern of weakness	Common cancer associations	Other features
Carcinomatous neuromyopathy	Pelvic girdle—symmetric	*Lung:* 15% men, 12% women. *Ovary:* 16%. *Stomach:* 7% men, 13% women	Wasting, EMG abnormality, and increase in muscle enzymes are not invariable
Dermatomyositis (+?PM)	Proximal limb. Truncal	Reflects underlying cancer frequency in local population	Response to steroids is usual
Myasthenia gravis (MG)	Frequently ocular and bulbar muscles involved	Thymus. Any	Muscle strength fluctuates (fatiguability). Responds to anti-cholinesterases
Eaton–Lambert myasthenic syndrome (ELMS)	Pelvic girdle muscles. Altered gait. Ocular muscles not affected	Small cell lung. Can occur up to 2–3 years after ELMS	Autonomic disturbances. EMG + poor response to anticholinesterase distinguish from MG
Oncogenic osteomalacia	Generalized. Develops insidiously	Small, discrete mesenchymal tumours in bone, soft tissues, and sinuses. Neurofibromatosis	Bone pain and bone demineralization. Hypophosphataemia and low circulating 1,25 OH vitamin D

abnormally increased bone turnover in the long bones. Radiographs often show periosteal elevation. HPOA complicates 20% of primary lung tumours, but it is associated with other malignancies.

- Polyarthritis may be the presenting feature of cancer. Most cases occur in those over 60 years old. Unlike RA, the arthritis associated with malignancy tends to be asymmetric, and does not cause erosions.
- **Eosinophilic fasciitis**, severe bilateral palmar fasciitis (often mistaken for scleroderma), and fasciitis associated with panniculitis have been associated with malignancy. Cases of 'shoulder–hand' syndrome (a form of reflex sympathetic dystrophy) that have been reported in association with malignancy probably reflect similar pathological processes.

Rheumatic diseases associated with an increased incidence of malignancy

There are a number of rheumatic diseases that are associated with an increased incidence of malignancy compared with healthy populations. These are dealt with briefly here and in more detail in Part 2 of this book:

- **Non-Hodgkin's lymphoma** is most strongly associated with RA. **Myeloma** and **paraproteinaemia** are also found in RA patients.
- The relative risk of colon cancer among RA patients is 0.77; this may be due to the use of chronic NSAIDs in this patient population, which may be protective.
- Use of cyclophosphamide is associated with an increased risk of lymphoma and bladder cancer. MTX may also be associated with an increased risk of lymphoma.
- Chronic AZA use is associated with an increased risk of skin cancer; patients taking AZA long-term should be counselled regarding sun protection and monitoring for skin cancer.
- Non-Hodgkin's lymphoma develops in a subset of patients with Sjögren's syndrome (4%). Its onset may be indicated by rapid enlargement of salivary glands, the appearance of a paraprotein, or decrease in circulating immunoglobulins or RF titre.
- Scleroderma has been associated with an increased risk of both lung cancer and non-Hodgkin's lymphoma.
- Dermatomyositis is probably associated with malignancy in adults, though convincing evidence for an association of polymyositis with malignancy is lacking. Neither is associated with malignancy in children.

Neurological disorders

These are discussed in detail in 📖 Chapter 2, p 19 in relation to anatomy and nerve root and dermatomal manifestations of entrapment neuropathy and inflammation (neuronitis/mononeuritis multiplex).

Part II

The clinical features and management of rheumatic diseases

Rheumatoid arthritis

Disease criteria and epidemiology for use in clinical trials

There is no exact definition or a pathognomic test for rheumatoid arthritis (RA). It is a common systemic inflammatory disease characterized by the presence of a destructive polyarthritis with a predisposition for affecting the small joints of the hands and feet and the wrists (although it can affect any synovial joint).The diagnosis rests on a composite of clinical and laboratory observations.

Diagnostic criteria are often developed for classification in the context of clinical trials and epidemiological work-they were not designed to diagnose patients with RA. Most criteria are dominated by signs and symptoms from the musculoskeletal system, but the disease has a number of extra-articular manifestations (eyes, lungs, skin for example). Examples of classification criteria include the simple New York criteria and 1987 ARA criteria (Table 5.1).

It is often difficult to apply these criteria to 'possible', 'early' or 'atypical' RA, and these criteria are best used for use in clinical trials of patients with established disease. Significant evidence, however, indicates that early treatment of rheumatoid arthritis greatly improves the long term outcomes associated with this disease, highlighting the importance of early diagnosis and therapy.

Table 5.1 The 1987 American College of Rheumatology criteria for the diagnosis of rheumatoid arthritis

	Criterion	Comments
1	Morning stiffness	Duration >1 hour lasting >6 weeks
2	Arthritis of at least three joints*	Soft tissue swelling lasting >6 weeks
3	Arthritis of hand joints	Wrists, MCPs, or PIPs lasting >6 weeks
4	Symmetrical arthritis	At least one area, lasting >6 weeks
5	Rheumatoid nodules	
6	Positive rheumatoid factor	
7	Radiographic changes	Erosions, particularly wrists, hands, and feet

At least four criteria must be fulfilled and there are no exclusion criteria.

*Possible areas: metacarpophalangeal joints (MCP), proximal interphalangeal joints (PIP), wrist, elbow, knee, ankle, metatarsophalangeal joints (MTP).

Incidence, prevalence, and morbidity

- The disease has a worldwide prevalence, and has been identified in all populations that have been examined. Figures for prevalence range from 0.2 to 5.3%, but the age distribution in developing countries may be a confounding factor and perhaps contribute to low figures in, for example, some parts of Africa.
- Data from the UK estimates a prevalence of 400 000 people, with an annual incidence of 12 000 (NICE, 2009).
- Accepting the difficulties involved in establishing an early diagnosis of RA, population studies on the incidence of the disease suggest figures of 3.4/10 000 in women and 1.4/10 000 in men. The incidence in men declines with age from age 45. In women, it increases until age 45, then plateaus and falls after the age of 75.
- RA is extremely heterogeneous with regard to severity and progression. Permanent remission can occur but is rare once joint damage has started. A distinction is sometimes made between cyclical disease and relentless progression but in practice it is perhaps more useful to consider widespread and limited chronic joint involvement.
- Around one-third of people with RA will stop work within the first 2 years of disease onset, and this increases with duration of disease.
- In the UK, the total costs of RA, including indirect costs such as social care and work-related disability range from £3.8-£4.8 billion per year, a significant cost to the UK economy (NICE, 2009).
- Life expectancy is reduced by approximately 7 years in men and 3 years in women. This is mainly due to cardiovascular disease, infections, respiratory disease, and RA itself. This figure would be expected to reduce given acknowledgement of the need to more aggressively manage cardiac risk factors and a reduction in vascular disease that might occur as a consequence of earlier intervention of inflammatory disease.

The clinical features of rheumatoid arthritis

General features
- Pain
- Morning stiffness
- Myalgia
- Fatigue
- Weight loss
- Joint pain with or without overt swelling or radiological evidence of joint erosions.

Patterns of joint involvement
- Synovitis of the small joints of the hands and feet with symmetry and sparing of the distal interphalangeal joints is the most characteristic feature of RA (Plate 6).
- A mono- or bilateral arthropathy of the shoulder or wrist may account for up to 30–40% of initial presentations.
- 5% of initial presentations involve the knee.
- Any synovial joint can become involved in RA. The hands, wrists, elbows, shoulders, and knees are involved most commonly, followed by the hip and temporomandibular joints. RA also affects the clavicular joints and the crico-arytenoid.
- Patients may also present with a tenosynovitis or bursitis. The diagnosis and management of these conditions is covered in ☐ Chapter 2, p 19
- Though presented often in textbooks as features of 'swan neck' and 'boutoniere', deformity of the digits appears late in disease and are features of chronic disease; they are not usually seen at initial presentation where signs of synovitis and joint damage may be subtle.
- Though often suspected, there is no absolute evidence that stress, whether physical or psychological, triggers the disease.

Pregnancy
- Beneficial effect on RA, especially during the last trimester.
- Symptoms usually return within 1–2 months postpartum and may be more severe than prior disease.
- Lactation has no effect.
- No evidence that RA patients have more medical complications during pregnancy per se. Therapeutics and pregnancy are discussed later in this chapter and ☐ Chapter 21, p545.

Organ disease in rheumatoid arthritis

See Table 5.2.

Lymph nodes

Lymph nodes are often enlarged but rarely palpable. In a few cases RA may present with widespread lymphadenopathy mimicking Hodgkin's disease. Biopsies will show reactive changes only.

Pulmonary disease

- Pleuritis (like pericarditis) is frequent but often mild. Like other pulmonary and cardiac manifestations, it is more common in older men.
- Pleural effusions with exudate.
- Rheumatoid pulmonary nodules are usually an asymptomatic finding in seropositive RA. Radiographically they are coin-shaped lesions that can be difficult to distinguish from malignancy. In patients in whom malignancy is clinically suspected, further imaging or tissue biopsy may be required.
- Diffuse interstitial fibrosis and alveolitis are rare associations. Methotrexate (MTX) is associated with the development of pneumonitis, often within the first year of treatment, though is less common than MTX-associated hepatic and haematological abnormalities. The underlying pathology is thought to be an immune-mediated hypersensitivity reaction rather than direct drug toxicity.

Cardiovascular disease

- Patients with RA suffer from increased cardiovascular disease, independent of the traditional risk factors. Inflammation is thought to play an important part in the development of atherosclerosis and the systemic inflammatory response in RA may explain the link.
- Cardiovascular mortality (ischaemic heart disease and strokes) is increased in patients with early and established disease and in women, a group traditionally at lower risk. A recent meta-analysis of 24 studies involving over 100 000 patients showed a 50% increase in cardiovascular mortality compared with the general population.[1]

Skin

- Raynaud's phenomenon (RP) may be present with infarcts, skin ulceration, and superinfection.
- Rheumatoid nodules occur in up to 30% of patients, and are found principally on the extensor surface of the forearm and over pressure areas throughout the skin. Nodules are not specific for RA but are useful in diagnosis and prognosis, correlating with seropositivity, disease activity, and progression.

1 Aviña-Zubieta JA, Choi HK, Sadatsafavi M, et al. (2008). Risk of cardiovascular mortality in patients with rheumatoid arthritis: a meta-analysis of observational studies. *Arth Rheum* **59**(12): 1690–7.

- Leucocytoclastic vasculitis also occurs and is seen as palpable purpura; most often this resolves spontaneously.
- Rheumatoid vasculitis can lead to large ulcerations on the lower extremities, although this is an uncommon manifestation.

Ocular involvement
- Painful scleritis, leading to scleromalacia.
- Episcleritis is benign and resolves.
- Uveitis and conjunctivitis are not associated with RA.

Table 5.2 Some organ disease in rheumatoid arthritis

Organ	Manifestation	Frequency (%)
Lymph nodes	Enlargement	>50
Spleen	Enlargement	25
	Felty's syndrome	<1
Lungs	Pleuritis	>30
	Nodules	5
	Fibrosis	Rare
Heart	Pericarditis	>10
	Myocarditis	>5
	Nodules	5
	Cardiovascular disease (RA is an independent risk factor)	Standardized mortality ratio: Male 1.3 Female 1.9
Muscle	Atrophy	Common
	Myositis	Rare
Bone	Osteoporosis	Common
Skin	Nodules	>20
	Vasculitis	1
Eyes	Sicca syndrome	10
	Scleritis	1
	Nodules	<2
Nervous system	Nerve entrapment	Common
	Mononeuritis multiplex	<1
	Cord compression	Rare

Neurological involvement

- Entrapment neuropathy secondary to synovitis is common. Median nerve compression can occur early in the disease. Other rarer examples include the ulnar nerve at the elbow, and the posterior tibial nerve at the tarsal tunnel.
- Mononeuritis multiplex, a peripheral and often bilateral neuropathy, can present acutely. A sudden onset of motor neuropathy can signal the presence of aggressive vasculitis and poor prognosis.
- Rheumatoid vasculitis classically occurs in patients with 'burnt-out' RA, but with high titre RF and a history of erosive arthritis.
- Cervical subluxation at the atlantoaxial level described in one-third of RA patients but is usually asymptomatic. Subluxation at lower levels is rare, but is more likely to cause pain and neurological symptoms. Incidence is decreasing with use of early and more aggressive disease-modifying therapy.
- Cervical myelopathy due to cervical instability can be fatal. Symptoms include paraesthesias, weakness, paralysis, sensory loss, incontinence, and syncope. Urgent imaging and neurosurgical referral are required if this is suspected.

Bone

- Cytokines, generated in inflammation, encourage bone resorption by osteoclast induction leading to peri-articular osteoporosis.
- Inactivity, nutritional deficiency, glucocorticoids, and pre-existing osteoporosis constitute additional risk factors for spontaneous fractures.

Tendons and ligaments

Spontaneous rupture is common, most often at the wrist, hand, and rotator cuff. More often, tenosynovitis and weakening of ligaments leads to joint instability and subluxation.

Infection

Anecdotal evidence that infections may trigger flares in RA.

RA patients are more susceptible to septic arthritis, often compounded by the use of immunosuppressive drugs (see later in this chapter). In such a situation, the usual signs of sepsis may be absent, delaying the diagnosis.

Secondary amyloidosis

Renal involvement is the most common type of organ failure, though the skin, liver, and GI tract are often affected. Intensive antirheumatic therapy now gives a more favorable outlook, with 80% 5-year survival rates.

Felty's syndrome

Association of splenomegaly and neutropenia in typically rather destructive RA. Systemic disease, hepatomegaly, and lymphadenopathy are also common, and the occurrence of RA in relatives is higher than expected. In uncomplicated cases, treatment should be conservative, splenectomy remaining controversial and often only transient in effect.

Large granular lymphocyte (LGL) syndrome

Associated with neutropenia and splenomegaly. LGL syndrome is differentiated from Felty's syndrome by the presence large granular lymphocytes and a clonal lymphocytosis. Clonality can be demonstrated through PCR of the T-cell receptor-gamma gene. The arthritis is typically less destructive than that seen with Felty's syndrome, though not always.

The evaluation and treatment of rheumatoid arthritis

- A clearly documented assessment is invaluable for the ongoing monitoring of the disease and treatment (Table 5.3).
- The ESR and CRP are useful measures periodically in the assessment of disease activity, and haematological and biochemical parameters will not only expose underlying organ disease, but are important in the regular monitoring of a number of drug treatments.
- Early erosive changes on plain radiographs of the hands and feet can be of great value in the assessment of patients with minimal clinical signs. Other imaging modalities such as ultrasound or MRI can also detect synovitis and erosions in the presence of minimal clinical signs and normal radiographs.
- IgM rheumatoid factor (RF) is of value in establishing the diagnosis, however, a low positive result can be misleading and a negative result should not alter a diagnosis made on clinical grounds. Only 70–80% of patients with RA will be RF positive. The RF need not be repeated regularly unless in patients whose initial result is negative or very low but clinically have signs suggestive of the disease. With time these cases may become strongly positive and their disease will require more aggressive management.
- Anti-cyclic citrullinated peptide (anti-CCP) antibodies are important surrogate markers for diagnosis and prognosis in RA. In both early and established disease, anti-CCP antibodies are more sensitive and more specific than RF. Anti-CCP antibodies may be detected in roughly 50–60% of patients with early RA. They are also a marker of erosive disease and may predict the development of RA in patients with non-specific inflammatory symptoms.
- The ultimate goal would be the complete remission of disease but this is rarely possible and initial assessment and decisions about treatment need to take account of the relative degree of both inflammatory and mechanical disease as well as their psychological impact.
- While a functional assessment is of value, particularly in respect to trial data, regular monitoring need not employ formal status questionnaires and often a global view from the patient, physician, or physiotherapist, is enough.
- The Disease Activity Score (DAS) is a composite score using tender and swollen joint count, ESR, and patient global assessment of disease activity using a 100 mm visual analogue scale. The DAS is used in clinical trials to assess response to treatment. Clinically, it is used more in Europe than in the United States.
- The DAS28 is calculated by surveying 28 joints (knees + upper extremities). It is calculated as follows:
- $DAS28 = 0.56 \star$ (number tender joints) $+ 0.28 \star$ (number of swollen joints) $+ 0.70 \ln(ESR)$ $+ 0.014$ Global assessment (in mm)

Table 5.3 Documenting the initial evaluation of RA

1	The duration of morning stiffness
	The degree of pain
	Fatigue
	Function (utilizing a score system such as Health Assessment Questionnaire—HAQ)
	Patient global assessment of disease activity
2	The distribution and number of painful joints, and the distribution and number of swollen joints, including periodicity
	The distribution and nature of mechanical joint disease noting loss of function, instability, and modifying factors
	The presence or absence of extra-articular disease
3	Radiographs of affected joints looking for erosive disease and mechanical damage
4	Laboratory tests
	ESR and CRP
	FBC
	Renal and liver function tests
	Urinalysis
	Rheumatoid factor
	Anti-CCP antibodies

- A multidisciplinary approach with physiotherapists, occupational therapists, podiatrists, social services, and surgeons is an important part of management (Table 5.4).
- In the UK both NICE and the British Society for Rheumatology have produced guidance for managing RA, both in early and established disease. The key features of the guidance are:
  - early referral to specialists and the multi-disciplinary team according to patient need;
  - the provision of an individualized care plan, early introduction of disease modifying therapies (combination therapies recommended, see later in chapter) with regular follow-up, monitoring of disease activity, and alteration in treatments as required.

Which drugs, when, and what to monitor? (Table 5.5 and
📖 Chapter 21, p 545)

NSAIDs

• Offer reliable but limited, relief of pain, swelling, and stiffness, improving
quality of life in the majority of cases. Adverse effects are, however,
common and sometimes life-threatening; awareness and patient
education is essential. Combinations of NSAIDs should be avoided.

Table 5.4 The main components in the treatment of RA

Modality	Examples
Education and counselling	Specialist nurse practitioner
	Self-care groups
	National organizations
Physiotherapy	Exercise
	Joint protection
Occupational therapy	Adaptation
	Aids
	Splints
Podiatry and chiropody	Orthotics
	Surgical shoes
Medication	Pain control
	Disease control
Non-medical pain management	Transcutaneous nerve stimulation
	Acupuncture
	Psychotherapy
	Surgery
Surgery	Joint replacement
	Arthrodesis
	Tendon release/repair

• Selective COX-2 NSAIDs are of similar efficacy to diclofenac or
naproxen, and may be of value in patients intolerant of NSAIDs. Many
agents in this class, however, have been withdrawn from the market
due to concerns regarding COX-2 inhibitors and increased risk of
myocardial infarction. Of concern is a study showing that even standard
NSAIDs are also associated with an increased risk of myocardial
infarction.

- These drugs should be used appropriately at the lowest possible dose and avoided for long-term use in all patients, particularly those with adverse cardiovascular or GI risk profiles (Table 5.6). Proton-pump inhibitors should also be considered as adjunctive therapy in appropriate patients, and wherever possible, safer alternatives, such as paracetamol, codeine, or compound analgesics, should be used.

Table 5.5 Pharmacotherapy of rheumatoid arthritis

Drug type	Examples
Pain relief	Simple analgesia
	NSAIDs
Disease-modifying drugs	Glucocorticoids (oral, IM, intra-articular)
	Methotrexate
	Sulfasalazine
	Hydroxychloroquine
	Leflunomide
Biologic therapies	Anti-TNF-α: etanercept, infliximab, adalimumab, certolizumab
	Anti B-cell: rituximab
	IL-1 receptor antagonists: anakinra (not approved by NICE)
	IL-6 antagonists: tocilizumab
For disease complications	Anaemia: iron, erythropoietin
	Osteoporosis: calcium and vitamin D, bisphosphonates, teriparatide
	Vasculitis: glucocorticoids, cyclophosphamide
	Amyloidosis: chlorambucil, anti-TNF-α therapies

Disease modifying antirheumatic drugs (DMARDs)

- NICE guidance now recommends combination therapy in early disease with MTX, at least one other DMARD [most commonly sulfasalazine (SSZ) and/or hydroxychloroquine (HCQ)] and short-term glucocorticoids, ideally within the first 3 months of onset of persistent symptoms and using rapid dose escalation titrated to patient response and side effects.[1]

1 National Institute for Health and Clinical Excellence. Rheumatoid Arthritis; the management of rheumatoid arthritis in adults. February 2009. www.nice.org.uk/CG79.

- Combination therapy has been to shown to be as safe as monotherapy and more effective in reducing disease activity and reducing joint damage. However, efficacy is unpredictable and variable in duration.
- Toxicity is an important concern and this should always be discussed with patients
- DMARDs are slow-acting, sometimes taking 3–6 months to have effect.
- Final choice of DMARDs is influenced by a number of factors including, patient compliance, convenience of administration, severity of disease, presence of other medical conditions, pregnancy, monitoring requirements and frequency, and nature of adverse events.

Table 5.6 Adverse reactions of NSAIDs

Organ/ complication	Occurrence	Comments
GI tract	Common	Gastritis, bleeding, and perforation. High risk in elderly and those with ulcer history
Renal	Common	Fluid retention, papillary necrosis
Hypertension	Common	Interference with drugs such as thiazide diuretics
Myocardial infarction	Increased risk in those with cardiovascular risk factors	COX-1 and COX-2 drugs
Pulmonary	Not uncommon	Exacerbation of asthma, pneumonitis (naproxen)
Skin	Not uncommon	Hypersensitivity, erythema multiforme
CNS	Not uncommon Rare	Tinnitus, fatigue, cognitive disturbance Aseptic meningitis
Hepatic	Uncommon	Drug-induced hepatitis
Haematological	Rare	Bone marrow dyscrasias

Methotrexate (MTX)

- Given weekly by mouth, sc or im injection.
- Toxicity (stomatitis, GI disturbance, and alopecia) may be reduced by the addition of folic acid daily, without loss of therapeutic effect. Parenteral administration is a useful option if oral treatment is not tolerated, and there is also some evidence of improved efficacy compared with oral administration.
- Pneumonitis is uncommon and pulmonary fibrosis (a rare complication of MTX) should not deter the physician from using MTX in aggressive systemic and skeletal disease. Rare, life-threatening, pulmonary toxicity can occur at any time but is most common in the first year and is not directly related to dose or duration of treatment. A chest X-ray should be taken before MTX is commenced.
- Mild drug-induced hepatitis is relatively common and is often corrected by the addition of folic acid. Overt liver disease is rare. Routine liver biopsy is not necessary, being restricted to assessment of patients with other liver disease and possibly patients with persistent liver function abnormalities in spite of discontinuing treatment.
- Liver function abnormalities fluctuate and may require the drug to be stopped for a short period if transaminase levels rise above 2–3 times the upper limit of normal, with possible re-introduction after a period of time when levels have normalized, with close monitoring. Patients are advised that they should abstain from alcohol use completely.
- Myelosuppression is rarely severe. Antifolate drugs such as trimethoprim, and folate deficiency increase the risk of toxicity. Renal impairment reduces MTX clearance and may lead to toxicity. Pregnancy and breastfeeding are contraindications to the use of MTX. Both men and women should wait 3 months after stopping treatment before trying to conceive a child. Diminished fertility caused by MTX is reversible.
- NSAID use is not contraindicated. There is the potential for interaction and hepatotoxicity, and close monitoring remains a prerequisite for commencing therapy.
- Patients having major operations are not advised to stop treatment before surgery as there is no evidence to suggest that this reduces the risk of post-operative complications such as wound healing or sepsis, and increases the risk of a disease flare. However, in practice surgeons often ask patients to stop 1–2 weeks prior to surgery and restart 1 week after surgery. This should be avoided as it may lead to loss of disease control and delay in recovery from the surgery.

Sulfasalazine and hydroxychloroquine

- Sulfasalazine (SSZ) and hydroxychloroquine (HCQ) are often used initially in mild RA, partly because of their relative safety and convenience. Both agents are generally well-tolerated and take effect within 1–3 months. Many clinicians now choose MTX first if there is evidence of early aggressive disease.
- Retinal toxicity and maculopathy are rare with HCQ. The risk increases with abnormal liver or kidney function, after a cumulative dose of 800 g, and in patients aged 70 years and over. The eyes should be checked formally yearly and the patient informed to report any visual disturbances.
- There is potential for accumulation of HCQ in the foetus during pregnancy, and for chromosomal damage, although in studies of SLE, no significant risk to the foetus has been found.
- SSZ has been used successfully in pregnancy. There have been case reports of congenital malformations, although the overall risk is considered very small.
- SSZ may cause leucopenia, pancytopenia, haemolysis, and aplastic anaemia. Serious bone marrow toxicity is, however, uncommon. It can also induce a hepatic transaminitis.
- SSZ can rarely cause a hypersensitivity reaction characterized by liver function test abnormalities, lymphadenopathy, and rash.
- Spermatogenesis can be affected by SSZ, but it is reversible. There does not appear to be an adverse effect on female fertility.

Leflunomide

- Leflunomide is also effective for the treatment of RA. It is an inhibitor of the enzyme dihydro-orotate dehydrogenase and shows anti-proliferative activity, inhibiting pyrimidine synthesis. It has a long half-life of 2 weeks.
- Leflunomide is used as monotherapy and in conjunction with other DMARDs.
- Initially, it was administered with a loading dose of 100 mg daily for 3 days followed by maintenance therapy with 10–20 mg daily. The loading dose was associated with gastrointestinal disturbance and diarrhoea in many patients, and clinicians now mainly use maintenance therapy doses from the start.
- It has been shown to reduce disease activity and joint damage in clinical trials, and many side-effects are similar to other DMARDs (myelosuppression, elevation of liver transaminases). Other side effects include diarrhoea and hypertension. Severe hepatitis is uncommon and occurs in the first 6 months of treatment. Regular blood monitoring of full blood count, liver function tests, and blood pressure are required.
- Interstitial pneumonitis is a recognized, but uncommon side effect, and any new or worsening respiratory symptoms should be investigated and the drug discontinued, and the drug should not be used in patients with existing interstitial lung disease.

- Leflunomide should not be initiated in female patients wishing to become pregnant in the near future.
- The long half-life has implications for drug withdrawal, particularly in female patients wishing to become pregnant; also in 'washout' before starting a trial drug or withdrawing for complications. Washout may require colestyramine for between 14 days to 6 weeks, followed by 2 blood tests to ensure drug levels are below 0.02 mg/L.

Other DMARDs

- Other DMARDs, including oral and IM gold, penicillamine, azathioprine, ciclosporin, and cyclophosphamide, have largely fallen out of favour due to the availability of more effective or less toxic regimens. Decisions should be based on discussion between the doctor and patient taking into account the risks and benefits. These agents, their side-effects and monitoring are detailed in Table 5.7.

Glucocorticoids

- IM and oral steroids are very effective in active RA, reducing active disease in an acute crisis or while waiting for a DMARD to take effect.
- Local steroid injections (📖 Chapter 21, p 545) are of value in symptom control both early in the disease and in an acute flare. The effect on joint recovery may be dramatic, but short-lived, with little impact on the overall process of RA, and should not be repeated any more than once every 3 months. It is sometimes of value to combine injections with a joint 'washout' in refractory cases. There is no evidence to suggest an increased risk of joint infection, as long as aseptic technique is used.
- High-dose systemic administration may reduce overall disease activity in the short-term, but adverse effects preclude its uninhibited use and it is best preserved for initial short-term use in combination therapy or in refractory RA and severe extra-articular complications.
- There have been reports linking glucocorticoid therapy to foetal congenital malformations, and there is little data on lactation. Prednisone, dexamethasone, and betamethasone appear to be safe, but should be used only when necessary.
- Long-term use of glucocorticoids may be associated with a wide range of consequences, including cataracts, premature coronary artery disease, accelerated osteoporosis, muscle atrophy, and increased risk of avascular necrosis. Appropriate bone protection therapy should be given to patients expected to be on glucocorticoid therapy for >3 months.

Anti-TNF-α therapy

- TNF-α is a potent pro-inflammatory cytokine whose levels are elevated in RA.
- At present, there are 4 agents available for the treatment of active RA, namely adalimumab (Humira®), etanercept (Enbrel®), certolizumab pegol (Cimzia®) and infliximab (Remicade®). Infliximab is a chimeric

Table 5.7 Monitoring guidelines for DMARDs in rheumatoid arthritis

Drug	Main toxicity	Other side-effects	Monitoring
Sulfasalazine	Myelosuppression	Stains body fluid, rash, hepatitis	FBC and LFT every 2 weeks until dose stable and thereafter every 3 months
Methotrexate	Myelosuppression	Hepatitis, pneumonitis, rash	FBC and LFT every 2 weeks until dose stable. Baseline CXR. FBC and LFT every 4–6 weeks. U&E every 6 months thereafter
Hydroxychloroquine	Macular damage	Visual disturbance	Ophthalmic review if visual disturbance
*Intramuscular gold	Myelosuppression	Rash, reversible proteinuria	FBC and urinalysis before every dose
*Penicillamine	Myelosuppression, drug-induced myasthenic syndrome	Rashes, proteinuria	FBC and urinalysis every 2 weeks until dose stable then monthly
*Azathioprine	Myelosuppression	Hepatitis	FBC every 2 weeks until dose stable then every 8 weeks. LFT every 3 months
Leflunomide	Myelosuppression	Hepatitis, diarrhoea, alopecia, skin allergies, hypertension	FBC every 2 weeks for 6 weeks then every 8 weeks. LFT and blood pressure every 12 weeks
*Ciclosporin	Hypertension, renal toxicity	Gum hyperplasia, hyperlipidemia, hyperuricaemia	Serum creatinine and BP every 2 weeks until the dose has been stable for 3 months. Thereafter serum creatinine and BP monthly. FBC, LFTs monthly until dose stable for 3 months and then 3-monthly. Serum lipids 6-monthly

FBC = full blood count; CXR = chest radiograph; LFT = liver function tests; U&E = urea and electrolytes. *Agents are no longer commonly used for RA.

human–murine anti-TNF-α monoclonal antibody, etanercept is a recombinant human TNF receptor fusion protein, certolizumab pegol is a pegylated Fab fragment of a fully humanized anti-TNF monoclonal antibody and adalimumab is a fully humanized complete anti-TNF-α monoclonal antibody. Infliximab is administered by slow iv infusion at 0, 2, 6, and every 4–8 weeks thereafter depending on response. Etanercept is administered by SC injection and can now be given once instead of twice weekly. Certolizumab pegol is given by sc injection at a dose of 400 mg in weeks 0, 2, and 4, followed by a maintenance dose of 200 mg every 2 weeks. Adalimumab is given by sc injection every 2 weeks.

- With all the above anti-TNF-α agents, co-administration with MTX is recommended when tolerated as this has been shown to increase efficacy, and use with infliximab also reduces the production of anti-infliximab and antinuclear antibodies.
- There is evidence that patients may respond to a second anti-TNF α if there is inadequate response to a first therapy. In revised NICE guidelines (2010), a second anti-TNF-α agent is recommended only if rituximab has not been effective or is contra-indicated.[1]
- In the UK, the NICE has published guidelines for the use of these drugs based on clinical efficacy, health-related quality of life and cost effectiveness. (Table 5.8)
- These therapies are not without their adverse events. Common reactions include headache, nausea, and injection-site reactions. Serious bacterial infections have been reported, and patients with active infection should have their treatment stopped. Patients at risk of recurrent infection should not use these drugs (e.g. in-dwelling urinary catheter, immunodeficiency states). Other reported side-effects include demyelination, worsening of heart failure, lupus-like syndromes, and bone marrow dyscrasias.
- Reactivation of tuberculosis has been reported mainly in infliximab and adalimumab patients (3 or 4 times increased risk compared with etanercept), and most commonly within 3 months of the beginning of treatment. Patients should be assessed for TB risk, and guidelines for assessing risk and managing *Mycobacterium tuberculosis* infection in patients due to start anti-TNF-α therapy have been published by the British Thoracic Society (www.brit-thoracic.org.uk).
- Ongoing concern about the long-term safety of these drugs, especially with regard to malignancy. It is well known that RA patients have 2 times higher risk of increased risk of developing lymphoma compared with the general population. Debate continues as to whether reports of lymphoma in RA patients on anti-TNF α therapy reflect a real drug effect or the known increased incidence of lymphoma in RA patients, but current evidence from the UK Registry suggests no increased incidence of lymphoma in patients with RA on anti-TNF-α therapy compared with RA controls. No increased risk has been found with other types of malignancy.
- Pregnancy, breastfeeding, sepsis, and malignancy are exclusion criteria, although there have been many reports of successful pregnancies in patients on anti-TNF-α therapy.

---

1 National Institute for Health and Clinical Excellence. June 2010. www.nice.org.uk/

Table 5.8 Summary of UK NICE/BSR Guidelines for the use of the first anti-TNF-α therapy in RA

1 Patients must satisfy 1987 ACR criteria for diagnosis of RA
2 A Disease Activity Score of >5.1 at 2 points, 1 month apart
3 Adequate trial of at least 2 standard DMARDs, one of which should be methotrexate. An adequate trial is defined as: <ul><li>treatment for at least 6 months, with at least 2 months at standard target dose (unless toxicity)</li><li>treatment for <6 months where treatment was withdrawn due to intolerance or toxicity, normally after at least 2 months of therapeutic doses</li></ul>
4 Exclusion criteria: pregnancy or breastfeeding. Active infection or high risk of infection. Malignant or pre-malignant states
5 Criteria for withdrawal of therapy: adverse events or inefficacy
6 An alternative anti-TNF-α therapy may be considered for patients in whom treatment is withdrawn due to an adverse event before the initial 6-month assessment of efficacy

(From NICE clinical guidance 79: Rheumatoid arthritis, and NICE technology appraisal guidance 130).

Interleukin-1 receptor antagonists: anakinra

Interleukin-1 (IL-1) is a pro-inflammatory cytokine. Anakinra is an IL-1 receptor antagonist that competes with IL-1 for binding. The agent is given by daily sc injection. Randomized controlled trials have shown it is more effective than placebo. Side-effects include injection-site reactions, blood dyscrasias, and infection. Anti-TNF-α therapies should not be used in conjunction and clearance is reduced in renal impairment. NICE has not approved its use in RA.

B cell depletion: rituximab

There is increasing evidence that B cells play an important role in the pathogenesis of RA. Rituximab is a chimeric monoclonal antibody against human CD 20 that is present on developing B cells prior to the plasma cell stage. Administration of rituximab leads to rapid CD20 positive B cell depletion in the peripheral blood. Normal B cell repopulation occurs within the next 3 months. Rituximab was first used in non-Hodgkins lymphoma. Randomized placebo-controlled trials have shown that in RF positive patients who have failed several DMARDs, a course of rituximab (2 infusions 2 weeks apart with corticosteroids) achieves a significant improvement in disease activity at 6 months compared with MTX alone. There is concern about persistent hypogammaglobulinaemia after repeated courses. A recent systematic review has shown no increase in serious infections with rituximab compared with placebo.[1]

NICE has recommended rituximab to be used with MTX in the treatment of severe RA who have had an inadequate response to other DMARDs and at least one other anti-TNF-α therapy.

---

1 Salliot C, Dougados M, Gossec L. (2009) Risk of serious infections during rituximab, abatacept and anakinra treatments for rheumatoid arthritis: meta-analyses of randomised placebo-controlled trials. *Ann Rheum Dis* **68**(1): 25–32. Epub 2008 Jan 18.

CTLA4-Ig: abatacept

Abatacept disrupts the CD80/86 co-stimulatory signal required for T-cell activation by competing with CD28 for binding. Abatacept is administered intravenously at weeks 0, 2 and 4, and then monthly thereafter, and is effective in patients who have previously failed MTX or TNF-α inhibitors. A recent systematic review has shown that the incidence of serious infections compared with placebo was equal.

In 2007, NICE did not recommend its use in RA, but the revised guidance in 2010 has allowed its use in patients who have had an inadequate response to a first anti-TNF-α therapy, and in whom rituximab has been ineffective or contraindicated.

Anti-interleukin 6 therapy: tocilizumab

Interleukin-6 is a potent pro-inflammatory cytokine. High levels have been found in serum and synovial fluid of RA patients, and levels correlate with disease activity. Tocilizumab is a fully humanized anti-IL6 receptor antibody and is given by monthly intravenous infusion. Studies have shown that it is effective in controlling disease and limiting radiographic progression in RA patients in whom MTX and anti-TNF-α therapies have been ineffective or not tolerated.

In 2010 NICE approved its use in the UK.

Experimental therapies in RA

Experimental therapies are detailed in Table 5.9.

Pregnancy and lactation

The use of anti-rheumatic drugs in pregnancy and lactation is summarized in Table 5.10 and discussed again in 📖 Chapter 21, p 545.

Table 5.9 Experimental therapies for the treatment of rheumatoid arthritis

Target	Principle
Cell cycle inhibitor	Temsirolimus
Ion channel blockers	Receptor antagonists
Cytokine inhibition	Anti-IL-6 antibody
	Oral TNF inhibitor
	Anti-IL-15 monoclonal antibody
B cells	Humanized anti CD-20 agents Anti-B cell stimulator protein (belimumab)
	Anti-BLyS/APRIL
	Anti TACI-Ig
Cell adhesion molecules	Humanized 4-1 and 4-7 monoclonal antibody (natalizumab)
Pro-inflammation	Fish/plant seed oils

Table 5.10 Antirheumatic drugs in pregnancy and lactation

Drug	Effects
Methotrexate	*Pregnancy:* teratogenic in experiments, protection with leucovorin. No adverse effects in low dose clinically (7.5 mg/week); termination not mandatory. Long-term follow-up data lacking, but drug better avoided or stopped.
	Lactation: no data and probably safe if dose not >7.5 mg/week.
Corticosteroids	*Pregnancy:* no convincing evidence of teratogenic effects; occasional neonatal adrenal suppression; better avoided but can be used or continued if indicated—prednisone dose preferably not >10 mg/day.
	Lactation: drug should be avoided on theoretical grounds, especially if dose >7.5 mg/day prednisone or equivalent.
Sulfasalazine	*Pregnancy:* isolated report of foetal abnormalities, but limited data and no convincing reports of teratogenic effects; drug can be continued.
	Lactation: inadequate data; probably safe if dose not >2 g/day.
Hydroxychloroquine	*Pregnancy:* adverse effects unlikely from limited data; termination not justified, drug can be continued.
	Lactation: inadequate data; probably safe.
Biologic therapies (including rituximab, TNF-α inhibitors, abatacept)	*Pregnancy and lactation:* contraindicated, primarily due to lack of data regarding outcomes.

Surgery in RA

- Damage to joints, with associated pain and loss of function remains a familiar feature of chronic RA. Surgical intervention may have a place in such situations, although certain procedures (e.g. shoulder replacement) may only be effective in reducing pain and may not necessarily improve function.
- Synovectomy is less frequently performed now, although tenosynovectomy is common, and a quick and safe relief of nerve entrapment.
- Common surgical procedures include:
  - decompression of the carpal tunnel;
  - reconstructive arthroplasty of hip and knee; less often the shoulder, elbow, and small joints of the hand;
  - corrective arthrotomies of the metatarsals;
  - stabilization of the cervical spine;
  - tendon release and transfer;
  - arthrodesis, particularly of the ankle joint.

- Patients should ideally be seen by a surgeon with expertise in dealing with patients with RA.

Management summary for treating RA

There remains a need for the development of early predictors of long-term outcome in RA, allowing better patient selection for early intervention.
  Poor prognostic indicators include:
- Early functional impairment.
- High RF and CCP titres.
- High ESR or CRP at diagnosis.
- Male gender.
- Radiographic evidence of erosions.
- Rheumatoid nodules.

Of all patients with RA:
- 20% will have mild disease.
- 75% moderate disease with relapses and remissions.
- 5% will have severe destructive disease.
- Patients are at risk of early cardiovascular disease. It is important to assess cardiovascular risk factors such as cholesterol, blood pressure, diabetes, corticosteroid use, smoking, etc., and modify them if possible.
- A multidisciplinary team is important in patient care and should be involved at an early stage.
- DMARD monitoring is needed to ensure patients do not suffer serious side-effects.
- Patients should be involved directly in any decisions about their care.

Polyarticular arthritis in children with a positive rheumatoid factor

- This subset of juvenile idiopathic arthritis (JIA—📖 Chapter 9, p 303) is clinically and genetically indistinguishable from adult RA. Approximately 25% of cases have a family history of seropositive RA.
- The disease usually presents as a polyarthritis (five or more joints) of the small joints of the hands and feet. In presentation before the age of 10 years there is often associated early involvement of the wrists, knees, ankles, and hindfeet as well. All other features of adult RA may be seen in children.
- Fever is rare.
- The ILAR criteria suggest that three consecutive positive tests for serum IgM RF should be taken twice over the course of 3 months before the diagnosis is made. This is because transient positive titres are seen in infection. It is also important to bear in mind that RF is also found in SLE (📖 Chapter 10, p 321), vasculitis (📖 Chapter 15, p 405), hypergammaglobulinaemia, and sarcoidosis (📖 Chapter 18, p 489). The clinical features may also appear similar to juvenile psoriatic arthropathy (📖 Chapter 8, p 281).
- Radiological changes with periostitis and local osteoporosis tend to occur early in the disease. One-third of cases progress to severe functional limitation within 10–15 years.
- Differences from adult RA include the problem of growth retardation, a tendency to early fusion of the carpal bones, and erosions at the distal interphalangeal joints.
- A few cases of aortic regurgitation and pericarditis have been reported. Pulmonary manifestations of RA are, however, relatively uncommon.
- In the few cases that have been followed through pregnancy, there appears to be an almost universal post-pregnancy relapse of the RA.
- Treatment of polyarticular JIA with positive RF in children is much the same as for adults. Early introduction of a DMARD is encouraged and most centres use MTX as first-line therapy. MTX is well-tolerated in children. Oral therapy is first-line, but sc administration is increasingly used, and has been shown to be effective in those with poor adherence or side-effects to oral treatment. A recent study using leflunomide found high rates of clinical improvement, but not as great as with MTX. If corticosteroid therapy is started, the preferred regimen is an alternate-day dosing.
- Cytotoxic agents tend to be spared for use in those with associated amyloidosis, vasculitis, pulmonary fibrosis, or aortic valve disease in the presence of active arthritis.
- Etanercept or adalimumab is appropriate for patients with active polyarticular disease who have been intolerant of, or not responded to, MTX.

Still's disease

Adult-onset Still's disease is an auto-inflammatory disease. The condition 'juvenile-onset Still's disease' is now usually grouped under juvenile idiopathic arthritis.

Typically affects 16–35-year-olds and presents with:
- Arthralgia.
- 'Salmon-pink' rash.
- Pyrexia.
- Fatigue.
- Lymphadenopathy.
- Elevated serum ferritin.
- Rare pericardial and pleural effusion.

Rheumatoid factor (RF) and anti-nuclear antibody (ANA) are classically negative.

Treatment of adult-onset Still's disease is similar to systemic JIA (Ⓜ Chapter 9, p 303).

Osteoarthritis

Introduction

Epidemiology and pathology

- Osteoarthritis (OA) is a chronic and dynamic disorder characterized by cartilage loss and bone remodelling.
- It is the most common condition to affect joints in humans. It is estimated that up to 8.5 million people in the UK have joint pain that can be due to OA, and that 15% of the UK population >55 years of age have symptomatic knee OA.
- UK prevalence of radiographic hand OA is estimated at 4.4 million people, radiographic significant knee OA affects 0.5 million people and >200 000 people have significant radiographic hip OA.[1]
- By 2020, OA is expected to be the fourth leading cause of disability worldwide.
- OA is a significant economic burden in the UK, with cost estimates of 1% of domestic Gross National Product, and 36 million working days lost.[2]
- Although there are recognized associations between OA, age, and trauma, advances in cartilage biochemistry and the recognition of crystal-associated disease have renewed interest in OA as a dynamic condition of cartilage loss (chondropathy) with a peri-articular bone reaction. At present, however, OA is assessed and managed clinically as a structural, rather than physiological condition, with an emphasis on established disease and also disease prevention using a holistic approach to care.
- Chondrocyte dysfunction leads to metalloproteinase enzyme release causing collagen and proteoglycan degradation. Synovial inflammation is present, with production of cytokines such as IL-1 and TNF-α that also induce metalloproteinase production.
- Macroscopic changes in OA include cystic bone degeneration, cartilage loss, and growth of irregular abnormal bone at joint margins (osteophytes).
- Microscopic changes include flaking and fibrillation of articular cartilage with variations in vascularity and cellularity of subchondral bone, leading to sclerosis and new bone formation.
- Most surveys of OA rely on radiographic features for definition and severity. These are problematic because correlation of radiographic change with clinical status, symptoms, and function can be poor; it is best at the hip and knee, but poor in the hand and spine. The correlation between pathology and radiology is shown in Table 6.1.
- There are various subgroups of OA and these are described below in the section on clinical features.

1 Arthritis and Musculoskeletal Alliance (2004). *Standards of care for people with osteoarthritis.* London: ARMA.

2 NICE (2008). *Clinical Guideline 59. Osteoarthritis: Care and management of osteoarthritis in adults.* London: NICE.

Risk factors

- Although no gender difference occurs in mild disease, severe disease favours women and patients older than 50 years. There is also a polyarticular form of hand OA—'nodal generalized OA'—that has a predilection for peri-menopausal women.
- OA of the hip is more common in Europeans than Asians or African-Americans.
- The Framingham study found that 27% of those aged 63–70 years had radiographic evidence of knee OA; this increased to 44% in those over 80 years old.
- A UK study showed 50% of adults >50 with radiographic knee OA had symptoms. Similar figures are seen in hip OA, but symptomatic hand OA in those with radiographic features has a lower prevalence of approximately 3–7%.
- Susceptibility factors include:
  - obesity (close association with new-onset and progression of knee OA, but not hip);
  - family history-particularly nodal generalized OA;
  - there is increased concordance for OA in monozygotic compared to dizygotic twins;
  - heritability estimates for common OA sites, such as hand, knee, and hip, are 40–60%, although specific susceptibility genes have not yet been identified;
  - high bone density; such as osteopetrosis (there is a negative correlation between OA onset and low bone density);
  - trauma;
  - femoral dysplasia (for hip OA);
  - hypermobility (rigorous studies required, although one recent large study suggests hypermobility is protective against hand OA);
  - low vitamin C and D levels are associated with progression of knee OA.
- Evidence regarding smoking and a protective effect on knee OA has been seen in some studies and remains controversial.
- Suggested risk factors for hip OA include previous hip disease (e.g. Perthes'), acetabular dysplasia, avascular necrosis of the femoral head, severe trauma, generalized OA, and occupation (e.g. farming).
- There is little evidence to link OA with repetitive injury from occupation or sports, such as running in those with normal joints, except perhaps knee-bending in men.
- Dockers and miners have a higher incidence of knee OA.

Table 6.1 Radiographic-pathological correlates in OA

Pathological change	Radiographic abnormality
Cartilage fibrillation, erosion	Localized joint-space narrowing
Subchondral new bone	Sclerosis
Myxoid degeneration	Subchondral cysts
Trabecular compression	Bone collapse/attrition
Fragmentation of osteochondral surface	Osseous ('loose') bodies

Clinical features of osteoarthritis

- The clinical features of pain and stiffness, functional impairment, and anatomical change, are interrelated, but often discordant.
- There are several potential mechanisms for pain; none are completely understood. Pain may arise from inflammatory mediators or intra-articular hypertension, stimulating capsular, periosteal, and synovial nerve fibres. Pain may also arise from enthesopathy or bursitis that can accompany structural alteration, muscle weakness, and altered joint use.
- Although stiffness is a common complaint in OA, prolonged early morning stiffness should lead the clinician to consider the presence of an inflammatory arthropathy.
- Bony enlargement and deformity, crepitus, restricted movement, joint instability, and 'stress' pain can also occur. Muscle weakness and wasting may be present.
- There are several subsets of OA that are worth noting. They are not absolute, and one set of characteristics may dominate the evolving disease at any one time. These subsets are:
  - primary OA—nodal generalized OA; erosive ('inflammatory') OA.
  - large joint OA (knee and hip); spinal OA.
  - secondary OA (Table 6.2).

Nodal generalized OA

- This common condition (Plate 6d) is characterized by:
  - polyarticular finger involvement;
  - Heberden's nodes (distal interphalangeal joint);
  - Bouchard's nodes (proximal interphalangeal joint);
  - predisposition to OA of knee, hip, and spine;
  - good functional outcome in the hands;
  - female preponderance;
  - peak onset around the menopause;
  - strong family history.
- There is a tendency to greater distal joint disease. The first carpometacarpal (CMC), metacarpophalangeal (MCP), and interphalangeal (IP) joints of the thumb are also often involved, as are the index and middle MCP joints.
- The more proximal joints of the hand and wrist are otherwise relatively spared.

Erosive OA

- This uncommon condition is characterized by:
  - hand interphalangeal involvement;
  - tendency to joint ankylosis;
  - florid inflammation (episodic);
  - radiographic subchondral erosive change.
- Unlike nodal OA, proximal and distal IP joints are equally involved and, less frequently, the MCPs.
- IP joint instability is common. Given the additional risk of ankylosis, functional impairment is more likely than nodal OA.
- The principal hallmark of the condition is subchondral erosive change that can lead to remodelling.

Large joint OA

- The knee is commonly affected and most frequently in the patello-femoral and medial tibiofemoral compartments; severe bone and cartilage loss at the latter site causes instability and the classic varus (bow knee) deformity.
- Subdivision of hip disease is usually made on the basis of local radiographic patterns. There are two principal groups:
  - Superior pole: common pattern, often unilateral, more common in men, and likely to progress
  - Central (medial): less common, usually bilateral, more common in women, and less likely to progress.
- Indeterminate 'concentric' radiographic patterns also exist.

Secondary OA

Secondary OA is seen in association with a wide variety of disorders as illustrated in Table 6.2.

Natural history of OA

- Progression in the knee may take many years. Cohort studies have found that radiographic deterioration occurs in one-third.
- Progression of hip disease is variable. A Danish study found that 66% of hips worsened radiologically over 10 years, although symptomatic improvement was common.
- Hand disease has the best prognosis, with episodic inflammatory phases associated with redness and swelling. Flares then reduce in frequency, and pain also improves. However, base of thumb OA has a worse prognosis than nodal OA.

Table 6.2 Secondary causes of OA

Trauma	Inflammatory arthritis
Metabolic/endocrine	**Crystal deposition disease**
Haemochromatosis	Calcium pyrophosphate
Acromegaly	Uric acid
Hyperparathyroidism	Hydroxyapatite
Ochronosis (alkaptonuria)	
Neuropathic disorders	**Anatomical abnormalities**
Diabetes mellitus	Bone dysplasia

The investigation of osteoarthritis

- OA is a clinical and radiological diagnosis. There are no specific laboratory tests.
- Joint space narrowing may be difficult to appreciate in early OA; as the disease progresses, other findings may appear, including osteophytes, subchondral bone sclerosis, and subchondral cysts.
- Radiographs correlate poorly with symptoms and clinical function. Many older patients will have radiographic changes consistent with OA, but will be asymptomatic.
- MRI may be better at identifying early loss of articular cartilage, but this and other imaging modalities have not been well validated for the evaluation of osteoarthritis.
- Laboratory tests (including synovial fluid analysis) may be useful to exclude other causes of joint pain, such as pseudogout.
- There are potential markers of tissue destruction and inflammation that may be of use clinically in the future. A profile of several markers with genetic analysis may in the future provide an individual assessment for disease development and response to therapy. Examples of markers include:
  - cartilage oligomeric matrix protein (COMP);
  - pyridinoline and bone sialoprotein;
  - metalloproteinases;
  - hylauronan.

The management of osteoarthritis

Successful management

Successful management centres on:
- A good history:
  - symptoms and impact on life;
  - functional disability;
  - functional requirements;
  - patient expectations;
  - psychological factors.
- A good examination:
  - extent of abnormality;
  - origin of pain;
  - degree of inflammation;
  - instability of joint;
  - muscle condition;
  - other medical, soft-tissue, and neurological disease.
- A multi-disciplinary approach. NICE have produced guidelines for management of OA in adults that emphasizes a holistic approach tailored to the patient's specific needs.[1] NICE identifies CORE treatments that should be offered to all patients, in addition to use of pharmacological and adjunctive treatments based on patient need.

Modalities for management

- Exercise is an important intervention, to build muscle strength, encourage weight loss, and improve endurance and joint proprioception.
- Advice alone is not as good as a specific program with follow-up.
- In more marked disease, support splints and walking aids, or other assistive devices may be necessary.
- Education has been shown in meta-analyses to have a significant effect on pain and function, but only 20% as effective as NSAID treatment.
- Weight management is a core treatment.
- Transcutaneous nerve stimulation (TENS) is recommended by NICE, although the evidence for long-term effectiveness of other treatments, such as acupuncture is poor and its use is not supported by NICE.
- Analgesia can be effective. Initial therapy should be with paracetamol in a regular dose of 1 g four times daily, with topical non-steroidal anti-inflammatory drugs (NSAIDs) used first in preference to oral NSAIDs, COX-2 inhibitors, or opioids. Topical capsaicin is also recommended.
- If the above are ineffective, then opioid or combination paracetamol/opioid preparations should be considered.
- NSAIDs/COX-2 inhibitors may be more effective in some cases, and may be of use for short periods during disease flares. NICE guidance emphasizes using them for the shortest time possible at the lowest dose, and with caution in older patients.

---

1 NICE (2008). *Clinical Guideline 59. Osteoarthritis: Care and management of osteoarthritis in adults.* London: NICE.

- Intra-articular injections of corticosteroids are very useful in treating disease flares with pain, and may result in sustained symptom improvement, although response duration is variable. There is no requirement to inject corticosteroid into a joint with an asymptomatic effusion. Many practitioners also add local anaesthetic, although there is no clear evidence that this improves the efficacy of the treatment. Most data is available for knee OA. Infection is rare (<1 in 10 000 incidence), but care should be taken to clean overlying skin, and injection through infected/psoriatic skin should be avoided. Other side effects to warn patients about are skin depigmentation and fat atrophy. It is advised that patients receive no more than 3 or 4 injections per year (☐ Chapter 22, p 589).
- The efficacy of intra-articular injection of hyaluronic acid derivatives (visco-supplementation) is controversial, although it may provide prolonged relief in some cases.
- Glucosamine and chondroitin sulphate are found in articular cartilage. Study evidence suggests that when given as oral supplements (glucosamine sulphate 1500 mg daily ± chondroitin sulphate) these agents have an analgesic effect in mild-to-moderate OA of the knee. There is little evidence for use in OA at other sites. NICE has not recommended use on prescription, although many primary and secondary care doctors would advise patients to obtain over-the-counter supplies for a period of 3 months to assess efficacy.
- There is some evidence that avocado/soybean unsaponifiable (ASU) supplementation, evening primrose oil, and omega-3 fish oils improve pain.
- The clinician should also seek ways to reduce the impact of disability. Options include:
  - occupational therapy: splints, tools, safe environment;
  - treat depression, anxiety, fibromyalgia;
  - coping strategies—behavioural therapy;
  - patient education.
- Arthroscopy and lavage/debridement should be offered only to those patients with knee OA who describe a clear history of mechanical locking, rather than giving way.
- For patients with activity-limiting significant osteoarthritis, joint replacement is effective in reducing pain, although function may not be restored. This approach requires good communication between health professionals and the patient to ensure that any referral to a surgeon is appropriate and reflects patient need.

Future therapeutic strategies

Research is focused not only with improving symptoms and outcome in OA, but developing disease modifying treatments with the hope of preventing ongoing joint damage. Approaches include:

• Inhibition of RANK ligand-mediated subchondral bone resorption using monoclonal antibodies.
• Bisphosphonates as anti-resorptive agents.
• Inhibition of cathepsin K, a potent protease involved in degradation of type I collagen in bone matrix.
• Large vitamin D supplementation studies are yet to be carried out.
• Diacerein, an IL-1 blocker, has been shown to reduce metalloproteinase production in knee OA subchondral bone osteoblasts. Further *in vivo* studies need to be performed.

The crystal arthropathies

The crystal arthropathies include gout, calcium pyrophosphate deposition disease (CPPD) or pseudogout, basic calcium phosphate (BCP) associated syndromes, and calcium oxalate arthritis.

Gout and hyperuricaemia

Epidemiology of gout

- In its most general sense, gout is a group of conditions characterized by hyperuricaemia and uric acid crystal formation. These clinical conditions include arthritis, tophaceous gout, uric acid nephrolithiasis, and gouty nephropathy. In its more commonly assumed definition, gout refers to the acute inflammatory arthropathy caused by uric acid crystal deposition.
- Gout is a relatively common condition, and is the most common form of inflammatory arthritis. In the UK 250 000 people per year consult their General Practitioner with a diagnosis of gout. Prevalence data from the United States on self-reported disease show figures of 13.6 per 1000 persons in adult men and 6.4 per 1000 persons for women. It is more common in the middle aged and elderly, and the prevalence may be increasing due to changes in lifestyle and diet.
- The risk factors for gout mirror those for hyperuricaemia, and are shown in Table 7.1.

The clinical features of gout

- The first stage of the condition is usually asymptomatic hyperuricaemia.
- Clinically, the first symptom is most often an acute, self-limiting, monoarticular inflammatory arthritis; up to 60–70% of attacks first occur in the big toe ('podagra'). Other frequently involved joints include the ankle, foot, knee, wrist, elbow (olecranon bursa), and the small joints of the hands. The axial large joints and spine are rarely involved. Some 70–80% of individuals will have recurrent attacks within 2 years.
- In the later stages of untreated disease, acute attacks are more often polyarticular, with shorter periods of remission, joint damage and deformity; these later stages are associated with loss of mobility, chronic pain, and formation of tophi (Plate 6).
- Tophi are deposits of urate embedded in a matrix composed of lipids, proteins, and calcific debris. Tophi are usually subcutaneous, but rarely occur in bone and other organs, such as the eye. The classic sites for tophi are the pinna of the ear, and bursa of the elbow and knee, Achilles tendon, and the dorsal surface of the MCP joints. Tophi are usually painless, although the overlying skin may ulcerate and become infected. Those most at risk of tophi are patients with prolonged severe hyperuricaemia, polyarticular gout, and the elderly with primary nodal OA (◻ Chapter 6, p 259) on diuretics.
- Hyperuricaemia by itself does not confirm a diagnosis of gout. Some clinicians will treat asymptomatic hyperuricaemia to prevent the onset of 'urate nephropathy', but this is controversial.

Table 7.1 The causes of hyperuricaemia and risk factors for gout

Primary gout	Male gender
	Age <40 years
	Obesity
	Family history
	Alcohol use and purine rich foods
	Renal insufficiency
	Hypertension
Inherited metabolic syndromes	X-linked HPRT deficiency (Lesch–Nyhan), X-linked raised PRPP synthetase activity. Autosomal recessive G6P deficiency (von Gierke's disease)
Uric acid overproduction	Cell lysis–tumour lysis syndrome, myeloproliferative disease, haemolytic anaemia, psoriasis, trauma; Drugs–alcohol, cytotoxic drugs, warfarin
Uric acid under-excretion	Renal failure
	Drugs–alcohol, salicylates, diuretics, laxatives, ciclosporin, levodopa, ethambutol, pyrazinamide
Lead toxicity	Renal impairment and altered purine turnover

HPRT = hypoxanthine guanine phosphoribosyl transferase—a salvage enzyme converting hypoxanthine back to precursors and therefore competing with its conversion to xanthine and then uric acid. PRPP = phosphoribosylpyrophosphate synthetase—a component enzyme in purine ring synthesis. G6P = glucose 6 phosphatase. G6P deficiency leads to increased activity of amido phosphoribosyl transferase and purine formation.

Investigation of gout

- Synovial fluid analysis remains the single most important diagnostic study. The diagnosis is made by the presence of typical, negatively birefringent, needle-shaped crystals seen with a polarized light microscope. The crystals may be extra- or intracellular. The absence of crystals does not rule out the diagnosis.
- Serum uric acid levels may be normal during an acute attack and may not reflect pre-attack levels. They cannot be used to exclude the diagnosis during an acute attack. Uric acid levels are of value in assessing the patient once the acute attack has subsided, either to establish the presence of hyperuricaemia or to monitor the effectiveness of therapies that lower serum urate.
- Radiographs are often normal during the early phase of the disease, except for the presence of soft tissue swelling. They are, however, useful for excluding other conditions such as trauma or infection (Table 7.2). Later in the disease, radiographs may demonstrate tophi near joints, tissue swelling, joint erosions, periosteal new bone formation, and joint deformity. Once these changes occur, gout may be misdiagnosed as RA (📖 Chapter 5, p 233) in some cases.
- Causes of hyperuricaemia should always be considered.

Table 7.2 Clinical conditions that can mimic gouty arthritis

CPPD disease (pseudogout)
BCP arthritis
Cellulitis
Infectious arthritis
Trauma
Rheumatoid arthritis
Psoriatic arthritis
Erythema nodosum
Reactive arthritis

The management of gouty arthritis

- The efficacy of any public health improvement measure for the prevention of gout is yet to be proven. It is reasonable to suggest that avoiding excess weight gain and alcohol, controlling hypertension, and avoiding exposure to diuretics and lead, may have some effect on decreasing the incidence of the condition.
- The management of gout should be seen as two phases: treatment of the acute attack, and treatment of chronic or tophaceous gout. The principal therapies for acute gout are NSAIDs, colchicine, and steroids. Many treatments are empiric, rather than evidence based.
- Traditionally indometacin has been the NSAID of choice in acute gout, but has no advantage over other NSAIDs or Coxibs. With treatment, symptoms should subside within 3–5 days.
- NSAIDs are contraindicated in renal insufficiency and should be used with caution in the elderly (who are often also taking aspirin) or those with GI risk factors. Evidence shows that NSAIDs decrease pain, swelling, and duration of attack.
- Colchicine can be very effective in acute gout, with a rapid onset of action. Oral colchicine, given at 0.5 mg bd for 5 days is very useful and can be well tolerated. It is often given in addition to NSAIDs (although there is no evidence to support this) or where NSAIDs are contraindicated. The 5-day dosage may be repeated for an acute attack after 72 h. Colchicine (iv) is not used due to the potential for bone marrow suppression. There are no randomized controlled trials comparing colchicine to NSAIDs.
- The true efficacy of oral and im corticosteroids in acute gout remains to be proven. Steroid regimens range from oral prednisone at tapering doses from 20–50 mg daily for an average of 10 days, to im triamcinolone 60 mg once only. A study comparing im triamcinolone with indometacin found no significant difference in time to recovery. Intra-articular steroids are useful if only one or two joints are affected.

In a case series from 1999, injection of triamcinolone acetonide into affected joints resolved all symptoms within 48 h.

- Corticosteroids should not be used if there is a possibility of septic arthritis.
- Drugs that decrease serum uric acid levels are the standard therapy for prophylaxis against repeated gout attacks, but should not be started after just one isolated attack. Allopurinol, a xanthine oxidase inhibitor, is the drug most commonly used, and the drug of choice in the presence of renal insufficiency, nephrolithiasis, or tophi. It should not be started during an acute attack of gout, as it is likely to make the situation worse. Equally, it should not be stopped during an attack if already on it.
- Allopurinol is usually given as a once daily dose of 300 mg. Patients, however, may require doses anywhere between 100 and 900 mg daily to achieve normal serum uric acid levels (i.e. < 5 mg/dL). The dose should be adjusted down in renal impairment. The onset of action of allopurinol is rapid, with effects seen as early as 4 days to 2 weeks.
- The most common side-effect of allopurinol is a hypersensitivity reaction with rash and fever. Rarely a severe reaction is seen with hepatitis, nephritis, and toxic epidermal necrolysis. In mild to moderate intolerance allopurinol can be reintroduced at very low levels, e.g. 10 mg, and built up slowly using desensitization regimens. Allopurinol can interfere with the metabolism of azathioprine and warfarin, augmenting their potential side-effects. During its introduction a patient may also experience an acute flare of gout. This may be treated with NSAIDs and/or low dose colchicine.
- Some patients may respond to a combination of allopurinol and a uricosuric agent (such as probenecid) when either alone has been ineffective. Uricosuric drugs should be avoided in patients with renal insufficiency or history of nephrolithiasis.
- Febuxostat is a non-purine xanthine oxidase inhibitor recently licensed in the UK. It appears to be more effective than allopurinol, and may be especially appropriate for patients who are allergic to allopurinol or have severe renal insufficiency.
- In patients who are unable to take allopurinol or a uricosuric drug, daily low-dose oral colchicine may be useful in preventing attacks. It is usually given in doses of 0.5 mg po once/twice daily. Serious side effects can still occur at this dose. This low-dose regimen may also be useful as prophylaxis against acute flares during the introduction of allopurinol.
- Fenofibrate is an established treatment for many lipid disorders. It also has the ability to decrease serum urate by increasing renal uric acid clearance. It may have a role (off label) in patients resistant or intolerant to other agents. It should be avoided in hepatic and biliary disease, hypothyroidism and pregnancy. Side-effects may include arthralgias and myalgias.
- Sulfinpyrazone is a uricosuric agent. It alters renal handling of urate by increasing urine excretion. Although effective and well tolerated, it is contraindicated in patients with renal stones and ineffective in those with renal insufficiency.

- Benzbromarone is another uricosuric agent available in Europe. It is effective in patients with renal insufficiency. Liver function must be monitored for drug-induced hepatitis; fulminant liver failure has been described.
- Patients with uric acid stones are best managed with adequate hydration, urinary alkalization, and allopurinol. This regimen is also effective in preventing calcium oxalate stones.
- Finally, gouty tophi may be amenable to surgical removal.

Calcium pyrophosphate dihydrate disease

- CPPD disease is the second most common form of crystal arthropathy. Our understanding of the pathophysiology of CPPD remains rudimentary, and consequently no specific therapies for this arthropathy exist.
- Several clinical syndromes are associated with CPPD; the features of the condition are heterogeneous, sometimes mimicking other rheumatic conditions. Definite associations with CPPD and chondrocalcinosis (i.e. calcification of fibro- and hyaline cartilage typically at the knee and wrist) include:
  - hypomagnesaemia
  - hypophosphatasia
  - haemochromatosis
  - Wilson's disease
  - hyperparathyroidism.
- Possible associations include:
  - gout;
  - ochronosis;
  - hypocalciuric hypercalcaemia;
  - diabetes mellitus;
  - X-linked hypophosphataemic rickets.
- These crystals are also found in the synovial fluid of patients with both acute and chronic arthritis. They are associated with advanced age, chondrocalcinosis, and a characteristic pattern of severe joint degeneration.
- There are several presentations of CPPD that afford at least some form of classification based on clinical features. It is not easy to categorize all cases, but the classification serves to point out the heterogeneity of the condition in acute, chronic, inflammatory, and non-inflammatory arthritis (Tables 7.3 and 7.4).

Laboratory investigations

- CPPD disease is defined by the presence of positively birefringent, rhomboid crystals on examination of synovial fluid under polarized light microscopy. The crystals may be intra- or extracellular.
- Radiographs of the affected joints may not be helpful in establishing the diagnosis. The presence of chondrocalcinosis increases the likelihood of CPPD disease. Radiographic clues that may help to distinguish CPPD from OA include:
  - axial involvement;
  - sacroiliac erosions;
  - cortical erosions of the femur;
  - osteonecrosis of the medial femoral condyle.
- Patients under the age of 60 years should be screened for secondary CPPD disease, i.e. serum calcium, magnesium, alkaline phosphatase, ferritin, iron, and iron binding capacity.

Table 7.3 The clinical presentations of CPPD disease

Type	Description	Frequency	Features
A	Pseudogout	25%	Acute pain and swelling, often a monoarthropathy of the knee, wrist, or shoulder. Rare in small joints
B	Pseudorheumatoid	5%	Polyarthritis. Synovitis. Joint flares out of phase with each other
C and D	Pseudo-osteoarthritis: C with attacks D without acute attacks	50%	Acute attacks on chronic symptoms
E	Asymptomatic	Unknown	Incidental chondrocalcinosis
F	Pseudoneurotrophic	Rare	Severe joint destruction neuropathy
Others	Tophaceous CPPD deposits		
	Spinal CPPD: 'Crowned dens syndrome' deposits around the atlantoaxial joint. Spinal stenosis. Cervical myelopathy		
	Tendon and bursa deposits		

Management of CPPD disease

- NSAIDs are the most commonly used therapy, but must be used with caution as the majority of affected patients are elderly.
- Joint aspiration and intra-articular corticosteroids are of benefit in acute flares of pseudogout. The role of oral steroids remains unclear.
- Low-dose oral colchicine (0.5 mg bd) may reduce the frequency of acute attacks in pseudogout.
- Rest, splinting, and eventual joint replacement may be helpful.
- Other therapies that have been tried include:
  - oral magnesium carbonate;
  - intra-articular glycosaminoglycan polysulfate;
  - intra-articular ^{90}yttrium and corticosteroid;
  - im gold or hydroxychloroquine for type B ('pseudorheumatoid') disease.

Table 7.4 Factors that may trigger acute pseudogout

Intercurrent illness, e.g. chest infection
Direct trauma to the joint
Surgery, especially parathyroidectomy
Blood transfusion and parenteral fluids
Institution of thyroxine replacement therapy
Joint lavage

Basic calcium phosphate associated disease

- Basic calcium phosphate (BCP) crystals include hydroxyapatite, octacalcium phosphate, and tri-calcium phosphate.
- These crystals are associated with several rheumatic conditions as shown in Table 7.5.
- The treatment of these conditions is as per CPPD disease (see ⬚ Calcium pyrophosphate dehydrate associated disease, p 276), with NSAIDs and colchicine principally.

Table 7.5 BCP associated conditions

Articular disease	Milwaukee shoulder syndrome (severe degenerative arthropathy, more common on the dominant side and in elderly women)
	Osteoarthritis (synovial fluid crystals found in up to 60% of OA patients)
	Erosive arthritis
	Mixed crystal deposition
Peri-articular	Pseudopodagra, calcific tendonitis and bursitis

Calcium oxalate arthritis

- This is an unusual form of arthritis. The crystals are positively birefringent and bipyramidal on polarized light microscopy.
- Radiographs and laboratory tests are not diagnostic.
- Treatment is as for CPPD disease.
- Several conditions are associated with calcium oxalate arthritis (Table 7.6).

Table 7.6 Conditions associated with calcium oxalate arthritis

End-stage renal disease on dialysis
Short bowel syndrome
Diet rich in rhubarb, spinach, ascorbic acid
Thiamine deficiency
Pyridoxine deficiency
Primary oxalosis: • Recessive trait • Early renal failure (age 20s) • Arthritis • Tendonitis

The spondyloarthropathies

Introduction

- The seronegative spondyloarthropathies are classically characterized by the following:
  - Sacroiliitis;
  - inflammatory back pain;
  - enthesitis.
- These diseases may also be accompanied by:
  - asymmetric peripheral arthritis;
  - extra-articular disease;
  - anterior uveitis.
- The group is made up of several conditions that often overlap. These are:
  - ankylosing spondylitis;
  - juvenile enthesitis-related arthritis;
  - psoriatic arthritis;
  - reactive arthropathy;
  - enteropathic arthritis;
  - undifferentiated spondylitis.
- The undifferentiated conditions include subsets of cases where features such as dactylitis, uveitis, or sacroiliitis exist without the full criteria for a diagnosis.
- Some physicians suggest that other diseases that may be associated with sacroiliitis should also be classified as spondyloarthropathies. These diseases include Whipple's disease and Synovitis-Acne-Pustulosis-Hyperostosis-Osteomyelitis (SAPHO) syndrome.
- Pathological changes are mainly at the insertion of tendons and ligaments into bone (i.e. enthesis), and extra-articular changes may also develop in the eye, aortic valve, lung, and skin.

Diagnostic criteria and clinical subsets

There is a general consensus that most criteria are too restricted given the wide spectrum of disease. For example, radiographic evidence of sacroiliitis in the absence of symptoms, or unilateral sacroiliitis with only dactylitis or uveitis, would be excluded by most criteria and yet could be part of the spondyloarthropathy spectrum. Criteria with acceptable sensitivity and specificity are shown in Table 8.1.

A variety of symptoms and signs are present and Table 8.2 highlights the differences between these conditions.

The specific expression of disease is a product of inter-related genetic and environmental factors. The precise link between triggers such as infection and pathogenesis, and the exact role of the HLA B27 molecule remains a mystery.

The HLA B27 molecule has an association with the spondyloarthropathies ranging between 50 and 95%. Interpretation of a positive result is complicated by the presence of this allele of the *HLA B* gene in up to 5–10% of the normal population. It may be useful to assess symptomatic first-degree relatives of HLA B27+ probands with ankylosing spondylitis (AS), for whom the risk of developing the same disease is approximately 1 in 3. However, most physicians would not advocate the routine use of this marker.

There are, however, a number of interesting observations in the study of HLA B27, which include the following:

I. HLA B27 is inherited as an autosomal co-dominant characteristic: 50% of first-degree relatives of probands with HLA B27 possess the antigen.

II. 5–10% of HLA B27 positive individuals develop AS over time and 20% of individuals with B27 develop a reactive arthropathy after contact with agents such as chlamydia or salmonella.

III. Only 50% of patients with psoriatic or enteropathic spondylitis are HLA B27 positive.

IV. Only 50% of non-Caucasians with AS are HLA B27 positive. This is considerably less than the prevalence of HLA B27 among Caucasians with AS (95%).

V. Relatives of probands with both sacroiliitis and HLA B27 frequently remain disease free.

VI. Concordance in identical twins is 70% vs 13% in non-identical twins.

VII. Uveitis is a common accompaniment of AS. HLA B27 is found in up to 40% of cases of uveitis, even in the absence of underlying rheumatic disease.

Table 8.1 Criteria for diagnosing spondyloarthropathies (Amor 1991)

Symptom(s)	Points
Clinical symptoms or past history of:	
1 Lumbar or dorsal pain at night or morning stiffness of the same areas	1
2 Asymmetrical oligoarthropathy	2
3 Alternating buttock pain	1
4 Dactylitis—sausage-like fingers or toes	2
5 Well-defined enthesopathic pain	2
6 Iritis	2
7 Non-gonococcal urethritis/cervicitis within 1 month of onset of arthritis	1
8 Acute diarrhoea within 1 month of onset of arthritis	1
9 Presence or history of psoriasis or inflammatory bowel disease	2
Radiological finding:	
10 Sacroiliitis	3
Genetic background:	
11 Presence of HLA B27 and/or family history of ankylosing spondylitis, reactive arthritis, uveitis, psoriasis, or chronic colitis	2
Response to treatment:	
12 Clear-cut improvement with NSAIDs	2

A patient is considered as having a spondyloarthropathy if the sum of the points is >6.

Reference: Amor B *et al. Ann Med Intern* 1991; **142**: 85–89.

Table 8.2 Comparison of the seronegative spondyloarthropathies

Feature	AS	REA	PsA	EA
Sex	>M	M=F	>F	M=F
Age onset (years)	20–30	Any age	Any age	Any age
Onset	Gradual	Sudden	Variable	Gradual
% HLA B27 positive	95		20 (50 if sacroiliac disease is present)	
Sacroiliitis	Always	Often	Often	Often
Peripheral joint disease	Lower limb > upper	Usually lower limb	Usually lower limb	Usually lower limb
Enthesitis	Present	Present	Present	Present
Uveitis	Common	Not common	Not common	Not common
Conjunctivitis	Not seen	Not common	Not seen	Not seen
Urethritis	Not seen	Rare	Not seen	Not seen
Skin disease	Not seen	Rare	Very common	Rare
Mucosal disease	Not seen	Not seen	Not seen	Not common

AS, ankylosing spondylitis; REA, reactive arthritis; PsA, psoriatic arthritis; EA, enteropathic arthropathy.

Ankylosing spondylitis

Epidemiology

- Few clinicians rely solely on the criteria; most would consider the diagnosis of ankylosing spondylitis (AS) in any case of symptomatic inflammatory back pain with radiographic evidence of sacroiliitis. The criteria for AS are shown in Table 8.3.
- The difficulty comes in recognizing early disease or subtle radiological change. There is often an insidious onset of back pain and morning stiffness that tends to improve with exercise. Occasionally, sacroiliitis is a chance finding in the absence of pain. More sophisticated investigations than the plain pelvic radiograph, such as magnetic resonance imaging, can detect early disease when X-rays are normal. Use of these imaging modalities should only be used in those with suspicious symptoms or signs of spondyloarthropathy.
- Patients are typically <40 years of age with a male to female ratio of approximately 3:1.
- The condition occurs more frequently in Caucasian populations. In American Indians, where HLA B27 prevalence is high, AS is particularly frequent, whereas the condition is less common in African-Americans, and rarer still in Sub-Saharan Africans, reflecting the declining prevalence of HLA B27 in these groups.
- Prevalence estimates in Caucasians range from 0.5 to 0.8 per 100 000 population in adults. This may be an underestimate as people with mild symptoms may not seek medical advice.
- As previously stated, HLA B27 typing has led to greater understanding of the spondyloarthropathies, but should not be considered a diagnostic test or necessary for the diagnosis of AS. Up to 5% of Caucasian patients with AS are negative for HLA B27.

Clinical features of AS

- The principal feature of the condition and allied diseases is *enthesitis*, i.e. fibrosis and ossification of ligament, tendon, and capsule insertions into bone (the entheses), mainly in the region of the discs and sacroiliac joints.
- Synovitis also occurs, typically in the larger peripheral joints (hips and knees in particular). 20–40% of patients have some degree of peripheral joint disease at some stage during their illness, in women more so than men. Approximately 50% of patients with adult AS will develop hip arthritis and some of these will need surgery.
- The standardized mortality ratio is 1.5; this increased mortality is due to cardiac valve and respiratory disease, amyloidosis, and fractures.
- Like other forms of chronic disease, AS patients have a significant risk of having to alter or give up work.
- Although recognized as typical of AS, few patients progress to the classical late 'bamboo spine'. When the spine does fuse (with 'syndesmophytes' bridging the gap between vertebral bodies) microfractures can occur leading to acute episodes of severe pain and spondylodiscitis, a term given to collapse of the vertebral end-plate and destruction of the disc–bone border. This process is usually

self-limiting, requiring rest and analgesia for up to 3 weeks. Most spinal disease is limited to chronic low-grade pain and stiffness with clinical evidence of a symmetrical reduction in spinal mobility.

- Patients may have insertional tendonitis at several other common sites including the Achilles tendon, intercostal muscles, plantar fascia, forearm flexor insertion into the lateral elbow epicondyle, and dactylitis of the hands and feet.

Table 8.3 Diagnostic criteria: Modified New York Criteria

Clinical criteria

- Low back pain and stiffness for >6 months, improving with exercise, but not relieved by rest

- Limitation of lumbar spine movements in sagittal and frontal planes

- Limitation of chest expansion relative to normal values for age and sex

Radiological criteria

- Greater than or equal to Grade II bilateral sacroiliitis

- Grade III or IV unilateral sacroiliitis

Combined diagnostic criteria

- Definite AS if radiological and clinical criterion

- Probable AS if 3 clinical criteria or a radiological criterion without signs or symptoms satisfying the clinical criteria

---

Van der Linden *et al.* Evaluation of diagnostic criteria for ankylosing spondylitis: a proposal for modification of the New York Criteria. *Arth Rheum*, 1984; **27**: 361–368.

Extra-articular disease in AS

- Constitutional features of fatigue, weight loss, low-grade fever, and anaemia are common. Fatigue as opposed to pain or stiffness can be the most troublesome symptom for many patients.

- Iritis occurs in up to 40% of cases, but has little correlation with disease activity in the spine. There are no known triggers for this condition and although self-limiting, topical, or systemic steroids may be required in severe cases. Iritis is usually unilateral.

- Upper lobe, bilateral pulmonary fibrosis is a recognized feature of the disease. Occasionally, the fibrotic area is invaded by aspergillus with changes mimicking tuberculosis. Treatment of the fibrosis is not effective. Pleuritis can occur as a consequence of insertional tendonitis of the costosternal and costovertebral muscles. Fusion of the thoracic wall leads to rigidity and reduction in chest expansion. Ventilation is maintained by the diaphragm; however, there is a three-fold increased risk of death from a respiratory cause compared with the normal population.

- Cardiac involvement includes aortic incompetence, cardiomegaly, and conduction defects. Of the 20% of patients with aortic valve disease, the majority are clinically undetectable.

- Neurological complaints are not a feature of AS, although nerve root entrapment or spinal cord/cauda equina compression can occur as a result of spinal fusion or fractures.
- Primary renal involvement is uncommon and if present may be due to co-existent medical conditions, NSAID use, or renal amyloidosis.
- Osteoporosis is an under-recognized finding. Estimates of prevalence range from 20–60%, increasing with age and disease duration, and disease is largely confined to the axial skeleton. Bone density scanning may be inaccurate in the lumbar spine due to the presence of syndesmophytes late in disease. Studies suggest that bone loss occurs early and during the acute inflammatory stage of the disease and that further bone loss, long-term, is rarely seen. Micro-fractures may occur with trauma, but the classical vertebral compression and wedge fractures of osteoporosis are rarely seen. Further work needs to be done to establish the need for, and efficacy of, current osteoporosis therapies for patients with AS.

Investigations in AS

- There is little correlation between any of the inflammatory markers and disease activity or clinical symptoms.
- Radiological evaluation is the most helpful form of investigation. Plain anteroposterior view radiographs are of the most value, but may not show early changes, and interpretation of sacroiliac joint radiographs during adolescence is often difficult. A false positive result is common due to projection artifacts. Early changes include loss of the subchondral sclerotic line. Changes may initially be asymmetric. Later findings include the more classical findings of subchondral sclerosis, erosions, and finally ankylosis. Radionuclide scanning may be sensitive, but is non-specific and may be more confusing than helpful. CT provides excellent views of the SI joints (in exchange for a higher radiation dose). MRI may demonstrate joint erosions, and also bone oedema and fatty change in marrow which are not detected by CT or plain radiographs.
- The main radiological features of 'primary' AS and that associated with inflammatory bowel disease are:
  - symmetrical sacroiliac changes;
  - ascending spread of disease;
  - facet joint involvement;
  - squaring of vertebrae;
  - syndesmophytes;
  - ossification;
  - osteitis pubis.
- It is said that AS associated reactive arthritis or psoriatic arthropathy (PsA), i.e. secondary AS, tends to differ in being far less severe radiologically, with often asymmetrical sacroiliac disease and random spinal involvement.
- It is important to differentiate syndesmophytes from osteophytes. Syndesmophytes are vertical; osteophytes are horizontal and occur in association with disc-space narrowing.
- AS should be distinguished from diffuse idiopathic skeletal hyperostosis (DISH). The two conditions are compared in Table 8.4.

Table 8.4 Differentiating diffuse idiopathic skeletal hyperostosis (DISH) and ankylosing spondylitis (AS)

Feature	DISH	AS
Age of onset (years)	Usually >50	Usually <40
Kyphosis	No	Yes
Reduced mobility	Occasionally	Very often
Pain	Common	Very common
Reduced chest expansion	No	Common
Radiological findings:		
Hyperostosis	Yes	Yes
Sacroiliac joint erosions	No	Yes
ALL ossification	Yes—common	No
PLL ossification	Yes—occasionally	No
Syndesmophytes	No	Very common
Erosive enthesitis	No	Very common
Non-erosive enthesitis	Very common	Common

ALL, anterior longitudinal ligament; PLL, posterior longitudinal ligament.

Disease status and prognostic indicators in AS

- There are validated self-administered instruments defining disease status in AS. Since one lacks the advantage of valuable laboratory tests, it is helpful that there is a good correlation between the self-reporting of symptoms and observed clinical status of patients with AS.
- Instruments for assessing disease status include indices produced by the Royal National Hospital for Rheumatic Diseases, Bath, UK, namely The Bath Ankylosing Spondylitis Functional Index BASFI), Disease Activity Index ASDAI), Metrology Index BASMI), and Radiology Index BASRI) (see Table 8.5). Several of these disease status scores are used in the UK for determining the introduction of anti-TNF-α therapy.
- It is difficult to define outcome for individual patients when considering prognosis. The main predictive factors of poor outcome in AS appear to be:
  - early hip involvement;
  - an ESR >30;
  - poor initial response to NSAIDs;
  - early loss of lumbar spine mobility;
  - presence of dactylitis;
  - oligoarticular disease;
  - onset <16 years;
  - low social–educational background;
  - sporadic disease rather than familial.

The treatment of ankylosing spondylitis

- General principles include the following:
  - patient education;
  - exercise;
  - physical therapy and hydrotherapy;
  - avoid smoking;
  - NSAIDs for spinal disease;
  - self-help groups.
- Emphasis is placed on the need to maintain posture and physical activity. Extension exercises are important as the natural history of the disease is towards flexion and loss of height. Physiotherapy and rehabilitation provide benefit in the short-term, but it remains unclear as to the benefits in the long-term. Spa treatment has been shown to improve function for up to 9 months, with subsequent reduction in health resource use. Spa therapy is expensive and not widely available.
- Fatigue may be a major concern, hampering exercise. In some cases, low-dose amitriptyline (📖 Chapter 21, p 545) at night may ameliorate this problem.
- For the majority of patients, NSAIDs remain the treatment of choice. The majority will be taking diclofenac or naproxen. Indometacin was widely used, but less so now because of its gastrointestinal side effects.
- Continuous, rather than intermittent NSAID (including COX-2 inhibitors) has been shown to slow radiographic progression of axial arthritis, but this did lead to an increase in adverse events, so patients on regular treatment should be reviewed regularly.
- Sulfasalazine (📖 Chapter 21, p 545) has been shown in meta-analysis to be efficacious when compared with placebo for peripheral joint disease only. However, improvement in symptoms and quality of life is often not dramatic, and sulfasalazine has a small role to play, perhaps mainly in peripheral inflammatory disease.
- Mixed results have been found with MTX. A Cochrane meta-analysis concluded that there is insufficient evidence to support the use of MTX. Benefit may be limited to patients with peripheral disease.
- Joint inflammation can be managed in acute, severe cases with intra-articular corticosteroids, as can dactylitis and tendonitis by local steroid infiltration. Care should be taken injecting around tendons, as rupture can occur. Injection around the Achilles tendon is not recommended. Systemic steroids are rarely used, although there is evidence that low dose iv therapy can produce a short-lived improvement in symptoms.
- NICE guidance has approved infliximab, etanercept and adalimumab (📖 Chapter 21, p 545) for use in patients with AS who satisfy the modified New York criteria, have a BASDAI score of at least 4 and a VAS pain score of at least 4–10 cm on 2 occasions, 12 weeks apart with no change in treatment **and** in whom conventional treatment with 2 or more NSAIDs at maximal tolerated doses for at least 4 weeks has failed to control symptoms. There is no requirement for use of MTX or other DMARDs.[1] Treatment should be assessed after 12 weeks.

1 NICE Technology Appraisal Guidance 143: Adalimumab, etanercept and adalimumab for ankylosing spondylitis. May 2008.

Table 8.5 Bath Ankylosing Spondylitis Disease Activity Index (BASDAI)

The assessment comprises 6 questions with an analogue score answer of 0 ('none') to 10 ('very severe') for each on a 10 cm scale.

The questions are:

1 How would you describe the overall level of fatigue/tiredness you have experienced?

2 How would you describe the overall level of AS neck, back, or hip pain you have had?

3 How would you describe the overall level of pain/swelling in joints other than neck, back, or hips you have had?

4 How would you describe the overall level of discomfort you have had from any areas tender to touch or pressure?

5 How would you describe the overall level of discomfort you have had from the time you wake up?

6 How long does your morning stiffness last from the time you wake up? (for this score the 10-cm scale is divided evenly so that 30 min lies at 2.5 cm, 1 h at 5 cm, 1.5 h at 7.5 cm, and 2 or more hours at 10 cm).

The score is calculated by adding each of the measures for question 1–4 to the mean of the sum of questions 5 and 6, and then dividing the whole by 5. The maximum score therefore is 10.

- Infliximab is given at a higher dose of 5 mg/kg (compared with 3 mg/kg used in RA). Etanercept and adalimumab are given in the same doses as RA.
- All TNF-α blockers reduce symptoms and spinal inflammation as seen on MRI, but larger and longer studies are needed to assess the effect on disease progression.
- Inevitably some patients require joint replacement, most commonly at the hip. Response to such surgery is usually excellent provided there are no major peri-articular contractures secondary to ankylosis. Surgery for spinal deformity is possible, but carries considerable anaesthetic and surgical risk and should be carried out in specialist centres.
- Topical steroid eye drops should be used to treat uveitis. If the symptoms persist for more than 3 days an ophthalmological opinion should be sought. Infliximab and etanercept have been used to treat resistant iritis.
- Any associated psoriasis, inflammatory bowel disease, or concern over reactive inflammation secondary to an infection should be treated accordingly.
- There is no treatment for pulmonary fibrosis associated with AS. Given the added potential concern of reduced chest expansion, patients should be advised not to smoke in an attempt to avoid further lung disease.
- Nevertheless, it is important to remember that the majority of patients have minimal functional impairment despite their disease, and lead full, active lives.

Psoriatic arthritis

Epidemiology and clinical features

- The association between psoriasis and an inflammatory arthropathy is well-recognized. It may affect any peripheral joint, as well as the axial skeleton and sacroiliac joints. Epidemiological studies support the notion of a distinct disease as opposed to the random finding of co-existing common conditions such as psoriasis and RA. Psoriasis affects 1–2% of the population, and 10% of these develop arthritis.

- The condition affects women and men equally, usually between the ages of 20–40.

- RF can be present in up to 10% of patients with psoriasis, 90% remaining seronegative, and most patients with psoriatic arthritis run a benign course. In about 20% of cases there is a chronic, progressive, and deforming arthropathy with an often asymmetrical pattern, including distal interphalangeal joint involvement, and specific radiological features that can distinguish it from RA.

- Nail lesions may be the only clinical feature that can identify patients with psoriasis destined to develop arthritis. These lesions occur in 90% of patients with psoriatic arthritis (PsA) and in 40% of patients with psoriasis alone. A comparison between PsA and RA (📖 Chapter 5, p 233) is made in Table 8.6. The joint symptoms most commonly occur after the diagnosis of psoriasis, but may pre-date or occur simultaneously in a minority.

- The clinical patterns of psoriatic arthritis are:
  - distal, involving the distal interphalangeal joints (DIP);
  - asymmetric oligoarthritis;
  - symmetrical polyarthritis, indistinguishable from RA;
  - spondylarthropathy.

- Arthritis mutilans is a classic but uncommon manifestation of psoriatic arthritis. Bone resorption leads to collapse of the soft tissue in the digits, creating 'telescoping fingers'. This can also be seen in severe RA.

- The radiological features associated with PsA that help to differentiate it from RA include:
  - absence of juxta-articular osteoporosis;
  - DIP disease;
  - 'whittling' (lysis) of terminal phalanges;
  - asymmetry;
  - 'pencil-in-cup' deformities;
  - ankylosis;
  - periostitis;
  - spondylitis.

- The patterns of arthritis may change over time in >60% of patients.

- It is not clear, however, if the patterns of disease have any prognostic significance and the changes and prognosis are variable.

- The frequency of spinal involvement can vary between 2% in isolated back disease, to 40%, when associated with peripheral arthritis.

- Dactylitis, swelling of the whole finger, occurs in over one-third of patients. Tenosynovitis and enthesitis are also common, particularly at the plantar fascia insertion and Achilles tendon.

Table 8.6 Comparison of psoriatic arthritis and rheumatoid arthritis

Feature	Psoriatic arthritis	Rheumatoid arthritis
Sex ratio	F = M	F>M
Symmetry of joint disease	Less common	Very common
DIP involvement	Common	Uncommon
Spine involvement	Common	Uncommon
Skin/nail changes	Common	Uncommon
Enthesopathy	Common	Uncommon
Ankylosis	Common	Uncommon
Osteopenia	Uncommon	Common

- Hyperuricaemia, probably related to high skin cell turnover, is not uncommon. In patients with psoriatic arthritis, the possibility of gout should be kept in mind.

Treatment of PsA

- This should include the treatment of the skin, as well as the joints and many patients are also under the care of a dermatologist.
- Patient education, physiotherapy, occupational therapy, and surgery all have a role to play akin to that already described above for RA and AS.
- Initial treatment in mild cases is with NSAIDs, adding a DMARD if inflammation and joint damage persist. Azathioprine, sulfasalazine, penicillamine, gold, and leflunomide may all be used with some effect; there are anecdotal reports of 'flares' of skin psoriasis with hydroxychloroquine (☐ Chapter 21, p 545). The most commonly used agent is MTX; it also can have a dramatically improving effect on the skin disease. Sulfasalazine may be more efficacious in those with both spinal and peripheral joint involvement.
- Oral and im steroids should be avoided, but intra-articular steroids may be used. Psoriatic plaques are colonized by bacteria, and injection through a plaque should be avoided for fear of introducing infection. Steroid taper may lead to a flare of pustular psoriasis.
- Etanercept, infliximab, and adalimumab are approved by NICE for the treatment of PSA and have positive effects on skin, as well as joint disease.[1] Patients need to have peripheral arthritis with 3 or more tender and swollen joints, *and* have not responded to at least two standard DMARDs alone or in combination. Doses are the same as those given in AS.
- Treatment should be assessed at 12 weeks using validated outcome measures such as the Psoriatic Arthritis Response Criteria (PSARC) measurements.

---

1 NICE Final appraisal determination. Etanercept, infliximab and adalimumab for the treatment of psoriatic arthritis (review of technology appraisal guidance 104 and 125), May 2010.

Reactive arthropathy

Clinical presentation

- Reactive arthritis is an aseptic inflammatory arthritis triggered by an infectious agent outside the joint. Risk of developing reactive arthritis is approximately 1–4%, and 20–25% in those who are HLA B27 positive.
- Spondyloarthropathies can be defined as 'reactive' if urethritis/cervicitis (sexually transmitted reactive arthritis—SARA) or diarrhoea (gut-associated reactive arthritis—GARA) are present. The features of the spondyloarthropathies can vary in the 'reactive' subgroup from one patient to another, and in the same patient at any given time in the course of the disease.
- The onset of reactive arthritis may be acute, with fever, weight loss, and diffuse polyarticular involvement. More often, however, there is limited joint synovitis and a low-grade, or absent fever.
- Mucocutaneous features include painless circinate balanitis of the glans penis, and pustular psoriasis of the palms or feet (keratoderma blennorhagica); these can be associated with a more severe outcome.
- Conjunctivitis is observed early. Uveitis is less frequent early in disease, often occurring in recurrent disease and between episodes of arthritis.
- Acute diarrhoea may precede the musculoskeletal symptoms by up to 1 month. The GI symptoms may be so mild as to be ignored by the patient and often the provoking agent has cleared from the gut before the joint symptoms arise. Several triggering agents have been isolated from stools and these include, *Shigella*, *Salmonella*, *Clostridium*, and *Yersinia*. Chronic diarrhoea does not appear to be associated with reactive arthritis. However, the demarcations can be blurred and some patients may have inflammatory bowel-associated arthropathies, or silent inflammatory lesions that appear to manifest as 'reactive-like' and are best described as undifferentiated spondyloarthropathy.
- Urethritis, prostatitis, or cervicitis may be present prompting suspicion of infection. Rigorous investigation is required to ensure pathogenic mycoplasma and ureaplasma are identified and eradicated. The most common non-gonococcal urethritis is due to *Chlamydia* (📕 Chapter 17, p 473).
- Recurrent or repeated infections do not always lead to a recurrence of arthritis and may occur in the absence of further sexual intercourse. There are some important differential diagnoses outside the spondyloarthropathies that include HIV-associated arthritis, Lyme disease, parvovirus arthropathies (📕 Chapter 17, p 473), and Behçet's disease (📕 Chapter 18, p 489).

Investigation and treatment of reactive arthritis

- The inflammatory nature of the condition can be confirmed by the presence of an elevated ESR and CRP. For therapeutic decisions in some cases, but mainly for epidemiological purposes, many tests can be done looking for a causative agent. Most screens are negative and in this sense there is merit in just taking a close history and limited investigation, rather than a full diagnostic work-up. If required, the clinician should request stool, urine, and blood cultures, urethral and vaginal swabs, and aspirate a swollen joint looking for cells, crystals (📖 Chapter 7, p 269), and infection. It may be helpful to enlist the expertise of colleagues in infectious diseases for the assessment of sexually acquired infections.
- The use of monoclonal antibodies, or DNA and RNA hybridization, in the search for products of triggering agents, is limited to research purposes. Likewise, tests for detecting antibodies to bacteria have no specific place in current clinical practice and do not have a predictive value on outcome.
- In the early stages of disease there are no radiological signs except in a very small number of cases where changes in the sacroiliac joints may be seen and probably pre-date presentation.
- There is no specific cure. NSAIDs and local corticosteroid injections are the mainstay of therapeutic intervention (📖 Chapter 21, p 545 and 📖 Chapter 22, p 589). If symptoms persist longer than 6 months and there is clinical evidence of ongoing synovitis and joint destruction then a disease-modifying agent, such as sulfasalazine, MTX, or azathioprine, should be considered.
- Taking account of all symptoms, the majority of patients are in complete remission at the end of 2 years, most within 6 months. The metatarsophalangeal joints and the heel often remain sites of persistent pain, and balanitis and keratoderma may persist, acting as markers of potential poorer prognosis. Other factors that may be predictive of poor outcome include oligoarthritis of the hip, persistently elevated ESR, B27 positivity, poor response to NSAIDs, dactylitis, and involvement of the lumbosacral spine.
- Aseptic urethritis and early conjunctivitis resolve quickly and spontaneously. Antibiotic therapy will clear underlying infections, but this may not have any effect on the duration of disease.
- Uveitis should be treated in the usual way with topical steroid drops and a referral to an ophthalmologist if there has been no response within 3 days.
- Patient education, particularly in the context of food hygiene and prevention of exposure to sexually-acquired infection, is important. Contact tracing is vital in cases of sexually transmitted infection.

Enteric arthropathy

Clinical presentation

- The arthropathies of ulcerative colitis and Crohn's disease have many similarities, and the combination of peripheral and axial skeletal disease, enthesopathies, mucocutaneous, and ocular disease fits neatly into the diagnostic realm of the spondylarthropathies.
- The exact pathology is unknown, but is thought to be due to impairment of the gut-mediated immunity and increased bowel permeability, allowing bacteria to pass through the bowel wall into the circulation.
- Mono- or asymmetrical oligoarthritis can be coincident with the onset of bowel disease or arise during the course of the disease. There is a close association between exacerbation of bowel and peripheral joint disorders, and enteropathic arthritis (EA) tends to remit after removal of diseased bowel tissue. The knees and ankles are most commonly involved.
- In contrast to peripheral arthritis, sacroiliitis is not clearly associated with either the onset or exacerbation of the bowel disease and may be present for years prior to the onset of colitis or ileitis.
- Other non-articular features to look for include:
  - uveitis (in about 10%);
  - erythema nodosum;
  - pyoderma gangrenosum;
  - aphthous stomatitis.
- Arthropathy associated with inflammatory bowel disease often improves with treatment of the bowel symptoms. Intra-articular steroids, azathioprine, sulfasalazine, and MTX can be used in resistant cases. NSAIDs should be used with caution as they can cause a flare of Crohn's disease. Anti-TNF-α therapies used in treatment of Crohn's disease may also improve joint symptoms.
- Enteric arthropathy may exist in patients with minimal or no gut symptoms. Presence of an asymmetric arthritis associated with oral ulcerations or erythema nodosum should trigger a colonoscopy with blind biopsies to evaluate for the presence of inflammatory bowel disease or Behçet's disease.

Spondyloarthropathies in childhood

Epidemiology and clinical presentation

- This umbrella term covers a heterogeneous group of diseases associated with HLA B27 that affect children under the age of 16 and produce a spectrum of symptoms in adulthood.
- The disease group includes:
  - enthesitis and arthritis syndrome;
  - juvenile ankylosing spondylitis;
  - juvenile reactive arthritis;
  - juvenile psoriatic arthritis (JPsA);
  - arthritis associated with inflammatory bowel disease
  - anterior uveitis.
- Using the International League of Associations for Rheumatology (ILAR) classification, the spectrum of diseases is called enthesitis-related arthritis (ERA).
- Incidence is estimated at 1.44 per 100 000 children. Prevalence has increased over the last 30 years.
- IgM RF and antinuclear antibodies are not found. 90% patients will be HLA B27 positive.
- The diagnosis is often more difficult in childhood as symptoms of back pain and radiological changes are uncommon. The diagnosis rests more often on the presence of lower limb large joint arthritis associated with enthesopathy, uveitis, psoriasis, or bowel pathology, and may be difficult to separate from JIA. The reader is referred to 📖 Chapter 9, p 303 for a description of the classification criteria for childhood arthropathies.
- Apart from an increased incidence of peripheral disease and rare axial symptoms, juvenile onset spondyloarthropathies resemble the adult forms. This lack of early axial disease may lead to initial misdiagnosis as oligoarticular JIA.
- The Rome and New York criteria for the diagnosis of adult AS have not been validated in children; nevertheless, a small proportion of children fit these criteria and are considered to have juvenile AS. Approximately 5–8% of children attending rheumatology clinics have AS. This compares with 75% having JIA. Juvenile AS commonly presents with lower limb large joint arthritis (often knees and ankles) with the early course often episodic. It also appears to differ from adult AS in the precocious destruction of the hip joint. The condition is reported more often in men than women, and 50% of cases go on to develop AS in adult life.
- Enthesitis and arthritis syndrome usually affects the feet and can be disabling. The disease is usually episodic, but some cases are chronic, resulting in bony erosions and joint ankylosis. Over 70% of patients with enthesitis syndrome will fulfill diagnostic criteria for AS after 5–10 years from onset.
- Childhood reactive arthritis and enteropathic arthropathy are essentially similar to adult disease.
- Treatment of ERA is with NSAIDs, adding DMARDs such as sulfasalazine or MTX in those with uncontrolled disease. Oral or iv steroids can be used to gain control in severe disease.

Juvenile spondyloarthropathy

- Juvenile spondyloarthropathy (JSpA) is defined in the ILAR criteria as either arthritis in the presence of psoriasis, or arthritis and at least 2 of:
  - dactylitis;
  - nail abnormalities (pitting or onycholysis);
  - family history of psoriasis confirmed by a dermatologist in at least one first-degree relative.
- The incidence of JSpA is estimated at 3 per 100 000, with a prevalence of 15 per 100 000.
- Oligo- or polyarthritis may occur and can affect large or small joints, the spine, and sacroiliac joints. Anterior uveitis is seen in 10–20%.
- JSpA, traditionally grouped with the spondylarthropathies, has greater clinical and laboratory similarity to JIA; important dissimilarities with the spondylarthropathies include a lack of association with HLA B27, and AS as an outcome.
- JSpA is also more common in women than men.
- Many patients will have persistent disease activity and may progress to polyarthritis over time.
- Childhood reactive arthritis and enteropathic arthropathy are essentially similar to adult disease.

Treatment of JSpA

- The principles of treatment include education, physical therapy, splints, orthotics, NSAIDs, and intra-articular corticosteroids for peripheral arthritis. Oral corticosteroids may be used for severe arthritis or enthesitis.
- Treatment of JSpA follows the paradigm of treating oligoarticular/polyarticular disease using NSAIDs, DMARDs such as MTX, and oral, iv or intra-articular corticosteroids.
- MTX has shown little effect in spondyloarthropathy patients without JSpA.
- Infliximab and etanercept have been used in refractory disease and appear to be as effective as in adult spondyloarthropathy treatment. They have also been used to treat uveitis.

Prognosis in JSpA

Remission rates vary widely in studies, with estimates of 10–20% in remission at 10 years. A large proportion of children will therefore have persisting disease in adult life, with associated disability.

Juvenile idiopathic arthritis

Introduction

- The classification of childhood onset arthritis has seen several changes over recent years. In this chapter we will discuss juvenile arthritis using headings and criteria from the International League of Associations for Rheumatology (ILAR.) The terms 'juvenile rheumatoid arthritis' (JIA) and 'juvenile chronic arthritis' (JCA) were discarded in the ILAR classification. The term 'juvenile idiopathic arthritis' was adopted to indicate arthritis present for at least 6 weeks and currently of no known cause in a patient <16 years.
- JIA is one of the most common chronic disorders of childhood, with an estimated UK incidence of 1 per 10 000, and prevalence of 1 per 1000.
- Studies suggest there is some a familial aggregation, however this may only account for 10–15% of the risk. Detail of the HLA and non-HLA genetic associations with JIA is beyond the scope of this text. An update can be found in Angeles-Han & Prahalad 2010 review.[1]
- The categories of JIA are:
  - systemic arthritis;
  - oligoarthritis (4 or fewer joints) ('persistent' or 'extended');
  - polyarthritis (rheumatoid factor positive and negative);
  - psoriatic arthritis;
  - enthesitis related arthritis;
  - undifferentiated arthritis.
- Where features of other rheumatic diseases are particular to childhood, these are discussed at the end of the relevant chapter.
  - rheumatoid factor positive polyarthritis (📖 Chapter 5, p 233);
  - psoriatic and enthesis related arthritis (📖 Chapter 8, p 281);
  - SLE (📖 Chapter 10, p 321);
  - back pain (📖 Chapter 20, p 525).
- For a review of classification of JIA we recommend Hofer et al. (2002.)[2] For an overview of the spectrum of paediatric and adolescent rheumatology we recommend Davies and Copeman (2006).[3]

General management principles in juvenile rheumatic diseases

- A multi-disciplinary approach is essential. Allied health professionals provide help with patient and family education, exercise, activities of daily living (home and school), maintenance of psychological well-being in patient and family, and advice on financial and disability support.
- Monitoring of height and weight is needed, and appropriate nutritional advice given if needed.

1 Angeles-Han S, Prahalad S (2010). The genetics of juvenile idiopathic arthritis: what is new in 2010? *Curr Rheumatol Rep* **12**(2): 87–93

2 Hofer M, Southwood T (2002). Classification of childhood arthritis. *Best Pract Res Clin Rheumatol* **16**: 379–96.

3 Davies K, Copeman A (2006). The spectrum of paediatric and adolescent rheumatology. *Best Pract Res Clin Rheumatol* **20**: 179–200.

- Ophthalmic input is required if uveitis is present.
- The dose of corticosteroid should be kept to the lowest possible to reduce the development of growth retardation. That said, higher doses of steroid are often required than in adults to gain initial control of disease. Bone density scanning or dual-energy X-ray absorptiometry (DEXA) should be considered and calcium and vitamin D should be given. Bisphosphonates should only be given under specialist guidance.
- A close connection with the child's school is needed. Fatigue is a common symptom and may require changes to the child's school timetable. It is important to continue education as much as possible during hospital admissions.
- Excellent communication skills are required to explain often complex treatments to patient and family. Coming to terms with a chronic disease is a difficult process and, again, will need a close working relationship between members of the multi-disciplinary team.
- The onset of adolescence brings new challenges. It is important to encourage the patient to be more active in decisions about disease management. Adolescence is a time of huge emotional and physical changes, and a chronic illness can make these changes more difficult. Discussion of personal issues such as sexuality, smoking, and alcohol require a good rapport with the patient. Parents should be encouraged to help develop the patient's independence in making treatment decisions, though this can be a long process. Adolescence is also the time to introduce the subject of transition from care by paediatric to adult health professionals. This is a gradual process and should be managed sensitively.

Oligoarthritis

- This is the most commonly encountered subset of the childhood chronic arthritides, accounting for 40–50% of all JIA.
- The condition is more common in girls than boys and presents before the age of 6 in most cases. Overall, the disease affects an estimated 30 per 100 000 children.
- ILAR classification criteria requires the presence of arthritis affecting 1–4 joints during the first 6 months of disease. The persistent subtype affects no further joints in the disease course. The extended subtype affects a total of >4 joints after the first 6 months of disease and can occur in up to 50% cases.
- Strong HLA associations with DRB1*08,11 and 13 and DPB1*02.
- The ILAR classification has the following exclusion criteria:
  - family history of psoriasis confirmed by a dermatologist in at least one first- or second-degree relative;
  - family history consistent with medically confirmed HLA B27 associated disease in at least one first- or second-degree relative;
  - a positive rheumatoid factor test;
  - HLA B27 positive male with onset of arthritis >8 years of age;
  - Presence of systemic arthritis (🕮 p 310).

Clinical features

- There are no specific signs, symptoms, or laboratory tests. Nevertheless, the clinical picture is often quite recognizable, and usually milder than conditions such as reactive or infective arthritis.
- Constitutional symptoms of fever, malaise, weight loss, and anorexia are not normally part of oligoarthritis.

Joint involvement

- Joint swelling, rather than pain, is the more common complaint.
- Stiffness may occur but rarely seems to limit function. Two-thirds of cases present with single joint disease, and a further 30% with 2 joints involved. There may be associated juxta-articular muscle atrophy. The child may simply present with a limping gait.
- The most common joints to be involved are the knee, ankle, and elbow. Small joints of the hands and feet are involved in <10% cases and does not predict progress to polyarticular disease. Shoulder and hip involvement is rare and should prompt a search for another condition, such as enthesitis-related arthritis. Patients may develop disease of the temporomandibular joint and cervical spine later in disease.
- A period of 2–5 years of active arthritis is a typical course for the condition. A patient who remains 'pauci-articular' for 5 years is unlikely to progress to polyarticular disease. A minority of cases will progress, but the criteria for judging this likelihood remains unclear; that said, some 40% of patients with concomitant uveitis develop polyarticular disease and therefore risk factors for uveitis might be considered partly as criteria for risk of polyarticular disease.

- Leg length discrepancy can occur due to unequal limb growth (Plate 20). When disease begins before 3 years of age there is a risk of the affected limb being longer. Flexing the knee on the affected side compensates for the discrepancy and this, in turn, will exacerbate any flexion contractures.
- Disease onset after the age of 9 years may result in a shorter affected limb; this is a consequence of early epiphyseal closure.
- Synovial cysts occur and respond to intra-articular steroid injections (which may have to be given under general anaesthetic). They can rupture, presenting as acute intense limb pain and swelling.
- Over 80% of children suffer little or no musculoskeletal disability at 15 years follow-up.

Eyes
- Uveitis is an important complication to be aware of. Up to 20% of cases develop a chronic, insidious, painless and potentially sight-threatening uveitis (most often anterior chamber).
- The risk of uveitis is associated with the mode of onset of arthritis and not the later extent of articular disease.
- Risk factors include:
  - female gender (female to male ratio up to 7.5:1);
  - young onset disease (mean age 4 years);
  - oligoarthritis, particularly the extended type;
  - positive antinuclear antibody.
- The uveitis is commonly asymptomatic, only 25% of patients complain of redness in the eye, pain, or visual disturbance. Up to two-thirds of patients have bilateral disease although not necessarily at the same time. As such, regular ophthalmic examination is required (Table 9.1).
- Uveitis and arthritis develop at different times. Uveitis may predate arthritis in up to 10% of cases. Otherwise, it is usually detected within 7 years (average 2 years) of the onset of arthritis.
- The main determinants of poor outcome of uveitis are the extent of initial disease at presentation, and uveitis documented before the onset of arthritis. Early intervention is probably the single most important factor in determining outcome.
- Chronic asymptomatic uveitis persisting into adulthood is recognized.
- Treatment is discussed in the next section.

Investigations in oligoarthritis
- There are no diagnostic tests.
- The acute-phase reactants are usually mildly raised.
- A persistent high ESR, with no other evidence of inflammation on other laboratory tests, might suggest the rare, congenital disorder hyperfibrinogenaemia. A high ESR should prompt a search for infection, occult inflammation, or malignancy, e.g. leukaemia.
- ANA are present in 40–75% of children. There is no evidence that ANA precede the development of the condition, or that titres correlate with disease activity.
- Rheumatoid factor is rare; positive in <5% of cases.
- Plain radiographs are valuable for assessing joint damage; however, the expertise of a paediatric radiologist familiar with normal variants of skeletal development should be sought.

- Clinical assessment and investigation should seek to exclude the common conditions of childhood rheumatic disease (Table 9.2).

Table 9.1 Uveitis surveillance: recommended frequency of slit-lamp examination

Condition	Frequency
Systemic onset	Yearly
Oligoarthritis and rheumatoid factor negative	
Onset before age 7:	ANA positive: 2–3-monthly for 4 years then 6-monthly for 3 years. Then yearly
	ANA negative: 6-monthly for 7 years. Then yearly
Onset after age 7:	6-monthly for 4 years. Then yearly

Table 9.2 The differential diagnosis of oligoarthritis

Condition	Examples
Monoarticular disease	Septic arthritis
	TB
	Trauma/haemarthrosis
	Patellofemoral pain
	Pigmented villonodular synovitis (requires tissue biopsy)
	Foreign-body synovitis
	Thalassaemia/sickle cell/haemophilia
Short-lived inflammatory arthropathy	Lyme disease
	Viral arthritis
	Reactive arthritis
	Post-streptococcal arthritis
The spondyloarthropathies	
Pain conditions	Hypermobility
	Complex regional pain syndromes
	Avulsion fractures
	Aseptic (avascular) necrosis
	Enthesitis
	Osteoid osteoma/bone pain

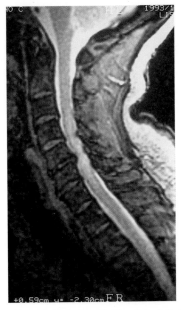

Plate 1 MR scan of the neck showing loss of height and signal affecting several discs with multisegmental spondylotic bars, compression of the cord from protrusion of the C5/6 disc and myelopathic changes (high signal) in the cord.

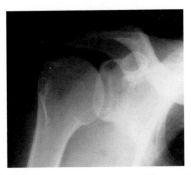

Plate 2 Patterns of radiographic abnormality in chronic SAI: sclerosis and cystic changes in the greater tuberosity.

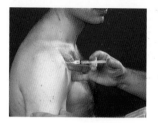

Plate 3 Injection of the glenohumeral joint via the anterior route.

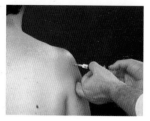

Plate 4 Injection of the subacromial space.

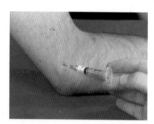

Plate 5 Injection of tennis elbow (lateral humeral epicondylitis/enthesis).

(a)

(b)

(c)

(d)

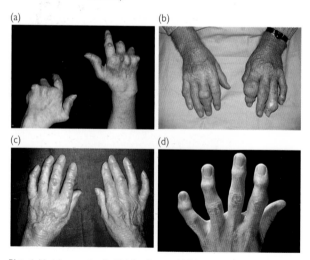

Plate 6 Nodules associated with joint diseases. (a) RA: typically over extensor surfaces and pressure areas. (b) Chronic tophaceous gout: tophi can be indistinguishable clinically from RA nodules though may appear as eccentric swellings around joints (image provided courtesy of Dr R. A. Watts). (c) Multicentric reticulohistiocytosis: nodules are in the skin, are small, yellowish-brown, and are often around nails. (d) Nodal OA: swelling is bony, typically at PIPJs and DIPJs.

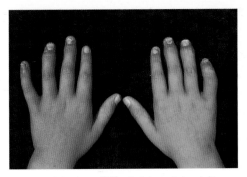

Plate 7 Dactylitis, nail changes, and DIPJ arthritis in psoriatic arthritis.

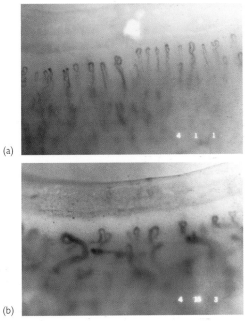

(a)

(b)

Plate 8 (a) Normal nailfold capillaries. (b) Nailfold capillaries in scleroderma showing avascular areas and dilated capillaries in an irregular orientation (original magnification ×65).

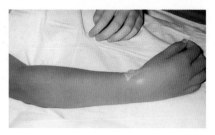

Plate 9 Diffuse arm and hand swelling in chronic regional pain syndrome (reflex sympathetic dystrophy) in a 13-year-old girl.

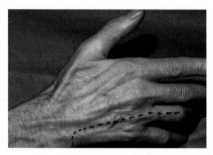

Plate 10 Slight flexion of fourth and fifth fingers as a result of an ulnar nerve lesion at the elbow. The area of sensory loss is indicated by the dotted line.

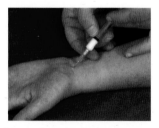

Plate 11 Injection of the carpal tunnel to the ulnar side of palmaris longus tendon.

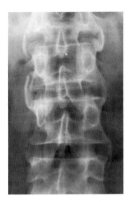

Plate 12 Psoriatic spondylitis: Non-marginal and 'floating' (non-attached) syndesmophytes.

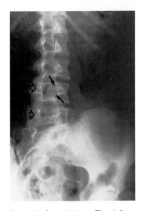

Plate 13 Spondylolysis. The defect in the pars interarticularis (black arrows) may only be noted on an oblique view. The patient has had a spinal fusion (open arrows).

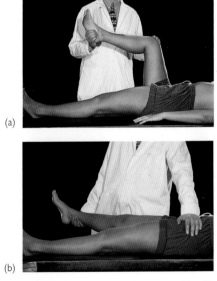

(a)

(b)

Plate 14 Testing passive hip flexion and rotational movements (a) and hip abduction (b). The pelvis should be fixed when testing abduction and adduction.

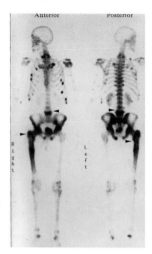

Plate 15 Bone scintigraphy (^{99m}Tc MDP) of a 65-year-old man with widespread bone pain and weakness suspected to have metastatic malignancy. Undecalcified transiliac bone biopsy confirmed severe osteomalacia. There was coincidental Paget's disease (arrowed lesions).

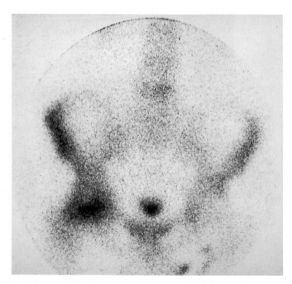

Plate 16 Bone scintigraphy showing osteonecrosis of the left femoral head (on the right-hand side as this an anterior view). Photopenia (an early sign) corresponds to ischaemia.

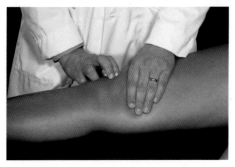

Plate 17 The 'patellar tap' test. Any fluid in the suprapatellar pouch is squeezed distally by the left hand. The patella is depressed by the right hand. It will normally tap the underlying femur immediately. Any delay in eliciting the tap or a feeling of damping as the patella is depressed suggests a joint effusion.

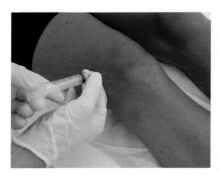

Plate 18 Injection of the knee (courtesy of Mrs Carey Tierney).

(a)

(b)

(c)

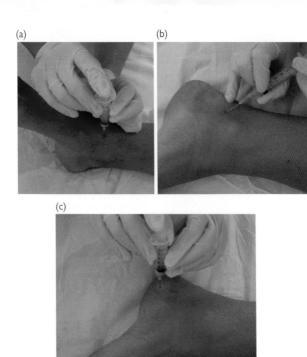

Plate 19 (a) Injection to ankle joint (b) Tarsal tunnel (c) Plantar fascia (three images courtesy of Mrs Carey Tierney).

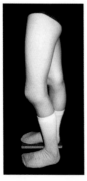

Plate 20 Increased growth of the left lower limb owing to chronic knee inflammation in (RF−) JIA.

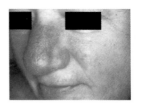

Plate 21 Lupus pernio presenting as a bluish-red or violaceous swelling of the nose extending onto the cheek.

Treatment of oligoarthritis

- The main principles are the maintenance of normal joint function during active disease, and the early treatment of ocular inflammation. A team approach is required.
- In those with only a few joints affected, NSAIDs or intra-articular steroid injections can be used.
- Intra-articular steroid injections may be useful in several situations:
  - the very young (unable to take oral medication);
  - marked persistent joint swelling;
  - synovial cysts causing limitation of movement.
- Cases with prolonged disease or extension to polyarticular disease require more aggressive treatment. Methotrexate (MTX) is the preferred choice. Oral or subcutaneous preparations are used. According to UK NICE guidelines, anti-TNF-α therapy with etanercept should be used with or without MTX in patients 4–17 years old with JIA affecting 5 or more joints in whom MTX has been ineffective or not tolerated.
- Motor development and activity is very important. There should always be assessment of growth, development, and social interaction. Physical therapy makes an important contribution to the overall management of the condition.
- Joint surgery is rarely necessary.
- Uveitis is treated with topical corticosteroids. Oral corticosteroids may be used for severe disease, but concerns remain regarding growth retardation. MTX, azathioprine (AZA), ciclosporin, mycophenolate mofetil (MMF), and anti-TNF-α agents have also been used depending on severity of disease. However, controlled studies of all these agents in uveitis are missing. The best evidence reaches 'level III,' i.e. expert opinion, clinical experience, or a descriptive study.
- Surgery may be necessary for cataracts, keratopathy, or glaucoma.

Systemic arthritis

- Systemic onset disease accounts for approximately 10–20% of juvenile arthritis.
- There is an equal sex incidence in systemic onset disease.
- The peak age of onset is 2–3 years.
- The non-articular features of the condition make a viral aetiology an attractive hypothesis, but there is little evidence for this.
- HLA studies demonstrate genetic heterogeneity with no clear associations.
- Systemic arthritis (SJIA) is increasingly recognized as an auto-inflammatory, rather than autoimmune disease, with abnormalities of innate immunological pathways being more significant, and a lack of autoantibody production.
- The inflammatory process is driven by IL-1 and IL-6. High levels are found in peripheral blood and synovial fluid of affected patients.

Clinical features

- While arthritis is required to confirm the diagnosis, true joint inflammation may not be present at the onset of disease; some patients have developed inflammation as late as 9 years after the onset.
- The ILAR classification criteria require the presence of arthritis with, or preceded by, a daily fever of at least 2 weeks duration in association with one or more of the following: an erythematous evanescent rash, generalized lymphadenopathy, hepatomegaly and/or splenomegaly, and serositis (Table 9.3).
- Most patients have arthritis at disease onset, and 50–60% will develop chronic persistent symptoms. In >75% of cases, the wrists, knees, and ankles are involved. Hip involvement occurs in about 50% of cases and is almost always bilateral, and associated with polyarticular disease. Hip and wrist joints are the most common sites of progressive destructive arthropathy, and one-third of patients with hip involvement will require hip arthroplasty.
- Tenosynovitis of the carpus and tarsus is common, and of the small joints, the hands are often affected more than the feet.
- Fever is the one extra-articular feature essential to making the diagnosis. The fever pattern is described as quotidian, often rising to 39°C before falling rapidly to normal, and typically in the late afternoon or early evening following a regular daily pattern. The patient often appears toxic during the fever, with chills and rigors, severe arthralgia and myalgia, and very often a rash. The fever should be present for at least 2 weeks and quotidian in character for at least 3 days to satisfy the diagnosis. Fever may persist for months even with treatment.
- The rash of systemic arthritis is a salmon-pink colour, most prominent over the chest, abdomen, back, and intertrigenous areas. The rash is usually macular, though occasional urticarial, with individual lesions 3–5 mm in diameter that may coalesce into larger ones. It has a tendency to come and go with the fever spike.
- Hepatomegaly, splenomegaly, and lymphadenopathy are common findings and usually asymptomatic. Mild elevation in serum

transaminases occurs frequently and is usually not significant clinically. This makes assessment of potentially hepatotoxic medications difficult. Chronic liver disease does not occur. It is, however, a feature of adult-onset Still's disease. Very rarely an acute fulminant liver failure occurs with encephalopathy, disseminated intravascular coagulation, and bleeding.

- Involvement of the serosal surfaces is one hallmark of systemic arthritis. Pericarditis, pleuritis, and sterile peritonitis are recognized manifestations of the disease; pericarditis is by far the more common of these. Most children will have echocardiographic evidence of pericarditis during systemic flares although <15% will be symptomatic. Pericardiocentesis may be required for large effusions. Rarely, the patient may have myocarditis, suggested clinically by persistent tachycardia, cardiomegaly, and congestive heart failure. There should always be a high index of suspicion in these cases as the mortality rate is high. Valvular disease is almost never seen. This may help to separate systemic arthritis from acute rheumatic fever with myocarditis.

Table 9.3 Clinical features of systemic arthritis

Frequency	Feature
Very common	Spiking fever (with chills and sweats)
	Evanescent rash
	Myalgia
	Arthralgia–oligo/polyarthritis—usually after first 6 months from onset
	Growth abnormalities
Common	Generalized lymphadenopathy
	Hepatosplenomegaly
	Polyserositis
	Anorexia
	Weight loss
Rare	Myocarditis
	Coagulopathy
	Eye disease
	CNS involvement
	Macrophage activation syndrome
	Primary pulmonary disease
	Renal disease
	Amyloidosis

- Abnormalities of growth are often as a consequence of hypercatabolism, poor nutrient intake, and concomitant use of corticosteroids. Suppression of disease activity and adequate nutrition are the most effective therapy. Growth hormone supplementation is reserved for patients whose growth is persistently below the third percentile on height charts and before epiphyseal fusion has occurred.
- Among the rarer features, CNS manifestations are dominated by irritability and lethargy during fever spikes; renal involvement may occur as a complication of treatment or indicate the onset of amyloidosis (☐ Chapter 18, p 489); and ocular involvement is distinctly unusual relative to other forms of JIA, although asymptomatic uveitis does occur.
- Amyloidosis (☐ Chapter 18, p 489) is a serious complication of all subtypes of JIA and is associated with significant morbidity and mortality. The most common cause of death with amyloidosis is renal failure (80% of cases in most series), followed by infection (10% of cases).
- Macrophage activation syndrome (MAS) has a strong association with sJIA and is caused by over-activation of macrophages causing a syndrome characterized by hepatosplenomegaly, pancytopenia, haemophagocytosis fever, lymphadenopathy, disseminated intravascular coagulation and liver failure. MAS requires immediate treatment with high-dose corticosteroid in the first instance. Ciclosporin has been used in addition for resistant cases, as well as intravenous immunoglobulin, plasmapharesis and anti-TNF-α agents.

Differential diagnosis

- The differential diagnosis of systemic arthritis should always be kept in mind.
- Infectious and post-infectious disorders, other inflammatory diseases, and malignancy have similar clinical manifestations.
- Features that may raise suspicion of another diagnosis include:
  - leucopenia, thrombocytopenia;
  - child looks ill even during afebrile episodes;
  - bony tenderness;
  - 'hard' hepatosplenomegaly/lymphadenopathy;
  - recent antibiotic use;
  - monoarthritis;
  - persistent diarrhoea;
  - marked weight loss.

Investigations in systemic arthritis

- There are no specific diagnostic tests.
- Characteristic haematological abnormalities include anaemia, thrombocytosis, and leucocytosis; the latter two abnormalities are hallmarks of the condition, so much so that normal counts raise suspicion about the diagnosis.
- Acute phase markers are usually increased; the ESR, CRP, gammaglobulins, ferritin and serum complement (this may help to differentiate the disease from SLE ☐ Chapter 10, p 321). The ESR may be normal or elevated in MAS complicating systemic arthritis.

- Hypoalbuminaemia may be multifactorial in aetiology (poor diet, reduced synthesis, intestinal leak), but should prompt the search for proteinuria, which, if 'heavy', would suggest amyloidosis and the need for renal or rectal biopsy, or scintigraphy using iodinated serum amyloid-P to detect deposits.
- Most children are seronegative for antinuclear antibody (ANA) and rheumatoid factor (RF). No antinuclear antibody specificities have been consistently identified.

The following tests are suggested for all patients in the initial diagnostic investigation of systemic arthritis:
- FBC and differential.
- U&E and LFTs.
- Coagulation screen.
- Serum immunoglobulins.
- Serum albumin.
- ANA titre.
- Blood cultures.
- Chest radiograph.
- Plain radiographs of selected affected joints.
- Abdominal and pelvic ultrasound.
- Electrocardiogram (ECG).
- Ocular slit lamp examination.

The following tests should also be considered:
- Muscle enzymes (📖 Chapter 14, p 385).
- Rheumatoid factor.
- Viral serology—parvovirus, adenovirus, etc. (📖 Chapter 17, p 473).
- Antistreptolysin antibody titres.
- Serum IgD.
- Urine catecholamines, e.g. homovanillic and vanillylmandelic acid.
- Joint aspiration (for monoarthritis).
- Tissue biopsy (including bone marrow aspirate).
- Echocardiogram.
- Upper gastrointestinal barium series.
- Isotope bone and/or gallium scan.

The radiological abnormalities seen are listed in Table 9.4.

The treatment of systemic arthritis

- The general approach to the management of the arthritis assumes the same principles as oligoarthritis.[1] However, there is increased drug-related toxicity in systemic JIA. This is seen with salicylates, NSAIDs, and DMARDs.
- Initial control of fever, joint pain, and serositis should be with NSAIDs; ibuprofen and naproxen are commonly used. The dose should be decreased in the presence of severe hypoalbuminaemia as the drugs are protein-bound. NSAIDs should be tried for at least 1 week before being deemed to have failed.

---

1 Weiss JE, Ilowite NT. (2005) Juvenile idiopathic arthritis. *Pediatr Clin N Am.* **52**: 413–42.

Table 9.4 Radiological abnormalities seen in systemic JIA

Feature	Percentage
Soft tissue swelling	80%
Joint space narrowing	50%
Growth abnormalities	50%
Erosions	40%
Subluxation	20%
Ankylosis	20%
Joint destruction	15%
Protrusio acetabulae	10%
Periosteal new bone	10%

- When NSAIDs fail to control symptoms, or symptoms are severe, regular or pulsed corticosteroid treatment is indicated. Steroids will control symptoms, but they do not limit the duration or alter the prognosis of the disease and should be used judiciously. The daily dose should be at least 1 mg/kg in divided doses.
- If symptoms persist past 4–8 weeks, MTX should be added, although MTX is not as effective in this situation as in oligoarticular JIA. Patients who have evidence of severe systemic disease (including anaemia, high fevers, severe serositis, malnutrition, or macrophage activating syndrome) should be treated simultaneously with glucocorticoids.
- If the patient does not respond, consideration should be given to the use of IL-1 or anti-TNF α therapy.
- Anakinra can be effective for the treatment of systemic arthritis, but the beneficial effect is often not sustained.
- Longer-acting agents such as Rilonacept, an IL-1 receptor fusion protein are being investigated in phase III trials in sJIA, and has been effective in treating other auto-inflammatory syndromes.
- Anti-TNF α therapies can be effective in systemic JIA, but often less so than in other JIA subtypes.
- Tocilizumab has been shown to be very effective, and trials are ongoing.
- Intravenous immunoglobulin or ciclosporin may also be considered for patients who have failed other treatment modalities.
- Bone marrow transplantation has been used in those with very severe disease, but has a significant mortality risk.

Rheumatoid factor negative polyarthritis in childhood

General points

- There are two subtypes RF negative (80%) and factor positive (20%).
- The RF should be checked on 2 occasions, 3 months apart. RF positive disease tends to occur most often in girls; it follows a pattern similar to adult RA (📖 Chapter 5, p 233).
- The arthritis usually affects 5 or more joints within the first 6 months of disease. There must be no psoriasis in the patient or in any first-degree relative.
- Polyarticular onset occurs in about 30% of all patients with JIA.
- In the ILAR criteria, polyarthritis with positive RF is excluded.

Clinical manifestations of RF-negative polyarthritis

- Extra-articular manifestations may be present; however, in general features like fever are low grade and of short duration, if present at all. In the very young, there may be a transient rash lasting 1–2 days early in the disease. There is generally no lymphadenopathy, hepatosplenomegaly, or visceral involvement.
- Rapidly progressive joint disease dominates the clinical manifestations. Swelling may limit mobility, resulting in local bone demineralization and muscle wasting. Chronic hyperaemia may induce local accelerated growth and cartilage fusion.
- Carpal fusion and tendonopathies are common in the hands, leading to classical features, such as boutonniere and swan-neck deformities. Flexion contracture is the first manifestation of elbow involvement, and the shoulders are commonly affected.
- In the lower limb, similar consequences are seen with tarsal fusion, tenosynovitis, and bursitis, flexion deformities of the knee, and flexion deformities and aseptic necrosis at the hip.
- Cervical spine involvement is common with features akin to RA; apophyseal joint fusion, instability, and risk of cord compression. There is often fusion of the apophyseal joints of C3–C5 leaving rigid segments that sublux above and below. Atlantoaxial subluxation, seen in RF-positive arthritis and juvenile ankylosing spondylitis, is rare in RF-negative polyarthropathy.
- Temporomandibular joint involvement is common, leading to reduced growth and micrognathia. Dental malocclusion may require surgery when growth is completed.
- Some specific features have led to a proposed subclassification of this condition (Table 9.5).

Table 9.5 Proposed sub-classification of RF-negative polyarthritis

Sub-classification	Percentage of cases	Characteristics
1 Positive for ANA—painful synovitis	About 40%	Female preponderance
		Most cases in very young (<3 years of age)
		Possible increased risk of eye disease
		Severe polyarthritis
2 With 'boggy' synovitis	15%	Mild pain
		Thick pannus
		Equal in sexes
		Functional impairment late
		Tenosynovitis common
3 'Dry' polyarthritis	15%	Little joint swelling
		Progressive stiffness
		Chronic muscle wasting
		Often referred late in to onset
4 With spondyloarthropathy	About 20%	Mid-childhood (8–10 years of age)
		Male preponderance
		At risk of spondylitis within 5–10 years

Laboratory investigations

The laboratory features are non-specific in RF-negative polyarthritis. The ESR, CRP, leucocyte count, and platelet count can be elevated or normal. A low red cell count is unusual and should prompt a search for an alternative diagnosis.

Treatment

* The management of this condition involves a common approach as discussed in the first two sections of this chapter, with adaptations according to the different subtypes shown.
* Treatment should start with a trial of an NSAID for 4–8 weeks, moving to a second NSAID for the same period of time if the first fails. Ibuprofen, naproxen, and diclofenac are commonly used.
* In non-responders to NSAIDs, intra-articular steroid injections may be necessary. Topical steroids should also be used from the onset with eye disease.
* DMARDs should also be introduced for at least 3 months.
* Methotrexate is the first-line drug of choice. Sulfasalazine may be used if there are features of spondyloarthropathy. Treatments should be continued for at least 6 months following remission; in a recently reported study, risk of relapse was no different after 12 vs 6 months therapy following remission, and sustained remission predicted by lower MRP8/14[1] biomarker levels.[2]
* Etanercept is used for patients intolerant of or unresponsive to, MTX. In the UK, Adalimumab is also now used with or without MTX for those with polyarticular JIA aged 13-17.
* In all cases surgery and rehabilitation play an important role in management, and physiotherapy and occupational therapy advice should be employed early.

---

1 Migration inhibitory factor-related proteins (MRP) -8 and -14 are associated with myeloid cell differentiation and belong to the S-100 family of calcium binding proteins. They are expressed in active inflammatory disease (not specific to JIA). MRP8/14 and MRP14 are generally associated with acute inflammation; MRP8 with chronic inflammation.

2 Foell D, Wulffraat N, Wedderburn LR, *et al.* (2010). Methotrexate withdrawal at 6 vs 12 months in juvenile idiopathic arthritis in remission: a randomized clinical trial. *J Am Med Ass.* **303**(13): 1266–73.

Chronic, infantile, neurological, cutaneous, and articular syndrome

- Closer scrutiny of paediatric inflammatory arthropathies has led to the description of syndromes that can be distinguished from systemic JIA. Among these syndromes is chronic, infantile, neurological, cutaneous, and articular syndrome (CINCA), different from JIA in its involvement of the central nervous system.
- The pathophysiology of this condition is auto-inflammatory. No immune complex, autoantibody, or immunodeficiency has been found.
- CINCA is also known as neonatal onset multisystem inflammatory disease (NOMID).
- CINCA/NOMID is one of the newly recognized cryopyrin-associated periodic fever syndromes (CAPS) and is an autosomal dominant syndrome caused by a mutation of the *NLRP3* gene on chromosome 1 that encodes the cryopyrin gene. The mutation causes excessive production of proteins that activate IL-1β.
- The first symptoms are often present at birth. Up to 50% of patients are born pre-term. Three-quarters of neonates (the rest usually within 6 months of birth) have a non-pruritic urticarial rash that resembles that of Still's disease. Intermittent 'flares' of the condition are associated with fever, and enlargement of the lymph nodes and spleen.
- Central nervous system and sensory anomalies are important manifestations of CINCA. Chronic aseptic meningitis may result in recurrent headaches, irritability, vomiting, and seizures. There may also be transient episodes of hemiplegia.
- Sensory anomalies are progressive. These include deafness and optic atrophy. Other eye involvement includes uveitis, chorioretinitis, keratitis, and conjunctivitis.
- The skull tends to have an increased cranial volume and there is delay in closure of the anterior fontanelle, and sometimes calcification of the falx and dura. Hydrocephalus is a late complication.
- Joint involvement is variable, but most often involves the knee. The main finding is an overgrowth of the epiphyseal plate, resulting in bony enlargement. Progressive contractures and loss of movement and function ensue. There is progressive growth retardation and, despite normal growth hormone profiles, a height below the third percentile is very frequent.
- Common morphological changes are also a feature. These include skull enlargement (often frontal bossing), a saddle-back nose, clubbing of the fingers and toes, and short and thick hands and feet.
- NSAIDs, MTX, corticosteroids, and other immunosuppressive agents have only partial benefit, and anti-TNF α therapies have not shown significant benefit.
- Blockade of the IL-1 receptor with anakinra and rilonacept results in dramatic improvement in the signs and symptoms associated with CINCA, but relapse occurs rapidly after treatment is stopped.
- Cankinumab, a long-acting humanized anti-IL-1β monoclonal antibody has been shown to be very effective for up to 2 months after a single dose, and further studies are ongoing.

Systemic lupus erythematosus

Introduction

- Systemic lupus erythematosus (SLE) is a complex clinical syndrome characterized by autoimmune-mediated, systemic inflammation that can affect multiple organs. This rubric encompasses a wide range of clinical manifestations of greatly varying severity.
- Prevalence varies worldwide, but USA studies give estimates of 100–240 per 10 000 and in Europe prevalence estimates range from 25–70 per 100 000.
- It is important to remember that there are variations in the incidence of clinical features between ethnic groups. With this in mind, the physician needs a keen sense of awareness of a variety of multisystem pathologies and to appreciate that SLE has taken on the mantle of syphilis as the great mimic of other conditions.
- The American Rheumatism Association (ARA), now the American College of Rheumatology, published its revised criteria for the classification of SLE in 1997 (Table 10.1). As stated in other sections of this book, criteria are for the classification of the disease for epidemiological and research purposes mostly and not as a diagnostic tool. In practice, however, these criteria naturally tend to form the cornerstone for clinical diagnosis.

Table 10.1 Revised criteria of the ARA for the classification of SLE

1	Malar rash	
2	Discoid rash	
3	Photosensitivity	
4	Oral ulcers	
5	Arthritis	
6	Serositis:	Pleuritis or pericarditis
7	Renal disorder:	Persistent proteinuria of >0.5 g/24 h or cellular casts
8	Neurological disorder (having excluded other causes):	Seizures or psychosis
9	Haematological disorders:	Haemolytic anaemia or
		Leucopenia $<4.0 \times 10^9$/L on 2 or more occasions
		Lymphopenia $<1.5 \times 10^9$/L on 2 or more occasions
		Thrombocytopenia $<100 \times 10^9$/L
10	Immunological disorders:	Anti-ds DNA antibody
		Anti-Sm antibody
		Antiphospholipid antibodies
11	Antinuclear antibody in raised titre	

SLE may be diagnosed if 4 or more of the 11 criteria are present either serially or simultaneously.

The clinical features of systemic lupus erythematosus

Lupus is 10–20 times more common in women than men, and most likely to develop between the ages of 15–40 years. It is commoner and often more severe in certain ethnic groups such as those of African-Caribbean, Indian subcontinent, Hispanic, and Chinese origin living in the USA and Europe than in white Caucasians. There are several non-specific features that are in common with many other chronic diseases. Of these, lethargy and fatigue are often the most disabling. Weight loss and persistent lymphadenopathy can also be seen in association with SLE.

Musculoskeletal

- Morning stiffness and polyarticular, symmetrical arthralgia or arthritis occur in 90% of cases. In most cases symptoms outweigh objective clinical signs, and overt joint damage from synovitis is confined to <10% of patients. Reversible subluxation of joints without erosive disease (Jaccoud's arthropathy) can also occur.
- Avascular necrosis occurs in 5–10% of patients; most cases being associated with previous steroid use.
- Myalgia is common, but true myositis in <5%, and myopathy may be a consequence of steroid treatment.

Skin

Approximately half of patients diagnosed with SLE will have the classic 'butterfly' rash over the nasal bridge and malar bones. The cutaneous manifestations of SLE are listed in Table 10.2.

Cardiovascular disease

- Pericardial disease is the most common component of heart involvement in lupus. Most cases are clinically silent; a mild pericarditis is more common than a clinically significant pericardial effusion. On echocardiography, pericardial thickening is seen more frequently than pericardial effusions.
- Although SLE can lead to life-threatening pericardial effusions or constrictive pericarditis, these manifestations are quite rare.
- Myocarditis is often asymptomatic, and may be present in 8–25% of patients. Clinical myocarditis (defined by combinations of tachycardia, dysrhythmias, a prolonged PR interval on electrocardiography, cardiomegaly, and congestive cardiac failure) is considerably less common. Histological studies suggest that a mild non-specific perivascular inflammatory infiltrate is a common feature.
- Corticosteroid therapy, although indicated for inflammatory cardiac disease, is itself an added risk factor for atherosclerosis given its propensity to induce hypertension, hypercholesterolaemia, and obesity.
- Systolic murmurs are common. The classic endocarditis described by Libman and Sacks rarely causes clinically significant lesions. Any valve vegetations identified in a patient who is febrile should raise the possibility of bacterial endocarditis.

- Cardiovascular disease in lupus patients is a recognized feature. Patients are 5–10 times more likely to have a coronary event than the general population. Women with SLE have a 5–6% increased risk of coronary heart disease compared to the general population, and those aged 35–44 years old are 50 times more likely to have a myocardial infarction than age-matched controls. Sub-clinical cardiovascular disease is also seen, with increased prevalence of carotid plaque and faster progression of plaque. The pathogenesis of early cardiovascular disease is multi-factorial including traditional risk factors (smoking, obesity, hypertension, diabetes mellitus, hyperlipidaemia, positive family history), lupus-related risk factors (disease activity and damage, steroid use, disease duration) and factors related to the inflammatory process (raised C-reactive protein and pro-inflammatory cytokine levels, elevated homocysteine levels). Reducing cardiovascular morbidity and mortality requires management of traditional risk factors, using antihypertensive agents and statins as appropriate, as well as minimizing corticosteroid use and achieving early and prolonged control of disease activity.

Table 10.2 Cutaneous manifestations of SLE

Frequency of occurrence	Feature
Common (20–50%)	Malar rash
	Photosensitive rash
	Chronic discoid lesions
	Non-scarring alopecia
Less common (5–20%)	Mucosal ulcers
Occasional (5%)	Peri-orbital oedema
	Bullous lupus
	Severe scarring alopecia
	Subacute cutaneous lupus
	Leg ulcers
	Panniculitis
	Cutaneous vasculitis

Pulmonary disease

- Because of the tendency for disease to be subclinical, chest radiographs and pulmonary function tests invariably indicate a greater degree of involvement than is evident clinically, and patients may present quite late in the disease process following a history of slow onset non-productive cough and increasing shortness of breath on exertion. Pulmonary function tests typically show both diminished total lung capacity and peak flow rates.
- Shrinking lung syndrome is associated with unexplained shortness of breath, initially exertional, but then at rest and on lying flat, small

lung volumes on chest X-ray, diaphragmatic elevation and restrictive pulmonary function tests in the absence of parenchymal lung disease. The exact cause is unknown and response to corticosteroids is good.
- Pleuritic pain/pleuritis is present in up to 60% of cases.
- Pleural effusions are a feature in one-third of patients, but they are usually small and clinically insignificant.
- Interstitial fibrosis, pulmonary vasculitis, and pneumonitis are found in up to one-fifth of lupus patients, but pulmonary hemorrhage is rare.
- Pulmonary hypertension is found in approximately 10% of patients with SLE, and is associated with Raynaud's phenomenon, vasculitis (Chapter 15, p 405), and antiphospholipid antibodies.
- Patients presenting with pleuritic pain and/or pulmonary hypertension should be investigated for the presence of pulmonary emboli and antiphospholipid syndrome (Chapter 11, p 343).

Renal involvement

- Assessment of blood pressure for hypertension, urine for protein, blood, and casts, and the serum creatinine and urea is an essential part of regular monitoring. Symptoms suggesting renal failure rarely become obvious until substantial damage has occurred. If early disease is suspected, the physician should consider a spot urine protein/creatinine ratio, which is more accurate that urine dipstick and more convenient than the conventional 24-h. urine collection for protein and creatinine. The glomerular filtration rate and renal function may also be assessed by nuclear medicine techniques.
- Renal biopsy should be considered when >500 mg proteinuria is detected. That said, there remain differences of opinion as to when and whether a renal biopsy is undertaken. Nephritis can transform from one type to another and the same biopsy may have more than one histological appearance. It must also be remembered that a renal biopsy has complications in itself.
- In 2003, the International Society of Nephrology (ISN) and Renal Pathology Society (RPS) released a new classification of lupus nephritis designed to standardize definitions. The 2003 ISN/RPS classification of lupus nephritis replaced the 1982 modified World Health Organization (WHO) classification:
  - *Class I:* minimal mesangial lupus nephritis;
  - *Class II:* mesangial proliferative lupus nephritis;
  - *Class III:* focal lupus nephritis (< 50% of glomeruli);
  - *Class III (A):* active lesions;
  - *Class III (A/C):* active and chronic lesions;
  - *Class III (C):* chronic inactive lesions;
  - *Class IV:* diffuse lupus nephritis (≥50% glomeruli), divided into diffuse segmental (IV-S) or global (IV-G) lupus nephritis;
  - *Class IV-(A):* active lesions;
  - *Class IV-(A/C):* active and chronic lesions;
  - *Class IV-(C):* chronic inactive lesions;
  - *Class V:* membranous lupus nephritis;
  - *Class VI:* advanced sclerosing lupus nephritis (≥90% globally sclerosed glomeruli without evidence of activity).

- Chronic, inactive lesions (glomerulosclerosis) are a poor prognostic feature.
- Although not uniformly agreed, it can be recommended that lupus patients with microscopic haematuria and/or proteinuria with an impaired glomerular filtration rate should be considered for renal biopsy. However, the information provided about prognosis should not be over-estimated and it is advised that the biopsy material be assessed in centres with a high degree of experience.

Haemopoietic involvement

- A high ESR is a common finding.
- A normochromic, normocytic 'anaemia of chronic inflammatory disease' presents in up to 70% of patients with lupus. Renal failure, NSAID-induced gastric bleeding, Coombs' positive, and microangiopathic haemolysis, and red cell aplasia, are factors that may contribute to the anaemia.
- Leucopenia and lymphopenia are common abnormalities of the white cell count in 50 and 80% of patients, respectively. A leucocytosis is rare, suggesting infection or steroid therapy.
- There are several forms of clinical thrombocytopenia. Chronic, indolent, and uncomplicated thrombocytopenia ($<100 \times 10^9$/L) is present in up to 20% of patients, particularly among SLE patients with antiphospholipid antibodies. A rarer acute and life-threatening severe thrombocytopenia is also recognized. This requires aggressive therapy initially with high-dose systemic steroids, and patients may require intravenous immunoglobulin. Some patients may also present with what initially appears to be an immune thrombocytopenia (ITP), later followed by other manifestations of lupus.

Nervous system disorders

- Features of neurological disease range from cognitive impairment (in up to 50% of patients) to psychoses and seizures (in 5–10% of patients over the course of their disease). Thromboembolic disease associated with antiphospholipid antibodies can cause major cerebrovascular damage (Chapter 11, p 343).
- Approximately 10% of patients will develop a sensory (or less often sensorimotor) peripheral neuropathy. Cranial nerve involvement is less common.
- Up to 70% prevalence of psychiatric illness has been quoted in the literature. However, this includes anxiety and depression, rarely separated in studies from the non-specific stresses associated with a debilitating and often painful disease, as opposed to the disease itself. This said, it does emphasize the degree of the problem, and that depression must be assessed and managed seriously in lupus.
- Whilst it is accepted that corticosteroids can induce psychiatric symptoms, in general it is felt the drugs given in lupus are not responsible for most of the psychiatric manifestations observed.
- Examination of the cerebrospinal fluid in neuropsychiatric disease should be performed as part of the initial evaluation of a new neurologic finding.

- Electroencephalography is often non-specific. Positron emission CT (SPECT and PET) is neither specific for, nor well-correlated with, central nervous system involvement. Magnetic resonance (MR) imaging with gadolinium is more sensitive than CT in detecting the small vessel vasculopathy associated with SLE.

Other clinical features

Other clinical features are listed in Table 10.3.

Table 10.3 Other clinical features of SLE

Vascular	Raynaud's phenomenon
	Cutaneous vasculitis
	Digital ulcers and gangrene
Gastrointestinal	Hepatomegaly (25%)
	Abdominal serositis (10–20%)
	Splenomegaly (10%)
	Mesenteric vasculitis (rare)
	Pancreatitis (rare)
Immunological	Hypergammaglobulinaemia (60%)

Antiphospholipid (antibody) syndrome and systemic lupus erythematosus

- Antiphospholipid antibodies include the lupus anticoagulant, anticardiolipin antibodies, and anti-β_2 glycoprotein-I antibodies.
- Antiphospholipid antibodies are present in up to one-third of patients with SLE.
- Although the presence of antiphospholipid antibodies alone is not sufficient to make this diagnosis, half of patients with SLE and antiphospholipid antibodies with eventually demonstrate evidence of hypercoagulability.
- The manifestations of SLE-associated antiphospholipid syndrome include:
  - venous and arterial thrombosis;
  - thrombocytopenia;
  - cerebral disease;
  - recurrent foetal loss;
  - pulmonary hypertension;
  - livedo reticularis.
- Some patients with antiphospholipid antibodies develop renal impairment (e.g. hypertension or proteinuria) due to multiple small thrombi.

Further details, including management, may be found in Chapter 11, p 343.

Pregnancy and systemic lupus erythematosus

- There is a disparity in the literature as to whether pregnancy is associated with an increased risk of lupus flare. However, pregnancy does not appear to worsen the long-term outcome of SLE.
- A USA study[1] has shown that lupus patients suffer more from gestational diabetes mellitus, hypertension, pulmonary hypertension, and renal failure and thrombotic episodes. Incidence of intra-uterine growth retardation, pre-term delivery and incidence of caesarean sections are also increased.
- Active disease greatly increases the risk of miscarriage and preterm birth.
- A major complication is pre-eclampsia. In the study above, it occurred in 22.5% women with lupus and 7.6% in healthy pregnant controls. Pre-existing renal disease may be an important risk factor.
- SLE is associated with an increased rate of foetal death late in pregnancy and overall approximately 10% of lupus pregnancies result in foetal loss.
- Anti-Ro antibodies are associated with foetal heart block and neonatal lupus.
- The antiphospholipid antibody syndrome and its associated complications during pregnancy is discussed in 📖 Chapter 11, p 343.
- Women who wish to conceive should receive appropriate counselling from specialists, and the discontinuation of teratogenic drugs can be discussed at this point. The manufacturer advises avoiding the use of hydroxychloroquine in pregnancy.
- Features of a high-risk pregnancy include increasing age, significant organ impairment/damage, active disease and high-dose steroids, and presence of antiphospholipid/Ro/La antibodies.
- Women at high-risk should be managed in a combined medical-obstetric clinic, and care should continue into the post-partum period, when flares and thromboembolic events can occur.

Drugs safety in pregnancy is discussed in 📖 Chapter 21, p 545.

1 Clowse MEB, Jamison M, Myers E, James AH (2008). A national study of the complications of lupus in pregnancy. *Am J Obstet Gynecol* **199**: 127.e1–127.e6.

Diagnosis and investigation of systemic lupus erythematosus

- The majority of investigations are aimed specifically at end-organ disease. Investigation in the form of radiographs, FBC, coagulation screen, ESR, CRP, renal and liver biochemistry, urinalysis, and blood pressure may lead to other tests, e.g. of haemolysis or pleuritic pain. The physician is directed to autoantibody and complement tests (Table 10.4).
- There are a variety of circulating autoantibodies to a range of nuclear, cytoplasmic, and plasma membrane antigens. Most patients (98% or more) will have antinuclear antibodies. Approximately 60% have elevated titres of dsDNA antibodies (detected as the immunofluorescent crithidia test or by specific ELISA or radioimmunoassay). Some patients have varying combinations of antibody profile that may change over the course of the disease. The antibodies, their prevalence and clinical association are shown in Table 10.4.
- Lupus is associated with deficiencies of the early classical pathway of complement (e.g. C1q, C1r, C1s, C2). The overall consequence is decreased clearance and increased deposition of complexes. Reduced levels of complement C3 and C4 are common in SLE, particularly at the time of a disease flare.
- A subset of patients will be 'serologically active but clinically quiescent', meaning they will have low complement levels and raised dsDNA titres, but no signs of active disease. Patients should always be treated on the basis of symptoms rather than blood tests alone.
- Some individuals may have high levels of RF and features of an erosive RA type disease. This 'overlap' syndrome is termed 'rhupus'. The mix of clinical features and autoantibodies is not peculiar to SLE and all the autoimmune rheumatic diseases are subject to the phenomenon of 'overlap' or 'undifferentiated' disease. In this situation a number of clinical features and antibodies common to several diseases are present. Treatment is determined by the end-organ disease that is present. The concept of 'mixed connective tissue disease' as a specific diagnosis, rather than 'undifferentiated' disease remains controversial.
- The assessment of disease activity is central to patient management. Several global activity indices have been produced that correlate well and are reliable. Awareness of changes in lupus activity, whether improvement of disease or not, is an essential part of decision-making and drug treatment. Global scoring systems such as the Systemic Lupus Erythematosus Disease Activity Index (SLEDAI) and the British Isles Lupus Assessment Group (BILAG) activity index are of some value, both in the context of clinical trials and long-term follow-up of patients.

- Equally constructive is the concept of an index of damage as distinct from disease activity. For example, a patient with shortness of breath may have an active but reversible pneumonitis or irreversible fibrosis; the distinction between disease activity and damage is important since the treatments are different. The SLICC (Systemic Lupus International Collaborating Clinics) damage index has been developed as a method of recording damage in patients with SLE. The reader is referred to two articles by Gladman et al.[1,2] as the background for current scoring system.

1 Gladman DD, Goldsmith CH, Urowitz MB, *et al.* (1994). Sensitivity to change of 3 systemic lupus eythematosus disease activity indices: international validation. *Journal of Rheumatology* **21**: 1468–71.

2 Gladman D, Ginzter E, Goldsmith C, *et al.* (1996).The development and initial validation of the Systemic Lupus International Collaborating Clinics/American College of Rheumatology damage index for systemic lupus erythematosus. *Arthritis and Rheumatism* **39**: 363–9.

Table 10.4 Autoantibodies of systemic lupus erythematosus commonly used in clinical practice

Autoantibody		Prevalence (%)	Associations
Intracellular:	DNA	40–90	Renal disease
	Histone	30–80	Drug-induced lupus
	Sm	30 (Africans, Caribbeans), 10 (Caucasians)	
	U1 RNP	20–30	
	rRNP	5–15	
	Ro/SS-A	25–40	Sjögren's syndrome, cutaneous lupus, congenital heart block
	La/SS-B	10–15	As Ro/SS-A
Cell membrane:	Cardiolipin	20–40	Pregnancy loss, thrombosis
	Red cell	<10	Haemolytic anaemia
	Platelets	<10	Immune thrombocytopenia
Extracellular:	RF	25	
	Complement C1q	50	

Drug-induced lupus erythematosus

- Many drugs have been implicated in causing drug-induced lupus erythematosus (DILE). Those definitely and most commonly associated with DILE are:
  - minocycline;
  - hydralazine;
  - procainamide;
  - isoniazid;
  - quinidine;
  - methyldopa;
  - chlorpromazine;
  - sulfasalazine;
  - anti-TNF-α drugs.
- Hydralazine-associated DILE is considered to be dose dependent, and procainamide, time dependent.
- Up to 90% of cases taking procainamide develop a positive ANA and 30% of these develop DILE.
- Renal, central nervous system, and skin features of SLE are rare in DILE. Other features of SLE such as articular, pulmonary, and serosal disease are common.
- In the majority of cases the condition subsides on withdrawing the drug. There is no contraindication to using these drugs in idiopathic SLE.

The treatment of systemic lupus erythematosus

- Several general measures are important:
  - rest as appropriate;
  - avoid overexposure to sunlight;
  - sunblock should be SPF 30 or greater, and should protect against both UVA and UVB;
  - control cardiovascular risk factors.
- Advice should include intake of calcium and vitamin D to maintain bone health. Patients on long-term steroids should be offered a bisphosphonate drug (assuming not contraindicated, e.g. premenopausal women, renal insufficiency) as prophylaxis against steroid-induced osteoporosis.
- Vaccinations, apart from 'live' vaccine (e.g. yellow fever, live polio) in patients on immunosuppressives, are not contraindicated though the degree of response differs from the healthy individual.
- Medium-to-high oestrogen contraceptive pills should be avoided. Progesterone only, the lowest oestrogen pill, or other methods of contraception are advised. Oral contraceptives should be avoided by women with SLE and antiphospholipid antibodies. Many patients tolerate hormone replacement therapy (HRT) but use in the menopause is controversial: there is a 20% increase in SLE flares among women taking HRT.

Reduction of cardiovascular disease risk factors

- Management of traditional risk factors (smoking, hypertension, diabetes).
- Statins for hypercholesterolaemia.
- Aspirin if antiphospholipid antibodies are present.
- Tighter control of SLE disease activity.

Table 10.5 outlines the common therapies used to treat the various clinical manifestations of SLE.

The management of SLE as an acute rheumatological emergency is discussed in 📖 Chapter 24, p 609.

New therapies in SLE

Rituximab

This anti-CD20 monoclonal antibody (in combination with intravenous corticosteroids and cyclophosphamide) was first used effectively in 2002 in patients with active systemic disease that had failed, or only had partial responded to conventional treatments. Subsequent open-label studies confirmed the efficacy of the drug, with benefits extending to 6 months. However, a recent randomized placebo-controlled trial failed to demonstrate that rituximab was beneficial to patients with moderate-to-severe SLE, although this could have been due to methodological issues and is still being investigated. Significant side-effects seen in this treatment group include infusion-related reactions and infection. Additionally, progressive multifocal leukoencephalopathy (PML) has been reported in association with rituximab in a small number of lupus patients, but PML is also seen in lupus patients who have never received rituximab. Nevertheless, patients should be counselled appropriately before commencing treatment.

Mycophenolate mofetil

Mycophenolate mofetil (MMF) reduces disease activity and mortality in mouse models of lupus. It has been studied in the management of lupus nephritis, where similar rates of remission, relapse, and infection were seen in comparison to the standard treatment of cyclophosphamide induction followed by azathioprine maintenance therapy. MMF was not associated with marrow suppression or amenorrhoea. MMF has also been seen to be effective in maintaining remission in lupus nephritis in comparison to long-term intravenous cyclophosphamide.

Autologous haemopoietic stem cell transplantation

Haemopoietic stem cell transplantation (HSCT) is used to treat haematological diseases, but has been used in patients with severe refractory SLE. The procedure is effective in inducing remission but is curative in <50%. Mortality is high and long-term effects are unknown. New autoimmune conditions have been reported after HSCT. It is currently used only in those with life-threatening SLE.

Other agents

- The efficacy of anti-TNF-α therapy in SLE is at present not clear. 16% of RA patients on these therapies develop double-stranded DNA antibodies, and 0.2% a transient lupus-like syndrome. A small, open label study has shown benefit in lupus nephritis, but further work needs to be done.
- Tocilizumab has been shown to improve disease activity scores and dsDNA antibody titres in open-label studies. It was approved for use in the UK in 2010.
- Epratuzumab, and anti-CD22 monoclonal antibody has been shown to reduce disease activity and seems to deplete a more 'lupus-specific'' set of B-cells than rituximab.
- Belimumab is a fully-humanized antibody that neutralizes the activity of the soluble B-lymphocyte stimulator (BLyS) is being studied in phase 3 trials.
- Abetimus sodium (LJP-394) is a B cell tolerogen made up of 4 identical strands of dsDNA that leads to serological improvement and a reduction in flares. Optimum-dose trials are ongoing.
- Pooled immunoglobulin (IVIG) may be of use in severely ill patients not responding to other therapies, and perhaps more so in situations where sepsis is the trigger and life-threatening. It may have a role in drug-resistant membranous and membranoproliferative nephritis, and has been used in severe immune thrombocytopenia and haemolytic anaemia with good effect.

Table 10.5 Recommendations for drug use in SLE

Symptom	Drug	Regimen
Arthralgia/fever	NSAIDs (caution with renal disease)	No special recommendation
Arthralgia/myalgia/lethargy	Hydroxychloroquine	400 mg daily; ophthalmic examination yearly, although the risk of untoward events is low.
Malar/discoid rash	Prednisolone, hydroxychloroquine, sunscreen	
Arthritis/serositis/myositis	Prednisolone, methotrexate, azathioprine	20–40 mg of prednisolone daily for 2–4 weeks, then reducing dose in 5 mg steps each week. Requires bone prophylaxis against osteoporosis if dose treatment for more than 3 months.
Autoimmune anaemia or thrombocytopenia (ITP)	Prednisolone, azathioprine, IVIG	60–80 mg prednisolone daily for 2 weeks, reducing in 10 mg steps per week after depending on response. 2.5 mg/kg azathioprine. ITP might also require immunoglobulin or splenectomy
Renal	Prednisolone, azathioprine, cyclophosphamide, mycophenolate	Severe disease may require monthly iv steroid and cyclophosphamide for 6 months then every 2–3 months for 2 years
Central nervous system	Prednisolone, azathioprine	Up to 80 mg daily
Raynaud's disease	📖 Chapter 13, p 363	

Prognosis and survival in systemic lupus erythematosus

- Many studies of the duration of disease and survival rates are confounded by inadequate attention paid to the ethnic group, age of onset, and socioeconomic status of individual patients. The number of patients lost to follow-up is also high. With the division of patients into those with or without overt nephritis, it is reasonable to state a 5-year survival in lupus of 90%. At 15 years, only 60% of those with nephritis will be alive compared with 85% of those patients without renal disease.
- A bi-modal mortality curve is considered to exist. Patients who die within 5 years usually have very active disease, requiring high doses of immunosuppressives. Those patients dying later tend to do so from cardiovascular disease, renal disease, and possibly infection.
- The combined effect of the disease and its treatment is to render the immune system prone to infection. It is often difficult to apportion responsibility to one or other. The possibility of infection must always be kept in mind and treated aggressively as outcome from sepsis can be very poor.
- Controlling risk factors for cardiovascular disease is important.
- Lupus itself increases the risk of all malignancies compared to the general population, particularly non-Hodgkins lymphoma. Cervical dysplasia is increased in lupus patients and regular monitoring should be emphasized. The exact contribution of disease activity, duration and immunosuppressive drug exposure to risk of developing a malignancy requires further research. Clinicians should be aware of this increased risk and be alert to investigating worrying symptoms promptly.

Childhood systemic lupus erythematosus

- This is a rare disease with an estimated incidence of 0.4 per 100 000. There are several features of childhood SLE that differ from the adult disease, though essentially the main features and treatment are in common. General management strategies (i.e. not including pharmacological agents) for child welfare are the same as those employed in the management of all paediatric arthritides—see 📖 Chapter 9, p 303.
- The overall prepubertal male to female ratio is 3:1, suggesting a higher male frequency in childhood SLE as compared with that seen in adults; the ratio reverts to the more classic adult ratio of 9:1 post-puberty.
- The disease is more common and severe in those of African-Caribbean and Asian origin.
- The main features at presentation are arthritis, myalgia, fever, and rash (all features with a frequency of approximately 60–80% of cases at diagnosis). Malar rash is present in 30% of cases at diagnosis, and renal disease at onset of disease is very common (up to 60%). True myositis with proximal weakness occurs in <10% of cases. Neuropsychiatric disease is present in up to 40% cases.
- Avascular necrosis is more common in children than adults with SLE (10–15% of cases), and is more common in SLE than other paediatric autoimmune rheumatic diseases where prolonged high-dose steroids are used.
- Raynaud's phenomenon is less common in childhood lupus and occurs in 10–20% of patients.
- Early atherosclerosis is also a feature of childhood disease, with studies estimating an incidence of myocardial infarction of 8% in patients with childhood-onset disease, occurring most commonly between 20-40 years old.[1]
- As in adult disease, hydroxychloroquine and NSAIDs can be used for mild skin and joint disease.
- Oral or iv corticosteroids are given for disease not responding to the above measures, or in moderate-to-severe multisystem disease. Growth retardation secondary to corticosteroids is a major concern, and the lowest possible dose of steroid should be used. Bone protection with calcium and vitamin D should also be given.
- Cyclophosphamide, azathioprine, methotrexate and mycophenolate mofetil are used as in adult disease. Case reports of successful autologous stem cell transplantation have been described.
- Management of traditional cardiovascular risk factors should use the same principles as in adult SLE.
- The 10-year survival for SLE in childhood is currently estimated at 85%.

---

1 Hersh AO, von Scheven E, Yazdany J, *et al.* (2009). Differences in long-term disease activity and treatment of adult patients with childhood- and adult-onset systemic lupus erythematosus. *Arth Rheum* **61**: 13–20.

Neonatal systemic lupus erythematosus

- This is a rare condition found in the newborn and characterized by subacute cutaneous lupus skin lesions, haemolytic anaemia, hepatitis, thrombocytopenia, and congenital heart block (CHB).
- It is associated with placental transmission of maternal Ro and La antibodies.
- The non-cardiac manifestations resolve within 1 year. Cardiac involvement often requires early pacemaker insertion, and mortality in the first 3 years of life is up to 30%.
- In women with anti-Ro/La antibodies there is a 5% chance of their first child being born with CHB; this rises to 15% with subsequent pregnancies.
- Foetal monitoring with echocardiography in the antenatal period is essential.

Chapter 11

The antiphospholipid (antibody) syndrome

Introduction

The antiphospholipid syndrome (APS) was first described in the 1980s and comprises arterial and venous thrombosis with or without pregnancy morbidity in the presence of anticardiolipin (ACL) antibodies or the lupus anticoagulant (LAC). It can be primary, or secondary to other autoimmune diseases, most commonly systemic lupus erythematosus (SLE) (⬚ Chapter 10, p 321).

APS can affect almost any body system or organ, and presents to many medical specialties, including rheumatology, dermatology, neurology, and cardiology.

Classification criteria were produced in 1999, and updated in 2006 to reflect the use of anti-β_2 glycoprotein-1 for diagnosis (Table 11.1).

Table 11.1 Classification criteria for the antiphospholipid syndrome

Clinical criteria	
Vascular thrombosis	1 or more clinical episodes of arterial, venous, or small vessel thrombosis in any tissue or organ, confirmed by objective criteria. Histopathology should show thrombosis without significant inflammation in the vessel wall
Pregnancy morbidity	1 or more unexplained deaths of a morphologically normal foetus at or beyond 10 weeks gestation
	OR
	1 or more premature births of a morphologically normal neonate at or before 34 weeks gestation due to pre-eclampsia, eclampsia, or placental insufficiency
	OR
	3 or more unexplained, consecutive, spontaneous abortions before 10 weeks gestation, excluding maternal anatomical or hormonal abnormalities, and excluding maternal and paternal chromosomal causes
Laboratory criteria	Medium/high titre of IgG and/or IgM isotype anticardiolipin antibody in blood on 2 or more occasions at least 12 weeks apart using standard assays
	Lupus anticoagulant present in plasma on 2 or more occasions at least 12 weeks apart
	Anti-β_2 Glycoprotein-I IgG or IgM in blood on 2 or more occasions at least 12 weeks apart using standard assays

Adapted from Miyakis S. *et al.* International consensus statement on an update of the classification criteria for definite antiphospholipid syndrome (APS). *J Thromb Haemostasis* 2006; **4**: 295–306.

Epidemiology and pathology

- Antiphospholipid (APL) is the overall term used. Patients may be classified in terms of the antibody present: anticardiolipin (ACL), lupus anticoagulant (LAC), or anti-β_2 glycoprotein-I.
- Antibodies are directed at protein–phospholipid complexes. Recently, antibodies to β_2-glycoprotein I (β_2GPI) have been found to be the main target antigen involved in the binding of anticardiolipin antibodies to anionic phospholipids.
- Case control studies estimate the prevalence of ACL in the normal population to be 1–4%. Prevalence in those >65 years increases to 12–50% depending on the study. Prevalence of ACL and LAC in SLE patients is estimated at 20–40% and 10–20%, respectively. These differences arise due to treatment history and the lack of uniformity of assay methods. Ethnicity also plays a role in the frequency and clinical importance of these antibodies.
- The LAC and ACL antibody tests are the most useful antibodies or identifying patients with the syndrome. The LAC test cannot be performed reliably if a patient is receiving heparin or oral anticoagulant. The ACL antibody assay is the most sensitive test available. The two tests can be discordant in up to 40% of cases and their unrelated behaviour in the course of disease and in the individual patient means that both assays are required to identify cases of APS.
- Apart from a clinical suspicion leading to a request for antiphospholipid antibody assays, a clue to their presence lies in finding a prolonged clotting time in assays for the 'internal pathway'-clotting cascade.
- The specificity of antiphospholipid antibodies probably differs in various disorders. Studies suggest that LAC and high titres of IgG ACL antibodies are associated with greater risk of thrombosis; the risk is much lower in patients with infection-related or drug-induced antibodies, which tend to be of the IgM isotype. 10% of patients with APS only have antibodies to β_2GPI. There is evidence that β_2GPI titre and simultaneous presence of ACL or LAC are associated with disease severity.
- The differential diagnosis of unexplained thrombosis includes genetic causes (e.g. protein C and S, and antithrombin III deficiencies) and drugs (including oestrogen, thalidomide, IVIG). However, these are usually associated with recurrent venous thrombosis. Most striking about APS is the feature of thrombosis in the setting of thrombocytopenia. The main differential diagnosis is thrombotic thrombocytopenic purpura. This is mainly a microvascular disorder most often associated with neurological features of confusion, seizures, and changes in consciousness level that can mimic the catastrophic form of APS.
- Only a third of all patients with APL/ACL ever experience thrombosis. After the first thrombotic event (either arterial or venous), recurrence is common, but can be prevented by treatment with warfarin.

Clinical features of antiphospholipid syndrome

Table 11.2 summarizes the main clinical features of APS and some of the less common findings.

Thrombosis

- Antiphospholipid antibodies are paradoxically associated with thrombosis, rather than haemorrhage.
- Vessels of all sizes, venous or arterial, may be affected without evidence of an inflammatory infiltrate, i.e. vasculitis. This distinction is important not only in trying to understand the pathogenesis of the disorder, but also in the choice of treatment. Unlike most clotting disorders, arterial thrombosis is a major feature of APS. The antibodies should be sought particularly in the younger stroke patient where they may account for up to 20% of cases.
- Widespread thrombosis is the feature of life-threatening 'catastrophic antiphospholipid syndrome'. In this situation the patient may present with acute medical collapse, severe thrombocytopenia, multi-organ failure (notably cerebral and renal), and adult respiratory distress syndrome.

Thrombocytopenia

This is common, although usually not severe enough to cause bleeding. ACL antibodies have been found in up to 30% of cases of presumed immune thrombocytopenic purpura (ITP). Some patients also develop a concomitant Coomb's positive haemolytic anaemia (Evan's syndrome).

Foetal loss

Recurrent spontaneous pregnancy loss is a common complication of APS. This can occur either as recurrent early loss or intrauterine foetal demise. Screening for the antibodies in the general population is not of value. Previous pregnancy history is of importance in determining the significance of a positive antibody titre.

Other features of antiphospholipid syndrome

- Transverse myelopathy, though rare, has a strong association with the presence of antiphospholipid antibodies.
- APS may be associated with multiple cardiovascular complications including accelerated atherosclerosis, valvular heart disease, and intracardiac thrombi. However, cardiac manifestations of APS result in significant morbidity for only 5% of patients. In a European cohort, myocardial infarction was the presenting feature of APS in 3% of patients, and was seen during follow-up in 5.5%. The prevalence of ACL in patients with myocardial infarction is estimated at 5–15%, but screening is not indicated, except in younger patients, those with other symptoms and signs of APS, and those with a family history of autoimmune disease. Mitral and aortic valve thickening and dysfunction is commonly seen on echocardiography, but significant morbidity is uncommon.

Table 11.2 Clinical features of the antiphospholipid syndrome

Feature	Subgroup	Frequency (%)
Major features:		
Thrombosis	Deep vein thrombosis	38.9
	Pulmonary embolism	14.1
	Arterial thrombosis, legs	4.3
	Arterial thrombosis, arms	2.7
	Stroke	19.8
	Transient ischaemic attack	11.1
	Valve thickening/dysfunction	11.6
	Livedo reticularis	24.1
Foetal manifestations	Early loss (<10 weeks)	35.4
	Late loss (≥10 weeks)	16.9
	Live birth	47.7
	Premature birth	10.6
Thrombocytopenia		29.6
Associated features:	Leg ulcers, livedo reticularis, thrombophlebitis	
	Heart valve lesions and myocardial infarction	
	Transverse myelitis, chorea	
	Pulmonary hypertension	
Less common findings	Splinter haemorrhages, digital gangrene, leg ulcers	
	Amaurosis fugax, retinal artery and vein occlusion	
	Renal artery stenosis/thrombosis	
	Ischaemic bone necrosis	
	Addison's disease	

Cervera R. *et al*. Antiphospholipid syndrome: Clinical and immunologic manifestations and patterns of disease expression in a cohort of 1000 patients. *Arth Rheum* 2002; **46**: 1019–1027.

Treatment of antiphospholipid syndrome

Treatment of APS is summarized in Table 11.3:

- There is no real evidence for the role of aspirin/warfarin in primary prevention. Modifiable risk factors should be reduced as much as possible (e.g. smoking and cholesterol reduction, and avoid oestrogens). Many clinicians however use low-dose aspirin in this group of patients.
- Studies suggest that lifelong and oral anticoagulation is an effective therapeutic option in the secondary prevention of thrombosis. In venous thrombosis with a transient or reversible risk factor however, 3–6 months treatment may be adequate. Care should be taken to maintain the international normalized ratio (INR) between 2 and 3. Randomized trials looking at high-intensity coagulation with an INR of 3–4 vs standard intensity treatment with an INR of 2–3 showed a slight increase in bleeding risk in the high-intensity group, and there was no clear reduction in thrombotic events with high-intensity treatment, so its current uses should not be recommended, with the exception of complicated cases where thrombosis is occurring despite warfarin therapy with an INR of 2–3.
- For arterial cerebral thrombosis, a recent review[1] suggests either warfarin, (INR 2–3) or clopidogrel or aspirin/dipyridamole depending on whether the thrombosis was cardioembolic or not.
- For arterial non-cerebral thrombosis, the same review suggests warfarin (INR 2–3) for non-cardiac thrombosis and aspirin/clopidogrel ± a stent in cardiac thrombosis.
- Mild thrombocytopenia need not be treated. Severe cases (<50 × 10^9/L) should be treated with oral corticosteroids in the first instance. In those failing to respond, gamma-globulin, danazol, and splenectomy have been used with varying success.
- The presence of antiphospholipid antibodies in pregnancy, in the absence of a history of thrombosis or foetal loss, is not an indication for anticoagulation. Many clinicians use low-dose aspirin in this setting.
- Pregnant women with a previous thrombosis should be on therapeutic dose low molecular weight heparin during the pregnancy (with regular monitoring for adverse effects), then converted to warfarin (INR 2–3) in the postpartum period.
- In patients with positive APL antibodies, but no thrombotic events, prophylactic heparin in the peri-operative period is recommended
- Women with APS on warfarin should be converted to standard heparin or low-molecular-weight heparins preferably prior to conception, although the reader should be aware that the latter may not be licensed for this purpose. Aspirin should also be introduced.
- Other advances have been the realization that high-dose immunosuppression is unwarranted and that combined care between rheumatology, obstetrics, and haematology, with judicious monitoring and timely intervention has a significant impact on outcome in pregnancy.

1 Giannikopoulos B, Krilis SA (2009). How I treat antiphospholipid syndrome. *Blood* **114**: 2020–30.

Table 11.3 The treatment of APS in those with a previous thrombosis

Clinical situation		Treatment
Asymptomatic		Observation and/or low-dose aspirin
Thrombosis	Deep venous—1st event	Lifelong warfarin (INR 2–3) OR
		3–6 months warfarin (INR 2–3) if additional transient/reversible risk factor
	1st stroke	Lifelong warfarin (INR 2–3) if cardioembolic
		Lifelong warfarin (INR 2–3) or clopidogrel or aspirin ± dipyridamole if non-cardioembolic
	Transient ischaemia	Low-dose aspirin
	1st non-cerebral arterial event	Lifelong warfarin (INR 2–3) if non-cardiac
		Aspirin/clopidogrel ± stent if cardiac
	Recurrent arterial/venous event, whilst on warfarin	Warfarin (INR 3–4) and low-dose aspirin or LMWH if unstable INR
	Catastrophic APS	iv heparin
		iv methylprednisolone plus
		plasmapheresis OR IVIG
Pregnancy	No previous history	Observation and/or low-dose aspirin
	Recurrent first trimester or second/third trimester foetal loss	Low-dose aspirin and LMWH
	Repeat foetal loss despite heparin and aspirin	Unknown
Thrombocytopenia	Mild (100–150 count)	Observe
	Moderate (50–100)	Observe
	Severe (<50)	Corticosteroids (as ITP), IVIG, immunosuppression (e.g. rituximab)

LMWH = low molecular weight heparin.

Adapted from Giannikopoulos B, Krilis SA. How I treat the antiphospholipd syndrome. *Blood* 2009; **114**: 2020–2030.

Catastrophic antiphospholipid syndrome

Introduction

- This rare variant of APS (<1% cases) affects small vessels and visceral organs and was first described in 1992. It is an important and serious condition that can present to many medical specialties.
- It can present in previously asymptomatic patients.
- The trigger is an infection in 20% cases. Other precipitating factors include trauma/surgery, malignancy, warfarin withdrawal in a patient with APS, pregnancy, and oral contraceptives.
- Catastrophic antiphospholipid syndrome (CAPS) is associated with other autoimmune conditions such as SLE (📖 Chapter 10, p 321), RA (📖 Chapter 5, p 233) and systemic sclerosis (SScl, 📖 Chapter 13, p 363).
- Despite these risk factors it is estimated that 45% cases have no known trigger.
- Mortality is high at 50% and most patients require the Intensive Care Unit.

Clinical features

- Diffuse peripheral and central thrombosis occurs leading to:
  - limb arterial and venous occlusion;
  - intra-abdominal organ infarction including renal failure;
  - pulmonary emboli and adult respiratory distress syndrome;
  - small vessel cerebrovascular disease;
  - aortic and mitral valve defects, and myocardial infarction;
  - other thrombotic complications, such as ovarian, testicular, and retinal vessel occlusion.
- Livedo reticularis, gangrene, and purpura are visible markers of the disorder on the skin.
- Bone marrow infarction has also been reported.
- Classification criteria have been produced.[1]
- Preliminary data from 300 patients in a CAPS registry[2] have shown the majority are female (72%), almost half had primary APS (46%) and a precipitating factor was found in 53%. Data from the registry also showed the most common sites are renal (71%), pulmonary (64%), cerebral (62%) and cardiac (51%).
- The presence of systemic immune response syndrome, in which pro-inflammatory cytokines are released from affected tissues, is also thought to contribute to morbidity and mortality.

1 Cervera R, Font J, Gomez-Puerta JA, et al. (2005). Validation of the preliminary criteria for the classification of the catastrophic antiphospholipid syndrome. *Ann Rheum Dis* **64**: 1205–9.

2 Cerevera R (2010). Catastrophic antiphospholipid syndrome (CAPS): update from the 'CAPS Registry'. *Lupus* **19**: 412–8.

Laboratory features

These include:
- Moderate-to-severe thrombocytopenia.
- Haemolysis with schistocytes.
- Disseminated intravascular coagulation.
- High levels of IgG ACL antibodies or presence of lupus anticoagulant.

The differential diagnosis

The clinician should consider the following conditions:
- Thrombotic thrombocytopenic purpura (red cell fragments more numerous than in CAPS).
- HELLP syndrome (haemolysis, elevated liver enzymes and low platelets).
- Haemolytic–uraemic syndrome.
- Cryoglobulinaemia.
- Vasculitis.

Treatment and prognosis

- Apart from techniques and therapies used in the intensive support of multiple organ failure, iv heparin, corticosteroids, plasmapheresis, and iv immunoglobulin (for 4–5 days at a dose of 0.4 g/kg/day) can be used.
- Case reports exist in single patients describing the use of prostacyclin, defibrotide (not licensed in the UK), fibrinolytics, and rituximab.
- Cyclophosphamide has been shown to be beneficial only in patients with APS and an SLE flare.
- Mortality remains >50% and 25% of survivors will develop further APS-related events.
- Recurrence of CAPS is very rare.

Sjögren's syndrome

Epidemiology and pathology

- Sjögren's syndrome (SS) is a chronic autoimmune disease of unknown aetiology, characterized by lymphocyte infiltration of exocrine glands resulting in xerostomia and keratoconjunctivitis sicca.
- The condition may be primary, associated with specific extraglandular (systemic) disease, or secondary, in association with a number of other autoimmune rheumatic diseases, including rheumatoid arthritis (RA, 📖 Chapter 5, p 233) and systemic lupus erythematosus (SLE, 📖 Chapter 10, p 321).
- It is also a disorder in which a benign autoimmune process can terminate in a lymphoid malignancy.
- The syndrome affects women more than men in a ratio of 9:1, and tends to occur at 40–50 years of age. It can, however, occur at any age.
- Population prevalence is estimated at 1%, similar to that of RA.
- The triggering of autoimmunity, and the development and continuation of an autoimmune response remain a great source of interest as much in SS as in other areas of autoimmune rheumatic disease. The links between environmental stimulus and immunogenetics, and the studies of humoral and lymphocyte activity may help to untangle the mechanisms whereby immunological dysregulation can lead to malignant transformation of B cells involved in the immune process.
- Epstein–Barr and retroviruses have been implicated in pathogenesis.
- HLA DR–3 is strongly associated.
- Antibodies to nuclear components Ro and La are found, and are thought to be formed when these antigens are exposed on the surface of apoptotic cells.
- Rheumatoid factor (RF) and antinuclear antibodies are also common and patients may be erroneously diagnosed with RA.
- Recently discovered autoantigens in SS include fodrin and muscarinic acetylcholine receptor M3.

The classification criteria for primary SS are listed in Table 12.1.

- To satisfy classification criteria for primary SS, either an abnormal labial gland biopsy or antibodies to Ro and/or La must be present.
- Exclusions include head and neck irradiation, hepatitis C, AIDS, preexisting lymphoma, sarcoidosis, graft vs host disease, anticholinergic drug use.

Table 12.1 Classification criteria for primary Sjögren's syndrome. For classification purposes, 4 of 6 criteria must be present

Criteria	Comment
Ocular symptoms	Dry eyes >3 months, sense of sand/gravel in eyes, or use of tear substitutes >3 times/day
Oral symptoms	Dry mouth >3 months, recurrent swollen salivary glands, frequent use of liquid to swallow
Positive Schirmer's test	
Low unstimulated salivary flow	Less than 0.1 mL/min
*Abnormal lower lip biopsy	
*Antibodies to Ro/La	

*One of these two criteria must be positive for this diagnosis.

Vitali C, et al. Classification criteria for Sjögren's syndrome; a revised version of the European criteria proposed by the American-European consensus group. *Ann Rheum Dis,* 2002; **61**: 554–558.

Clinical manifestations of Sjögren's syndrome

Glandular disease

- The initial manifestations can be non-specific and 8–10 years can elapse before the diagnosis is established.
- Typical initial features of 'sicca' syndrome include subjective dry eyes (xerophthalmia) in >50% at presentation, dry mouth (xerostomia) in 40%, and parotid/salivary gland enlargement in 25%. The prevalence of these manifestations increase with the duration of disease. There may be concurrent corneal and conjunctival damage (keratoconjunctivitis sicca), and dental caries from poor tear and salivary flow, respectively.
- A number of other conditions can lead to a dry mouth or parotid/salivary gland swelling, and these should be borne in mind during assessment.
- Some causes of xerostomia/ophthalmia include:
  - age (frequent in the elderly);
  - drugs—psychotropic, parasympathetic, antihypertensive, diuretics;
  - dehydration;
  - psychogenic;
  - irradiation;
  - congenital gland malformation or absence.
- Some causes of parotid gland enlargement include:
  - neoplasia;
  - bacterial and viral [mumps, influenza, Epstein–Barr virus (EBV)];
  - Cytomegalovirus (CMV), human immunodeficiency virus (HIV), coxsackie A infection;
  - recurrent parotitis/chronic sialadenitis;
  - sarcoidosis;
  - endocrine—diabetes mellitus, acromegaly.

Extraglandular (systemic) disease

Extraglandular disease is seen in one-third of patients with primary SS. The main symptoms are fatigue, low-grade fever, myalgia, and arthralgia (Table 12.2).

Joints

Joint pain is common; radiographs rarely reveal pathological changes. Non-erosive arthritis is more frequent in patients with Raynaud's phenomenon, and the latter can pre-date SS by many years. In contrast to SScl (Chapter 13, p 363), Raynaud's in SS is not associated with digital ulceration and infarcts.

Table 12.2 The incidence of extraglandular manifestations of primary Sjögren's syndrome

Condition	Frequency (%)
Arthralgia/arthritis	37
Raynaud's phenomenon	16
Cutaneous vasculitis	12
Pulmonary disease	9
Lymphadenopathy	7
Peripheral neuropathy	7
Renal disease	6
Autoimmune hepatitis	2
Lymphoproliferative disease	2
Myositis	1

Skin

- The skin may be involved with itchy annular erythema, alopecia, and hyper/hypopigmentation. A hypersensitivity vasculitis may also develop.
- Vascular involvement in SS affects small- and medium-sized vessels. The most common manifestations are purpura, urticaria, and skin ulceration. Skin vasculitis in SS is more benign and treatment with corticosteroids is not always needed.

Pulmonary disease

Pulmonary function abnormalities are seen in 25% patients, although they are not usually clinically significant. Lymphocytic infiltration occurs around bronchioles, leading to a picture of cryptogenic organizing pneumonia. This responds well to corticosteroids.

Renal disease

- Overt renal disease is found in 10% of patients with primary SS.
- An abnormal urine acidification test is found in up to 40% of cases but distal tubular acidosis (📖 Chapter 16, p 431) complicated by concurrent renal stones is relatively uncommon. Fanconi syndrome is also uncommon.
- Glomerulonephritis is rare and seen mainly in those with SS/SLE overlap. In many cases a consistent finding is cryoglobulinaemia and hypocomplementaemia.

Gastrointestinal and hepatobiliary disease

- Dysphagia due to dryness of the pharynx and oesophagus is common. Chronic atrophic gastritis may occur due to lymphocytic infiltration similar to that seen in the salivary glands.

- Subclinical hyperamylasaemia is a common finding in up to 25% of cases and there may be a close link between 'autoimmune cholangiitis' of SS and primary biliary cirrhosis (PBC). Sicca syndrome is found in approximately 50% of cases of PBC.
- Transaminitis may be due to hepatitis C. Hepatitis C can cause a Sjögren's-like disease often in association with a 'mixed' cryoglobulinaemia.

Neuromuscular disease

- Peripheral sensory neuropathy is the most common neuromuscular feature of SS, and may require measurement of epidermal nerve density by skin biopsy to confirm the diagnosis.
- Mononeuritis multiplex as a consequence of vasculitis is well recognized as is the isolated involvement of cranial nerves, particularly the trigeminal and optic nerve.
- Specific involvement of the central nervous system remains a controversy. Multiple sclerosis-like syndromes may be seen.
- Myalgia is common; myositis is rare, but responds to immunosuppression (📖 Chapter 14, p 385).

Lymphoproliferative disease

- Patients with SS have approximately a 16% increased risk of developing a lymphoma, compared to age, sex, and race-matched normal controls. The lymphomas are primarily B cell in origin, usually expressing the monoclonal IgMk, and of two major types, either highly undifferentiated, or well-differentiated immunocytomas.
- The clinical picture is diverse. The approach to therapy should be determined by the stage and histological grade of the disease.
- The salivary glands are the main site of lymphomatous change. The presence of lymphadenopathy, organomegaly, or persistent, painful, and continuously enlarged salivary glands, in the absence of infection, should raise suspicion and warrants biopsy. Other organs and systems may be affected including the reticuloendothelial system, lungs, kidneys, and GI tract.
- Risk factors include monoclonal gammopathy, cryoglobulins, hypocomplementaemia and major salivary gland swelling.

Cardiovascular system

Anti-Ro and La antibodies cross the placenta and can cause foetal congenital heart block. Mothers with these antibodies have a 1 in 20 risk. Foetal heart rate monitoring in specialist centres is needed. Oral dexamethasone given to mother's early following detection of heart block may reverse the condition. Neonatal lupus is also seen, its most common manifestation being a florid rash.

Other pathology in SS

- Over 50% of patients have antithyroid antibodies and altered thyroid biochemistry without necessarily overt clinical symptoms.
- Non-bacterial interstitial cystitis due to an intense inflammation of the mucosa can cause frequency, nocturia, and perineal pain.

- Mild normochromic, normocytic anaemia is common. Leucopaenia is seen in 15–20% of patients with SS. The ESR is often raised, but the CRP usually normal.

Other autoimmune diseases

In a recent retrospective case review of 114 patients with primary SS, 33% had an additional autoimmune disease, 6% two diseases, and 2% three diseases. Hypothyroidism was most common condition seen.

Investigation of Sjögren's syndrome

- Common laboratory findings in primary SS are detailed in Table 12.3.
- To evaluate the glandular component of the disease, various tests are used. Setting a cut-off point between the normal and abnormal individual is difficult.
- Salivary flow rates (sialometry) can be measured for whole saliva or separate secretions from different salivary glands, with or without stimulation. Patients with overt SS have decreased flow rates. This technique is simple and effective, but can be confounded by concomitant use of drugs with anticholinergic properties.
- Anatomical changes in the ductal system can be assessed by radio contrast sialography. This can, however, be painful and there is some controversy as to its sensitivity and specificity.
- Scintigraphy, with uptake of ^{99}Tc, may provide a functional evaluation of all the salivary glands by observing the rate and density of uptake and the time for it to appear in the mouth after iv administration. Scanning has a high sensitivity but low specificity. Neither sialography nor scintigraphy are suggested as routine investigations.
- Schirmer's test is used for the evaluation of tear secretion. Strips of filter paper 30 mm in length are slipped beneath the inferior eye-lid by a fold at one end of the strip. After 5 min the length of paper that has been made wet by the tears is measured; wetting of <5 mm is a strong indication of diminished tear secretion.
- A labial gland biopsy is often essential to the establishment of a diagnosis of SS, particularly when the patient lacks anti-Ro or anti-La antibodies:
  - Because there is a risk of (transient) sensory nerve damage, the biopsy should be performed by a surgeon with experience in the technique;
  - At least 4–6 glands must be harvested, since the pathologic process is focal;
  - Biopsies should not be performed if there is mucosal inflammation overlying the biopsy site or there is a past history of therapeutic head and neck irradiation;
  - The biopsy must be scored as to the number of lymphocytic foci (i.e. aggregates of 50 or more lymphocytes) that surround ducts or blood vessels, and are adjacent to histologically-normal acini;
  - A score of 1 or more foci per 4 mm^2 is compatible with SS. However, focal lymphocytic sialoadenitis can also be seen in hepatitis C, HIV, graft versus host disease and patients with autoimmune disease in the absence of sicca.

Table 12.3 Common laboratory findings in primary SS

Finding		Frequency (%)
General	Anaemia	20
	Thrombocytopenia	13
	Leucopaenia	16
	Raised ESR	22
	Monoclonal gammopathy	22
	Hypergammaglobulinaemia	22
Cryoglobulinaemia		9
Serology	ANA	74
	Rheumatoid factor	38
	Ro/SS-A	40
	La/SS-B	26
	ANCA	6
	Antimitochondrial	5

Garcia-Carrasco M, *et al*. Primary Sjögren syndrome: Clinical and immunologic disease patterns in a cohort of 400 patients. *Medicine* 2002; **81**: 270-80.

Treatment of Sjögren's syndrome

Table 12.4 summarizes the treatment options for Sjögren's syndrome.

Table 12.4 The treatment of Sjögren's syndrome

Condition	Treatment
Dry eyes	Artificial tears
	Topical ciclosporin drops
	Punctal occlusion (plugs)
	Treatment of Meibomian gland dysfunction (with warm compresses)
Dry mouth	Frequent sips of water and good oral hygiene
	Sugar-free lozenges/lemon drops
	Artificial saliva
Sicca manifestations	May improve with the cholinergic agent pilocarpine (side-effects include flushing/sweating), *or* cevimeline (not licensed in the UK) (fewer side-effects)
Vaginal dryness	Patients may respond to propionic acid gels. Rigorous treatment of infection. Advice on lubricants, etc., if there is pain with intercourse
Salivary gland	Infection—tetracycline (500 mg 4 times/day) and NSAIDs. Persistent pain and swelling—biopsy
Arthralgia	Hydroxychloroquine 200–400 mg/day
Systemic vasculitis	Necrotizing vasculitis and glomerulonephritis—prednisone and/or cyclophosphamide. Leucocytoclastic vasculitis—no specific therapy
Liver disease	Cholestasis may respond to ursodeoxychoic acid 10–15 mg/kg/day
Chronic erythematosus candidiasis	Topical nystatin, miconazole, or ketoconazole
Interstitial lung disease	Prednisolone, cyclophosphamide

Other treatments

- There is no evidence that azathioprine, low dose steroids, ciclosporin, infliximab or methotrexate are useful.
- Hydroxychloroquine normalizes ESR and immunoglobulin levels, but has no effect on salivary flow rates. Many clinicians use it to treat fatigue, myalgia, and arthralgia.
- Rituximab, in limited studies to date may improve symptoms in an SS patient treated for lymphoma.
- Oral interferon alfa improves salivary flow, but long-term use may be limited.

Systemic sclerosis and related disorders

Epidemiology and diagnostic criteria

- Scleroderma is a spectrum of rare disorders ranging from limited to generalized, non-systemic to systemic, and environmental to autoimmune rheumatic disease. Generalized scleroderma, systemic sclerosis, predominantly affects women and is associated with production of collagen, widespread microvascular damage, and inflammation.
- The spectrum of scleroderma and scleroderma-like syndromes includes:
  - Raynaud's phenomenon—primary, secondary;
  - scleroderma (localized)—morphoea, linear, *en coup-de-sabre*;
  - scleroderma (systemic)—limited cutaneous, diffuse cutaneous, scleroderma sine scleroderma;
  - chemical induced—environmental, occupational, drugs;
  - scleroderma-like disease (Table 13.1)—metabolic, immunological, localized sclerosis, and visceral disease.
- There is no single diagnostic test for systemic sclerosis (SScl), although there are specific autoantibodies. For the purpose of separating it from other autoimmune rheumatic diseases and identifying case profiles, preliminary criteria were developed in 1980 by the American Rheumatism Association. These criteria have a 97% sensitivity and specificity, but are less sensitive for the largest subset of patients with limited cutaneous disease, failing to identify 10% of such cases.
- Currently the most widely used classification (Table 13.2) defines 2 subsets divided into limited cutaneous (lcSScl) and diffuse cutaneous (dcSScl). Over 60% of cases are in the 'limited' subset, where visceral involvement is late, some 10–30 years after onset of Raynaud's. The term 'limited cutaneous' is now preferred to CREST (**c**alcinosis, **R**aynaud's phenomenon (RP), o**e**sophageal dysmotility, **s**clerodactyly, **t**elangiectasia), although this acronym is a useful reminder of the common characteristics of lcSScl.
- As a minimum, a patient must have RP and a positive antinuclear antibody (ANA) to consider a diagnosis of SScl.
- dcSSCL is more serious, of rapid onset, and associated with organ failure often within the first 5 years of presentation.
- Clearly, these models will continue to change and develop as knowledge of pathogenesis advances and immunological findings are matched to clinical subsets.

Table 13.1 Scleroderma-like syndromes

Metabolic/ inherited	Carcinoid syndrome	Scleroderma-like lesions can be found with malignant carcinoid; their presence is associated with a poor prognosis.
	Acromegaly	Associated with skin puffiness that can mimic early scleroderma. Acromegaly-skin also associated with increase in sebum and sweat absent in SScl.
	Phenylketonuria	Phenylalanine-restricted diet may improve skin changes.
	Amyloidosis	Plaques from direct dermal infiltration can mimic SScl; more common are alopecia, ecchymoses, and nail dystrophy.
Immunological/ inflammatory	Chronic graft vs host disease	Skin changes favour the trunk, hips, and thighs, but can affect the entire body. Associated with pruritis and hypopigmentation.
	Eosinophilic fasciitis	Associated with painful induration of the skin, hypereosinophilia, and hypergammaglobulinaemia. Early skin changes described as 'peau d'orange'.
	Overlap/ undifferentiated autoimmune rheumatic disease	Mixed connective tissue disease (MCTD) is associated with RNP-positivity, and is sometimes classified as a form of scleroderma. Polymyositis-scleroderma overlap syndromes are associated with antibodies to the PM/SScl complex.
	Scleroedema	Occurs with diabetes, monoclonal gammopathies, and after certain infections (e.g. strep throat). Unlike SScl, can occur without Raynaud's phenomenon.
	Scleromyxoedema	Waxy induration of the skin along the forehead, neck, and behind the ears. Not associated with Raynaud's phenomenon.
	Nephrogenic fibrosing dermopathy	Rapid induration of the skin and other organs associated with exposure to gadolinium-based contrast used for MRI.

Continued

Table 13.1 *(Cont'd)*

	Idiopathic pulmonary fibrosis	Patients diagnosed with idiopathic pulmonary fibrosis should be evaluated for the presence of Raynaud's, capillary loop dilatation, and other signs of SScl.
	POEMS	Polyneuropathy, organomegaly, endocrinopathy, M-protein, and skin changes. Hyperpigmentation is most common, but acrocyanosis/skin thickening are seen.
Acquired	Lipodermatosclerosis	Hyperpigmentation and induration of the lower extremities associated with chronic venous insufficiency.
	Eosinophilic myalgia syndrome and toxic oil syndrome	Acute syndrome caused by exposure to L-tryptophan and aniline-denatured rapeseed oil, respectively. Largely of historical interest.
	Bleomycin exposure	Used as a model to study scleroderma.

Table 13.2 The classification of systemic sclerosis

1 'Prescleroderma'	Raynaud's phenomenon, nail-fold capillary changes
	Disease-specific antinuclear antibodies: • Antitopoisomerase-1 (Scl-70) • Anticentromere (ACA) • Nucleolar
2 Diffuse cutaneous SScl	Skin changes within 1 year of Raynaud's. Truncal and acral (face, arms, hands, feet) skin involvement
	Tendon friction rubs
	Early, significant organ disease: • Interstitial lung disease • Oliguric renal failure ('scleroderma renal crisis') • Myocardial disease • Gastrointestinal disease
	Nail-fold capillary dilatation and/or 'drop out'
	Scl-70 antibodies in up to 60% of patients

Table 13.2 *(Cont'd)*

3 Limited cutaneous SScl	Raynaud's phenomenon for many years
	Acral skin involvement
	Late incidence of pulmonary hypertension with or without interstitial lung disease
	Skin calcification and telangiectasia
	Nail-fold capillary dilatation and/or 'drop out'
	ACA antibodies in 70–80% of patients
4 Scleroderma sine scleroderma	Raynaud's
	No skin involvement
	Presentation with lung fibrosis, renal crisis, cardiac or gastrointestinal disease
	Antinuclear antibodies may be present

- The three principle pathologies in scleroderma are:
  - *Raynaud's phenomenon*: a vasculopathy is found that manifests clinically as Raynaud's phenomenon, and pathologically as endothelial cell injury. Vascular injury may be the primary event either by vasomotor instability or microvascular intimal proliferation and vessel obliteration. Intravascular pathology in the form of increased platelet activity, red cell rigidity, and thrombosis may also be a factor;
  - *inflammation* occurs early in scleroderma, and may no longer be present at the time of diagnosis. Clinically, this active phase of scleroderma is associated with oedematous (not indurated) skin and the presence of tendon friction rubs (which can be felt by placing the hand over the tendon during active or passive range of motion);
  - *fibrosis* is the hallmark of several diseases and in SScl it is widespread and non-organ-specific. Excess deposition of collagen and extracellular matrix protein is found in the skin and internal organs of patients with SScl. Current research focuses on the role of several proteins including endothelin-1 and transforming growth factor-β.
- Several chemical agents have been implicated in the development of scleroderma, including:
  - silica;
  - organic chemicals;
  - aliphatic hydrocarbons—vinyl chloride, naphtha;
  - aromatic hydrocarbons—benzene, toluene;
  - drugs;
  - hydroxytryptophan, carbidopa, fenfluramine, bleomycin.
- These exposures likely explain only a very small fraction of patients who develop scleroderma or similar conditions.

Cutaneous features of scleroderma and their treatment

Scleroderma—'localized' skin changes

- This is distinct from SScl in its absence of vasospasm, vascular, and organ damage, and the distribution of skin lesions.
- Morphoea may be 'circumscribed' with just 1 or 2 lesions or 'generalized'. The rash is often itchy, violaceous, or erythematous, and progresses to firm 'hide-bound' skin with hypo- or hyperpigmentation, and subsequent atrophy. The 'circumscribed' condition tends to resolve within 3–5 years and treatment is often unnecessary. The acral parts are spared, the trunk and legs being most often involved. The 'generalized' form can be disfiguring, leading to contractures, ulceration, and occasionally malignancy. Generalized morphoea may respond to PUVA. Corticosteroids, penicillamine, methotrexate, intralesional interferon, or iv immunoglobulin may also be effective.
- Guttate morphoea is a variant with small 10-mm diameter papules and minimal sclerosis, resembling lichen sclerosus et atrophicus. The lesions usually localize to the neck, shoulders, and anterior chest wall.
- Linear scleroderma describes a band-like pattern of sclerosis, often in a dermatomal distribution. The sclerotic areas often cross over joints, and are associated with soft tissue and bone atrophy, and growth defects. Treatment is similar to generalized morphoea as above. Physiotherapy and appropriate exercises may help to minimize growth defects in the childhood form.
- *En coup-de-sabre* is linear sclerosis involving the face or scalp, and associated with hemi-atrophy of the face on the same side. The lesion assumes a depressed appearance reminiscent of a scar from a sabre.

Scleroderma/systemic sclerosis—'diffuse' skin changes

- The changes in the skin usually proceed through three phases of early, classic, and late. In the early stage there may be non-pitting oedema of the hands and feet, most marked in the mornings and often associated with RP. The skin then becomes taut, the epidermis thins, hair growth ceases, and skin creases disappear and the 'classic' changes of scleroderma become more pronounced. The classic changes remain static for many years.
- The late phase may evolve at any time. Truncal and limb skin softens such that it can be difficult to know that a person ever had sclerosis. However, the hand changes rarely resolve and continue to show the ravages of fibrosis and contractures. During this phase of the disease digital pitting scars, loss of finger pad tissue, ulcers, telangiectasia, and calcinosis can occur.
- All patients with SScl will have some involvement of the face and the digits (although this involvement may be mild). Skin thickening limited to the fingers, but sparing the proximal upper extremities is called *sclerodactly*.
- *Limited scleroderma* (lcSScl) is associated with skin involvement limited to the hands and face. This form of SScl, also known as CREST, can lead to pulmonary arterial hypertension in the absence of pulmonary fibrosis.

- *Diffuse scleroderma* (dcSScl) is associated with taut hypo- or hyperpigmented skin involvement proximal to the elbow, knee, or clavicle. In this group there is a preponderance of visceral involvement (such as pulmonary fibrosis) in the first 5 years of symptoms.
- A practical scheme for assessing dcSScl and lcSScl by dividing the disease into early and late stages is shown in Table 13.3.

Raynaud's phenomenon (Table 13.4)

- The overall prevalence of this phenomenon is between 3 and 10% of the population worldwide, variation depending on climate, skin colour, and racial background in particular. In SScl RP is present in approximately 95% of cases.
- The classical features are episodic pallor of the digits (due to ischaemia), followed by cyanosis (due to deoxygenation), and then redness and suffusion with pain and tingling. The last stage of redness is a reactive hyperaemia following the return of blood. Continuous blueness/cyanosis with pain is not characteristic of RP.
- Symptoms that might suggest secondary RP include an onset in men, patients older than 45 years, symptoms all year round, digital ulceration, and asymmetry.
- The antinuclear antibodies discussed earlier should be sought nail-fold capillaroscopy should be performed (Plate 8). Pathological changes seen on capillaroscopy include nail-fold capillary dilatation, haemorrhage, and drop-out. Both have a high predictive power for detecting those patients likely to develop SScl.
- Conservative measures should be directed at keeping the core body temperature warm.

Table 13.3 Characteristic findings in early and late systemic sclerosis

Diffuse cutaneous features	Early onset (<3 years from onset of disease)	Late onset (>3 years from onset of disease)
Constitutional	Fatigue, weight loss	Minimal
Vascular	Raynaud's (often mild)	Severe Raynaud's. Telangiectasia
Cutaneous	Rapid progression involving arms, face, and trunk	Stable or some regression
Musculoskeletal	Arthralgia, myalgia, stiffness	Flexion contractures
Gastrointestinal	Dysphagia and 'heart burn'	More severe dysphagia. Midgut and anorectal disease
Cardiopulmonary	Myocarditis, pericarditis, lung fibrosis	Progression of established disease/pulmonary hypertension
Renal	Maximum risk of scleroderma renal crisis	Crisis uncommon after 4 years

Limited cutaneous features	Early onset (<10 years from onset of disease)	Late onset (>10 years from onset of disease)
Constitutional	None	Digital ulceration or gangrene
Vascular	Severe Raynaud's. Telangiectasia	Stable, calcinosis
Cutaneous	Mild sclerosis on face	Flexion contractures
Musculoskeletal	Occasional joint stiffness	More severe symptoms common. Midgut and anorectal disease
Gastrointestinal	Dysphagia and 'heart burn'	Slow progressive lung fibrosis. Pulmonary hypertension.
Cardiopulmonary	Rarely involved	Right-sided heart failure
Renal	No direct involvement	Rarely involved

Table 13.4 The treatment of Raynaud's phenomenon

Treatment	Examples	Comments
Non-pharmacological	Hand warmers. Protective clothing	Universally helpful
	Evening primrose oil	Effective in clinical trials
	Fish-oil capsules	
Parenteral vasodilator	Nifedipine or amlodipine	Calcium channel blockers can be effective, but may cause oedema, hypotension, headache, etc.
	Sildenafil	
	Losartan	
	Topical glyceryl trinitrate	High rate of discontinuation due to side effects
	Prostacyclin	For severe attacks, digital gangrene, and prior to hand surgery
Surgery	Chemical or operative lumbar or digital sympathectomy. Debridement. Amputation	

Systemic features of the disease, investigation, and treatment

The gastrointestinal tract (Table 13.5)

- The GI tract is probably the most commonly involved system in SScl. Over 90% of all patients with lcSScl and dcSScl develop oesophageal hypomotility, with >50% of patients with lcSScl having serious disease.
- The cause of gastrointestinal dysfunction in SScl is not entirely clear. Possible contributing factors include neural dysfunction, tissue fibrosis, and muscle atrophy. In the earliest stages of neural dysfunction most patients are asymptomatic.
- Prokinetic drugs, such as metoclopramide may help some patients with oesophageal hypomotility.
- Many patients develop reflux oesophagitis. Simple advice such as raising the head of the bed, taking frequent small meals, and avoiding late night snacks, may help. Patients often require high-dose proton-pump inhibitors.
- Small bowel disease with hypomobility can lead to weight loss and malabsorption; bacterial overgrowth may exacerbate the situation requiring rotational courses of antibiotics and the use of prokinetic drugs. Ultimately, the small bowel may fail, necessitating total parenteral nutrition.
- Atony and hypomotility of the rectum and sigmoid colon may cause constipation and incontinence, best managed with bulking agents, although severe cases may need limited surgery or the use of implantable sacral stimulators.
- Anaemia due to vascular lesions in the GI mucosa is now widely recognized. The classic appearance in the stomach is now called gastric antrum venous ectasia (watermelon stomach), and these lesions may be treated by argon laser therapy if blood loss is significant, although this is not curative.

Pulmonary disease (Table 13.6)

- Pulmonary disease ranks second to oesophageal in frequency of visceral disease. With the improvements in management of renal disease, pulmonary disease is now the major cause of death in SScl.
- The major clinical manifestations are parenchymal lung disease (interstitial lung disease, organizing pneumonia, and traction bronchiectasis) and pulmonary vascular disease (isolated pulmonary hypertension, pulmonary hypertension associated with interstitial lung disease, and pulmonary oedema). Far less common conditions include pleurisy, aspiration pneumonia, drug-induced pneumonitis, and spontaneous pneumothorax.

Table 13.5 Common gastrointestinal disorders in systemic sclerosis

Site	Disorder	Investigation	Treatment
Mouth	Caries, sicca syndrome	Dental radiographs	Oral hygiene. Artificial saliva
Oesophagus	Hypomotility	Barium swallow	Metoclopramide
	Reflux		High-dose proton pump inhibitors
	Strictures	Endoscopy	Dilatation
Stomach	Gastroparesis		Metoclopramide
	Gastric ulcer	Barium swallow. Endoscopy	Proton-pump inhibitor
Small bowel	Hypomotility	Barium follow-through	Metoclopramide
	Malabsorption	Hydrogen breath test	Pancreatic supplements. Low-dose octreotide. Nutritional support, antibiotics
		Jejunal aspiration/biopsy	If serologic evidence of coeliac disease is present
		Stool cultures	
Large bowel	Hypomotility	Barium enema	Stool bulking agents
Anus	Incontinence	Rectal manometry	Surgery. Neurostimulator

Table 13.6 Cardiopulmonary disorders in systemic sclerosis

Disease	Frequency	Investigation	Treatment
Lung disease:			
Pulmonary fibrosis	Most common in dcSScl (Scl-70+)	Chest radiograph, lung function tests, high-resolution chest CT scan	Controversial; consider corticosteroids and cyclophosphamide
Pleurisy	Uncommon	Chest radiograph	NSAIDs. Low-dose oral prednisolone
Bronchiectasis	Rare	Chest CT scan	Antibiotics. Physiotherapy
Pneumothorax	Rare	Chest radiograph	Chest tube, pleurodesis
Pulmonary hypertension	10–15% overall	Doppler echocardiogram. Catheter studies	Endothelial 1 receptor antagonists (bosentan), prostacyclin sildenafil. Anticoagulation. Long-term oxygen therapy
Cardiac disease:			
Dysrhythmias and conduction defects	Common, but rarely symptomatic	ECG. 24-h ambulatory cardiac monitor	Dependent on rhythm—drugs, pacemaker
Pericarditis	10–15% overall	Echocardiogram	As pleurisy, above
Myocarditis	Rare		Prednisolone, cyclophosphamide. Diuretics
Myocardial fibrosis	30–50% of dcSScl		Controversial; consider diuretics, ACE inhibitors

- Interstitial lung disease often develops insidiously and established fibrosis is currently untreatable. Early diagnosis is therefore vital. Most centres would now treat active disease with oral corticosteroids and either oral or iv cyclophosphamide, although the data are controversial.
- The plain chest radiograph is not a sensitive test for early fibrosis. Lung function tests can be discriminatory. The single-breath diffusion test [diffusion capacity for carbon monoxide (DLCO)] is abnormal in >70% of early cases and lung volumes are often decreased. In the case of a low DLCO and normal lung volumes, the clinician should think of pulmonary hypertension.
- High-resolution CT scanning now plays a major part in detecting and following interstitial lung disease and should be performed whenever possible.
- Fibrosis tends to be associated with dcSScl and Scl-70 antibodies, and PAH with lcSScl and anti-centromere antibodies.
- Recent studies suggest a prevalence of PAH of 12–15% in SScl. Right heart catheterization is the gold standard method of diagnosis, but screening using this method is not practical. Annual echocardiography by experienced practitioners, lung function tests, and clinical assessment are essential to help detect subclinical disease.
- Treatment of PAH associated with SScl has developed rapidly over the last 5–10 years. Continuous parenteral prostacyclin improves symptoms and pulmonary artery pressures, but not mortality. Studies are in progress using subcutaneous and nebulized prostacyclin. Bosentan, an oral endothelin receptor antagonist, improves function and is now an accepted treatment. Sildenafil inhibits phosphodiesterase type 5, and enhances relaxation of vascular smooth muscle, as well as inhibiting their growth. A recent double-blind placebo-controlled study of patients with idiopathic or connective tissue disease associated pulmonary hypertension found that sildenafil significantly improves 6-min walk times and mean pulmonary artery pressure.

Cardiac disease

There are many cardiac manifestations including pericardial effusion, arrhythmias, and myocardial fibrosis. Heart block has been reported, but is rare. Many cases are subclinical and careful monitoring is needed. More epidemiological research is needed in this area.

Renal disease

- Renal disease has been superseded by lung disease as the main cause of death in SScl due to the impact of ACE inhibitors in the treatment of hypertensive renal crisis. However, it remains a major, life-threatening complication of SScl.
- Both epithelial and endothelial damage occur before becoming clinically detectable.
- The most characteristic pattern of involvement is the renal hypertensive crisis, generally occurring with dcSScl within the first 5 years of disease onset. In high-risk patients the incidence may be as high as 20%, and associated with micro-angiopathic haemolytic anaemia, encephalopathy, and convulsions. Mortality may reach 10%.

- A more insidious pattern of renal involvement is also reported in which there a slow decline in glomerular filtration rate is accompanied by proteinuria. This is very uncommon, but probably reflects a more benign vascular and fibrotic process.
- Hypertension should be treated with angiotensin-converting enzyme inhibitors (ACE-I) and calcium-channel blockers.
- Dialysis may become necessary. It is important to know that considerable recovery of renal function can be made after an acute crisis and that decisions involving renal transplantation should be withheld for up to 2 years.
- Corticosteroids are known to increase the risk of renal crisis in dcSSdl. Doses >20 mg prednisolone daily should be avoided.
- Other associated risks for hypertensive renal crisis include rapidly progressive skin disease, diffuse cutaneous disease, and the presence of antibodies to RNA polymerase III.

The management of scleroderma renal crisis as an acute rheumatological emergency is discussed in 🕮 Chapter 24, p 609.

Other organ involvement

Table 13.7 summarizes the involvement of other organs in SSCL.

Malignancy

It has been suggested that there is an increased incidence of all malignancies in SScl patients. Potential causes include immunosuppressive drug use, increased incidence of cancers in scar tissue and oncogene over expression. However, as these patients are closely monitored, there may be ascertainment bias. Further work is needed in this area.

Table 13.7 Other organ involvement associated with systemic sclerosis

Organ	Effect	Frequency
Thyroid gland	Spectrum of autoimmune disease. Hypothyroidism common	20–40%
Liver	Primary biliary cirrhosis	3% of lcSScl*
Nervous system	Trigeminal neuralgia	5%
	Carpal tunnel syndrome	3%
	Sensorimotor neuropathy	
	Autonomic neuropathy	
Genital	Cavernosal artery fibrosis causing impotence	Up to 50%

* Antimitochondrial antibodies found in up to 25% of patients with SSCL and anticentromere antibodies found in 10–20% of patients with primary biliary cirrhosis.

Antifibrotic and immunosuppressive therapies for systemic sclerosis

- Apart from the specific therapies alluded to in the sections on skin and systemic disease above, a number of general systemic therapies are under investigation, although none have demonstrated marked benefit.
- Currently no treatment can induce complete remission of the disease. Some therapies can offer partial relief and control of end-organ damage. The evaluation of treatments is extremely difficult given the complexity, heterogeneity, and episodic nature of the disease, as well as the paucity of patients.
- Penicillamine was been widely used in the past, but a single randomized controlled trial has shown no benefit.
- Novel potential antifibrotic therapies may develop through understanding more about anti cytokine antibodies that block fibroblast activation (e.g. anti-TGF-β), or by antagonists/gene translocations that influence pre- and post-translational modification of collagen.
- Both antimetabolite and alkylating immunomodulatory agents have been used, particularly in early dcSScl. The majority of these therapies are currently being evaluated in controlled trials (Table 13.8).
- Halofuginone, a type I collagen synthesis inhibitor has shown beneficial effects in treating scarring and has been used to mixed effect in bleomycin-induced scleroderma. Further work is needed to assess its use in SScl.
- A recent open label study of minocycline suggests this agent does not work.
- Studies are currently under way looking at the effect of anti-TNF-α agents in early skin disease that is mainly inflammatory in nature.
- Autologous stem cell transplant has been performed in severe disease, but has a high mortality rate. Its place in treatment strategies needs further research.

Table 13.8 Anti-metabolite and alkylating immunomodulatory agents being evaluated for use in treatment of SScl

Agent	Comment
Cyclophosphamide	Efficacy from trial data on lung fibrosis. Often given with steroids
Mycophenolate	Improvement in skin disease
Methotrexate	Control trial demonstrated no benefit in dcSScl
Anti-thymocyte globulin	Possible benefit in diffuse disease, high morbidity
Pooled gammaglobulin	Limited data
Plasmapheresis	Equivocal and anecdotal
Ciclosporin	Beneficial on skin sclerosis
	Watch for renal crisis
	Reduce dose if on calcium-channel blockers
Chlorambucil	Anecdotal and control trial failed to show superiority over placebo
Plasmapheresis	Equivocal and anecdotal
Photopheresis	Limited data; mixed results

Summary—the approach to systemic sclerosis

Diffuse cutaneous systemic sclerosis

History and physical examination generally establishes the diagnosis and autoantibody profiles may identify poor prognosis. The extent of visceral disease should be assessed by baseline investigations as follows:

- Urea and electrolytes.
- Creatinine clearance and urinary protein (repeat annually).
- Barium swallow/GI endoscopy depending on symptoms.
- Chest radiograph at baseline.
- Lung function tests (annually).
- Electrocardiogram (annually).
- Doppler echocardiography (with estimate of pulmonary artery pressure), repeat annually.
- High-resolution CT lung scan if lung function abnormal.
- Given the paucity of patients, it is important to be aware of local or national centres of expertise and patient suitability for clinical trials.

Limited cutaneous systemic sclerosis

By the time of presentation physical signs are usually diagnostic. Investigations are as above and treatment is mostly symptomatic, concentrating on vascular (RP and pulmonary hypertension) and gastrointestinal (GI) disease, with annual review.

Prognosis

- SScl has the highest case-specific mortality of any autoimmune rheumatic disease. Estimates of 5 years mortality in scleroderma range from 34 to 73%. Standardized mortality ratios have been estimated at 3–4 times expected. Logistic regression modelling suggests 3 factors—proteinuria, elevated ESR, and low carbon monoxide diffusion capacity—are >80% accurate at predicting mortality >5 years.
- Patients with renal crisis have been estimated to have a 50% mortality, although the use of ACE inhibitors and renal replacement therapies may have reduced this.
- Anti-topoisomerase and anti-RNA polymerase antibodies have also been associated with SScl-related mortality.
- Advances in the understanding of mechanisms leading to pulmonary hypertension has led to new therapies that, with time, may show significant impact in slowing disease progression.

Scleroderma-like fibrosing disorders

Eosinophilic fasciitis

- This is an uncommon idiopathic condition that is characterized by the rapid spread of skin changes over the extremities. Skin initially takes on a 'peau d'orange' appearance, which is replaced by induration.
- Like SScl, flexion contractures and Raynaud's phenomenon may be present. Unlike SScl, the epidermis is spared (i.e. superficial wrinkling is intact) and nail-fold capillary microscopy is normal.
- The condition may resolve spontaneously. Otherwise, 70% of cases respond to corticosteroids.
- The condition may be a paraneoplastic phenomenon. It is over-represented in women and in the haematological malignancies in this respect. The paraneoplastic condition often fails to respond to steroids and resolves on successful treatment of the underlying malignancy.
- Methotrexate or mycophenolate mofetil may be helpful, but this has not been well studied.

Nephrogenic systemic fibrosis

- Nephrogenic systemic fibrosis (NSF) is also known as nephrogenic fibrosing dermopathy, the current nomenclature reflects the systemic nature of this disease, which can lead to fibrosis in the muscles, myocardium, lungs, kidneys, and testes.
- NSF is characterized by the presence of skin induration, nodular plaques, and flexion contractures in the absence of RP.
- Lesions develop over days to weeks, and initially favour the lower extremities.
- The majority of patients will have end-stage renal disease and a history of exposure to gadoliunium-based contrast.
- Histologically, NSF lesions are characterized by collagen bundles surrounded by fibroblast-like epitheliod or stellate cells, and mucin deposition, which can extend into the fascia and muscles.
- Response to immunosuppressive agents is disappointing. Early institution of physical therapy to prevent contractures and muscle wasting is important. Pain management may be especially challenging.

Scleromyxoedema

- This is characterized by waxy induration of the skin along the forehead (glabella), the neck, and behind the ears.
- Unlike SScl, scleromyxoedema may also affect the middle of the back, which is generally spared in scleroderma.
- Scleromyxoedema can be associated with oesophageal dysmotility and myopathy; case reports have also demonstrated an association with severe neurological sequelae, including encephalopathy, seizures, coma, and psychosis.
- This condition may respond to intravenous immunoglobulin.

Scleroedema

- Scleroedema is a scleroderma-like disorder associated with doughy induration of the skin along the back, neck, face and chest.
- Unlike scleroderma, the extremities are typically spared.
- This disorder is generally seen in association with poorly controlled diabetes, monoclonal gammopathy, or following certain infections, such as streptococcal pharyngitis.
- Prognosis depends on the underlying aetiology. Scleroedema that occurs after infection may resolve spontaneously. Scleroedema associated with diabetes may improve with better glucose control.
- For some patients, ultraviolet light therapy (such as UVA-1, PUVA and photophoresis) may be beneficial.

Idiopathic inflammatory myopathies: polymyositis and dermatomyositis

Epidemiology and diagnosis

- The idiopathic inflammatory myopathies are characterized by proximal muscle weakness and evidence of autoimmune-mediated muscle breakdown. These disorders include:
  - polymyositis;
  - dermatomyositis;
  - juvenile dermatomyositis;
  - myositis associated with neoplasia;
  - myositis associated with connective tissue disease;
  - inclusion body myositis.
- Polymyositis (PM) and dermatomyositis (DM) are the most common forms of 'idiopathic inflammatory myopathy' (IIM), the latter distinguished by the presence of a characteristic rash. Overlap syndromes with other autoimmune rheumatic diseases occur in 15–20% of cases.
- These conditions are rare. PM has an estimated incidence of 2–8 per million. Incidence increases with age and is highest between the ages of 40–65 years. The male to female ratio is 2:1, but is lower in myositis associated with malignancy and higher during the childbearing years (5:1). A small amount of evidence suggests that the incidence in African-Caribbeans compared to white Caucasians is 3–4:1.
- The uncertainty about aetiology makes classification of these conditions difficult. However, a modification of Bohan and Peter's classification (1975) shown in Table 14.1 serves this purpose at present.
- There are a number of secondary causes of myositis and myopathies. These will be discussed later in this chapter.
- The criteria for the diagnosis of PM and DM are shown in Table 14.2.
- Mimics of IIM and other causes of a raised CK should always be considered, particularly in apparently 'immunosuppressant resistant' cases (Table 14.4).

Table 14.1 Modification of Bohan and Peter's classification of PM and DM

1	Primary idiopathic polymyositis
2	Primary idiopathic dermatomyositis
3	1 or 2 above, with malignancy
4	Juvenile poly(dermato)myositis
5	Overlap syndromes with other autoimmune rheumatic diseases
6	Inclusion-body myositis
7	Rarer myositis: granulomatous, eosinophilic, focal, orbital
8	Drug-induced

Table 14.2 Criteria for the diagnosis of poly/dermatomyositis

1	Compatible weakness. Symmetrical proximal muscle weakness developing over weeks or months
2	Elevated serum muscle enzymes, creatine kinase, and aldolase
3	Typical electromyographic findings: myopathic potentials (low amplitude, short duration, polyphasic) fibrillation, positive sharp waves, increased insertional activity, complex repetitive discharges
4	Typical muscle biopsy findings
5	Dermatological features of DM: • Gottron's papules, involving fingers, elbows, knees, and medial malleoli • Heliotrope sign around the eyes • Erythematous and/or poikilodermatous rash

Clinical features of polymyositis and dermatomyositis

Myositis

- Muscle weakness is the main clinical feature in both conditions and is almost universal, tending to develop insidiously over months, but occasionally developing with great speed.
- The weakness is usually symmetric and diffuse, involving the proximal muscles of the neck, shoulders, trunk, hips, and thighs, the lower limb muscles tending to be clinically symptomatic first.
- Weakness of the distal muscles is rare, but can occur late in the disease. The face and ocular muscles may also be involved.
- Shortness of breath may be a consequence of diaphragmatic and intercostal muscle weakness (as well as other causes that will be discussed later), and should be looked for.
- Myalgia occurs in about 50% of cases; it can be mild and sometimes difficult to distinguish from polymyalgia rheumatica.
- There may be atrophy in chronic disease, more so in PM than DM, and contractures may occur in disease of long duration.
- Often the distinction between autoimmune rheumatic disease overlapping with PM/DM versus an autoimmune rheumatic disease with myositis as a manifestation can be very difficult. The relative severity of clinical symptoms and the serological picture may be of help.

Cutaneous disease

- The rash of DM commonly precedes the weakness by weeks to months. The rash may parallel the weakness or remain independent, persisting after the myositis resolves. Erythematous or violaceous papules or plaques (Gottron's papules) or macular patches (Gottron's sign) may occur over the metacarpophalangeal and proximal (occasionally distal) interphalangeal joints. Occasionally, these lesions may be found on the extensor surfaces of the knees, wrists, elbows, or medial malleoli. The rash is present in up to 80% of cases.
- A macular eruption may involve the upper chest, neck, shoulders, extremities, face, and scalp. This may develop into poikiloderma, hyper- or hypopigmentation with atrophy and telangiectasia. Typical features include the 'V' sign at the base of the neck anteriorly, and the 'shawl' sign at the back of the neck and across the shoulders.
- The heliotrope rash, found in 30–60% of cases, is a purple/lilac coloured suffusion around the eyes, often associated with peri-orbital oedema. It is characteristic, but not pathognomic.
- Some patients have typical cutaneous DM, but do not develop overt myositis. The term 'amyopathic DM' is applied. The same risk of malignancy and systemic complications remains.
- Calcinosis, cutaneous vasculitis, and ulceration, rare in adults, are more common in juvenile DM.

Malignancy

- Studies suggest a modest increase in malignancies within 1–2 years of onset in DM. The malignancy may pre-date, peri-date, or post-date the onset of myositis. In the majority of cases, cancer and myositis have an independent course.
- The largest population studies suggest the presence of malignancy to occur in 15% of cases of DM (relative risk in men 2.4, in women 3.4) and 9% of cases of PM (relative risk in men 1.8, and in women 1.7). Cancer deaths in studies suggest an increase in DM, but not PM, supporting a true association with DM, rather than a study bias due to intensive searching. The highest risk appears to be in men older than 45 years with DM who lack myositis autoantibodies or overlap autoimmune rheumatic disease.
- Tumours frequent in the general population are frequent in PM and DM. There does, however, appear to be an increase in ovarian, breast, lung, stomach, colon, and bladder cancers out of proportion to that of other tumours.
- The extent of investigation is controversial. Thorough physical assessment should always include rectal, pelvic, and breast examination. Specific investigations should include a chest radiograph, urinalysis, prostate-specific antigen in men, faecal occult blood testing, mammography, and cervical smear, and probably pelvic ultrasound and CA 125 levels in women. Further bowel investigations are open to debate and determined by individual patient symptoms. Remember that an elevated ALT may be from muscle and need not indicate liver pathology.
- Malignancy manifesting as paraneoplastic myopathy and its investigation is discussed in 📖 Chapter 4, p 193.

Systemic manifestations

Table 14.3 shows the systemic manifestations of PM and DM.

Clinical features potentially pointing towards an alternative diagnosis to idiopathic inflammatory myopathy

- Certain features in the history and clinical presentation might suggest a non-inflammatory myopathy. It is important to identify features that may point towards storage diseases, genetic myopathies and neuropathy (Table 14.4 and 14.6). These include:
  - family history of myopathy;
  - drug history;
  - weakness/cramp worsened by exercise or dietary changes (e.g. fasting, carbohydrate intake);
  - muscle atrophy, hypertrophy, or myotonia;
  - fasiculation and other neurological signs;
  - facial/scapulo-humeral involvement.

Assessment of disease activity and damage

- Disease activity measures contain variations on the following information:
  - patient and physician global disease activity scale;
  - duration of active disease;
  - severity at onset;
  - muscle strength measure;
  - physical function measures (Health Assessment Questionnaire;)
  - patient quality of life measures (e.g. Short Form-36);
  - laboratory tests results;
  - quantitative muscle atrophy (e.g. by MRI);
  - damage to different organs/musculoskeletal system/skin (including ulceration and calcinosis).
- Several activity and damage measures are available e.g. MYOACT (Activity) and MYODAM (Damage),[1] and Myositis Disease Index (MDI); the latter recently demonstrated to have good construct and validity in adult and juvenile myositis.[2]

1 Isenberg DA, Allen E, Farewell V, *et al.* (2004). [International Myositis and Clinical Studies Group (IMACS)]. International consensus outcome measures for patients with idiopathic inflammatory myopathies. Development and initial validation of myositis activity and damage indices in patients with adult onset disease. *Rheumatol (Oxf.).* **43**(1): 49–54.

2 Rider LG, Lachenbruch PA, Montore JB, *et al.* (2009). Damage extent and predictors in adult and juvenile dermatomyositis and polymyositis as determined with the myositis damage index. *Arth Rheum* **60**(11): 3425–35.

Table 14.3 Systemic manifestations of PM and DM

Organ/system	Features
General	Fatigue, malaise, weight loss
	Fevers—in 40% overall
	Raynaud's phenomenon
Pulmonary	Due to muscle weakness: aspiration pneumonia, respiratory failure (low TLC, VC, high RV)* (common)
	Due to local disease: interstitial fibrosis, pulmonary vasculitis, pulmonary hypertension (common)
	Due to treatment: hypersensitivity pneumonitis, opportunistic infection
Gastrointestinal	Oesophageal dysphagia—in 30%
	Striated muscle dysfunction
	Cricopharyngeal dysfunction
	Low oesophageal dysfunction
	Stomach and bowel dysmotility[†]
Cardiovascular	Cardiomyopathy—<5%
	Pericardial effusion—up to 20%
	Hypertension and ischaemic heart disease (common)[1]
	Heart block—rare
	Dysrhythmias—uncommon
Skeletal	Arthropathy
	Deformity, mild erosive arthritis
Renal	Very rare. Possible myoglobinuria

* TLC = total lung capacity; VC = vital capacity; RV = residual volume.

† Intestinal vasculitis, perforation, and pneumatosis cystoides intestinalis, features of juvenile DM, are very rare in the adult.

1 Limaye VS, Lester S, Blumbergs P, Roberts-Thompson PJ (2010). Idiopathic inflammatory myositis is associated with a high incidence of hypertension and diabetes mellitus. *Int J Rheum Dis* **13**(2): 132–7.

Investigation of polymyositis and dermatomyositis

The investigation of potential malignancy in DM has been discussed earlier in this chapter and is covered in principle in 📖 Chapter 4, p 193. Specific investigations for PM/DM include the following:

Muscle enzyme levels

- Serum levels of enzymes released from damaged muscle may be helpful both in diagnosis and monitoring of the disease; creatine kinase (CK) is most widely used, although aldolase may be more sensitive in some cases.
- There are a number of causes of a high CK level (Table 14.4), and levels, particularly in DM, may not be increased despite active myositis and may be influenced partly by muscle bulk, i.e. relative chronic muscle atrophy. The latter is difficult to assess since measures of muscle mass do not necessarily correlate well with degree of inflammation, although atrophy on MRI may be a useful indicator of damage/severity in some cases.

Muscle biopsy

- All patients should have a muscle biopsy to confirm the diagnosis and to exclude conditions that may resemble IIM.
- There is an argument for not doing so in the patient with proximal weakness, elevated enzymes, typical EMG changes, a rash of DM, confirmed myositis-specific autoantibodies, or an overlap autoimmune rheumatic disease and myositis-associated autoantibodies. For most patients, however, it is important to remember that the mimics are more common than the inflammatory myopathies themselves. Therefore, Patients with a clinical diagnosis of PM/DM who do not respond to immunosuppressive treatment as expected may benefit from a biopsy in order to confirm a diagnosis.
- A needle biopsy may be adequate in some cases. However, an open biopsy gives the best picture of muscle architecture and is required for certain functional enzyme studies:
  - *dermatomyositis*: perivascular inflammatory infiltrate (B lymphocytes, CD4 T lymphocytes) with capillaritis;
  - *polymyositis*: intramuscular inflammatory infiltrate (CD8+ T lymphocytes) with muscle fibre degeneration and replacement with fat;
  - *inclusion body myositis*: basophilic intracellular vacuoles ('inclusion bodies').
- Optimal processing and evaluation, minimizing risk of artifact, requires co-ordination with the pathologist prior to the biopsy taking place.

Table 14.4 The causes of a raised creatine kinase

Cause	Examples
Strenuous prolonged exercise	
Muscle trauma	
Diseases affecting muscle	Myositis
	Metabolic (e.g. glycogen storage)
	Dystrophy
	Myocardial infarction
	Rhabdomyolysis
Drugs (also Table 14.7)	Necrotizing myopathy (statins, ciclosporin, labetolol, alcohol
	Induction of myositis (L-tryptophan, L-dopa, phenytoin, lamotrigine, hydroxycarbamide)
	Amphiphillic [(hydroxy)chloroquine, amiodarone]
	Microtubule (colchicine, vincristine)
	Inhibition of CK excretion (barbiturates, morphine, diazepam)
Metabolic abnormalities	Hypothyroidism
	Hypokalaemia (including drug-induced (diuretics, laxatives, steroids)
	Ketoacidosis
	Renal failure
Normal variants	Ethnic group (often higher normal values in the Black population)
	Increased muscle mass
	Technical artifact

Autoantibodies in myositis

- A high antinuclear antibody (ANA) and myositis-specific autoantibodies (MSA) favour PM/DM over other myopathies. The various associations with autoantibodies are shown in Table 14.5.
- A modest correlation with the anti-synthetase antibody anti-Jo-1 antibodies is observed, but the usefulness of titres as an index of disease activity is not established.
- Other rarer anti-synthetase antibodies, like anti-Jo-1, are associated with interstitial lung disease, arthritis, Raynaud's phenomenon, and 'mechanic's hands' (i.e. dry, cracked skin across the digits); so-called anti-synthetase syndrome (ASS). Each accounts for <5% of myositis cases and antibodies include anti-PL-7, anti-PL-12, anti-EJ, and anti-OJ. anti-Ha, anti-KS, and anti-Zo are rare.
- Anti-SRP antibodies herald an acute-onset, severe illness, often with little evidence of inflammation on biopsy. These patients require aggressive immunosuppression.
- Anti-Mi-2 and anti-CADM-140 are found in 10–20% of cases of DM.
- Anti-p140 (anti-MJ) is found in up to 25% of cases of juvenile DM and associated with calcinosis.

Electromyography

- Electromyography (EMG) and nerve conduction studies cannot establish the diagnosis of PM/DM with certainty, but can demonstrate a myopathic process, and help to exclude other neuropathies and certain myopathies. Table 14.6 gives the differential diagnoses of myopathy and Table 14.7 lists other drug-induced myopathies.
- 90% of patients will have abnormal EMG studies.
- Early findings include low-amplitude, short-duration, polyphasic potentials, with early recruitment and full interference patterns (i.e. more fibres are required to achieve a given force). The latter features are in contrast to neuropathies where there is decreased recruitment and interference. With time, re-innervation of denervated fibres leads to high-amplitude, long-duration, polyphasic potentials.
- Other features include spontaneous activity in up to 75% of cases, fibrillations, and repetitive discharges akin to myotonia, but of constant amplitude and starting and stopping abruptly.

Imaging

- Magnetic resonance imaging (MRI), ultrasound, computed tomography (CT), ^{99}Tc, and thallium have been used to assess the distribution of disease.
- MRI with T2-weighted images and fat suppression or short tau inversion recovery (STIR) is best at identifying areas of muscle inflammation, atrophy, or fatty infiltration.

Table 14.5 Antibodies in PM/DM

Antibody class	Antibody subclass	Percentage of PM/DM	Myositis subgroup
Myositis-specific:		In total 30–40	
Anticytoplasmic	Anti-Jo-1	20	Antisynthetase syndrome
	Anti-PL-7/ PL-12/OJ/EJ	<5 each	
	Anti-SRP	4	PM
Antinuclear	Anti-Mi-2	8	DM
	Anti-56 kDa	90	All
Myositis-associated:	Anti-PM-Scl	8	PM/DM–scleroderma overlap
	Anti-U1-RNP	12	PM/DM overlap syndromes
	Anti-U2/ U5-RNP	<2	PM
	Anti-Ro and Anti-La	5–10	Systemic lupus. Sjögren's syndrome

- On MRI, active myositis results in the appearance of muscle oedema. When evaluating a patient for weakness, MRI may be particularly useful in distinguishing weakness due to active inflammation from weakness due to previous damage or glucocorticoid myopathy (which would not be expected to show muscle oedema).
- Because involvement of muscles may be patchy, MRI may also help identify an optimal site for muscle biopsy.

Table 14.6 The differential diagnosis of myopathy

Agent	Examples
Infectious diseases:	
Viral	Retroviruses
	Picornaviruses (entero.)
	Adenoviruses
	Influenza
	Hepatitis B and C
Bacterial	Pyomyositis
	Lyme myositis
	Tuberculosis
Protozoa	Toxoplasmosis
	Trypanosomiasis
Parasites	Trichinosis
	Cysticercosis
Fungal	Candida
Idiopathic:	
• Inclusion body myositis	
• Autoimmune rheumatic disease	
• Other disorders	Granulomatous myositis
	Eosinophilic myositis
	Focal/orbital myositis
Other myopathies:	Dystrophies and congenital myopathies
	Enzyme deficiencies and lipid storage disorders
	Carcinomatosis
	Rhabdomyolysis
	Neurological: motor neuron disease, myasthenia gravis, Guillain–Barré syndrome
	Endocrine: hypo/hyperthyroidism, cortisol excess
	Metabolic: hypocalcaemia, hypokalaemia
	Malnutrition
	Drugs

Table 14.7 Drug-induced myopathy

Clinical picture	Examples
Drugs implicated in autoimmune myopathy	Penicillamine
	Cimetidine
	L-tryptophan
	Zidovudine
Myopathy with weakness, myalgia, and high CK	Colchicine
	Hydroxychloroquine
	Lipid-lowering agents
	Ciclosporin
	Vincristine
	Carbimazole, propylthiouracil
	Alcohol
	NSAIDs—rare in aspirin
Rhabdomyolysis picture	Alcohol
	Illicit drugs—cocaine, heroin
	Amphetamines
	Barbiturates
	Statins (particularly high dose)
	Anaesthetics—malignant hyperthermia
	Psychotropics—neuroleptic-malignant syndrome

Other tests

- The ESR is elevated in 50% of cases, but correlates poorly with disease activity and response to therapy. The CRP is not specific; high levels would suggest a concurrent infection.
- Complement levels in PM/DM are usually normal.
- Proteinuria may be the result of myoglobinuria.
- Serial spirometry for respiratory muscle weakness may be required.

Treatment of polymyositis and dermatomyositis

- Treatment should be started promptly pending completion of investigations, particularly in acute onset weakness, dysphagia, respiratory insufficiency, and systemic complications.
- Corticosteroids form the cornerstone of therapy, and 90% of patients will have at least a partial response.
- Most patients, however, will also require treatment with a steroid-sparing agent to maintain disease remission and to minimize corticosteroid-exposure.
- There is a lack of randomized placebo-controlled trials in treatment of PM and DM.
- An exercise program helps improve fatigue and muscle strength. Exercise should be used with caution during periods of disease activity, but there is no evidence that it causes prolonged worsening in muscle enzyme levels or inflammation.

Corticosteroids

- Oral prednisolone at 60–80 mg/day is continued until a decline in CK and/or a substantial improvement in muscle strength is seen. Severe cases (or extraskeletal involvement) may be treated with iv methylprednisolone 1 g/day for 3 days before starting oral prednisolone. High doses may be required for months and a bisphosphonate should be considered early as prophylaxis against steroid-induced osteoporosis. Adequate calcium and vitamin D intake should always be maintained.
- Most patients will respond to treatment, but this can be slow and partial. The CK is often seen to change faster than any apparent improvement in strength. Failure to respond may be due to one of several reasons:
  - incorrect diagnosis;
  - hereditary myopathy or 'inclusion-body' myositis;
  - steroid myopathy;
  - permanent loss of strength;
  - unresponsive to steroid therapy.
- When the initial goals have been reached, the dose of steroid should be tapered gradually over a 6-month period.

Immunosuppressive agents

- Methotrexate (MTX) and azathioprine (AZA) have demonstrable efficacy in retrospective analysis and, in the case of AZA, a controlled study:
  - MTX 10–25 mg by mouth or 7.5–25 mg subcutaneously per week
  - AZA 2–3 mg/kg/day
- AZA may be a better option for patients with interstitial lung disease or hepatitis, but may take longer to show effectiveness. Studies have shown a synergistic effect of MTX and AZA where a single drug has failed.

- Ciclosporin is a useful therapy in patients where MTX and AZA have been ineffective or not tolerated. It has been used in combination with MTX or iv gammaglobulin.
- Cyclophosphamide has had variable results and is used in resistant cases or in those cases where there is severe extraskeletal involvement such as vasculitis or lung disease.
- Tacrolimus has been used in refractory patients with anti-synthetase syndromes, with improvement in muscle strength, lung function, and cutaneous manifestations. It can be given as an ointment.
- Mycophenolate mofetil (MMF) and chlorambucil are also used.
- There are several reports of improvements in clinical and laboratory measures in patients with refractory PM/DM after receiving infliximab or etanercept.
- In open label studies, rituximab has been used in refractory DM with clinical improvement.
- Monoclonal antibodies against complement component C5 (eculizumab) are also being used in the treatment of DM.

Intravenous gammaglobulin (IVIG)

IVIG is obtained from healthy donor serum and contains a large antibody pool. There is increasing evidence of the efficacy of this treatment in both PM and DM. High-dose regimens in the form of 2 g/kg/day for 2–5 days each month have been advocated. However, the effectiveness of each treatment is of limited duration (6–8 weeks), tapering, and maintenance regimens are empirical and tachyphylaxis may occur. It can be used safely in immunocompromised patients and there are no reports of transmission of infectious diseases. Further studies are needed to refine the place and optimum treatment dose.

Treatment of extramuscular disease in polymyositis and dermatomyositis

- The rash of DM may respond to the treatment of the myositis. If lesions persist, hydroxychloroquine at 200–400 mg/day or topical tacrolimus may be of benefit. Photosensitivity can respond to sunscreens. Topical steroids are often not successful.
- The treatment of amyopathic DM is controversial. Sunscreens and hydroxychloroquine can be used and in some severe cases steroids or immunosuppressives are justified for the cutaneous disease. If treatment is withheld due to an absence of myositis, the patient should be followed closely, especially in the first 2 years after onset, to avoid delay in treatment should myositis develop.
- Calcinosis, principally a problem in juvenile disease, is difficult to treat. Treatment of the disease may help to prevent calcinosis, but it does not affect established calcinosis. Inflammation may respond to colchicine and surgical resection may help for accessible deposits.
- Physical therapy and passive exercises help prevent contractures, though active exercise is discouraged in the acute period of muscle inflammation.
- Interstitial lung disease is managed as in other autoimmune rheumatic disease, with oral steroids and oral or iv cyclophosphamide.

- Distal oesophageal dysmotility does not generally respond to immunosuppression, but measures similar to treatment of reflux may help.

Drug-induced myopathy

- Tables 14.4 and 14.7 list the drugs that commonly cause a myopathy.
- Recently most attention has been given to HMG-CoA reductase inhibitors (statins) used in lipid reduction therapy. These drugs are widely prescribed. In large-scale trials, myalgia has been noted in 11% of patients and significant myositis with elevated CK levels in 0.5%. Myalgia and cramp are the most common symptoms reported, and may be exacerbated by the use of other drugs (ciclosporin and fibrates) or other diseases (hypothyroidism). Patients presenting with muscular symptoms should have their muscle enzyme levels checked and the drug stopped or reduced in dose.

Prognosis in PM and DM

- PM and DM are diseases with a high mortality and morbidity. One retrospective study estimated a mortality rate of 22%, mostly due to malignancy and pulmonary disease.
- The use of prolonged immunosuppressive therapy increases the risk of infection, which may be with unusual organisms. Case reports have described atypical mycobacterial infections in patients with long-standing PM/DM.
- A worse prognosis is associated with increasing age, bulbar muscle, and cardiopulmonary involvement.

Inclusion-body myositis (IBM)

- This is a distinct disorder that comprises 20–30% of idiopathic myositis. It usually begins after the age of 50 years and is 3 times more common in men. The difficulty in distinguishing it from PM and its insidious onset can lead to considerable delay in diagnosis.
- Early in the disease course, there is a significant inflammatory component that may partially respond to glucocorticoids.
- Distal weakness and wasting can be as common as proximal, often involving the lower limbs before the upper, and sparing the face.
- Unlike PM/DM, IBM can present with diminished hand-grip strength, in addition to proximal muscle weakness.
- Dysphagia is a feature in 40% of cases and myalgias in 20%.
- An open biopsy (as opposed to needle biopsy) is essential to diagnose IBM. A needle biopsy may not be sufficient to allow the recognition of important clues that point away from other forms of myositis.
- Patients do not respond to treatment, as well as do those with PM. Immunosuppression may lead to reduction in muscle enzyme levels without improvement in strength or function.
- Treatment usually begins with high-dose corticosteroid for 3 months, adding in MTX or AZA if there is clinical improvement. If there is continued decline in strength or function, immunosuppression should be discontinued.
- Weakness will progress in most patients but this is often very slow. Patients may need assistance with daily activities within 10 years and some may be wheelchair bound within 15 years of onset of symptoms.
- Interferon beta may be efficacious in the treatment of inclusion-body myositis.

Polymyositis and dermatomyositis in children

- The primary clinical feature of both juvenile DM (JDM) and PM (JPM) is chronic, progressive, proximal muscle weakness.
- Fulfillment of the criteria of Bohan and Peter is needed to establish the diagnosis (Table 14.8). In addition to the rash, 3 of the other 4 criteria need to be met for DM. These criteria are 30 years old and need to be revised not least because biopsy and electromyography are performed less and less, given that they are invasive painful procedures and autoantibody profile, immunogenetic profile, and MRI used to define disease and prognosis.
- The conditions are rare; incidence values for JDM and JPM range form 2.5–5 per million.
- JDM is 10–20 times more common than JPM.
- The childhood peak for the disease is 5–9 years of age, with 25% of cases presenting at less than 4-years of age. Some specialists consider the younger age of onset a poor prognostic factor.
- Children of African or Asian origin may be at increased risk of chronic myositis. In the United States, Caucasian children with DM are reported more frequently, with a male to female ratio of 2:1. In the United Kingdom, Ireland, and China the ratio is in the order of 5:1.
- JDM is a systemic disease, most commonly affecting the gut, lungs, and nervous system. This is thought to be due to vasculitis that is more marked than in adult disease. Like adult disease it is a potentially life-threatening condition.
- Approximately 70% of cases of JDM have either myositis-specific or myositis-associated antibodies (Table 14.5). The clinical associations with these antibodies are the same as those seen in adult disease.
- The increased frequency of malignancy seen in adults with DM within 2 years of onset of disease is not seen in childhood DM or PM.
- Fever, abdominal pain, dysphagia, dyspnoea and peripheral arthritis are seen. Skin ulceration is seen in 20% of patients and can be severe and disabling. Lipodystrophy is a recognized skin finding. Calcinosis, is more common in childhood (10–30% of patients) and the outcome of this ranges from spontaneous resolution to chronic deposition and flexion contractures. Calcinosis is difficult to treat and causes long-term morbidity.

Pathogenesis

- Several infectious agents have been associated with the onset of JDM, which may also explain some temporal, seasonal, and regional differences in disease onset. The most prominent agents to date have been RNA picornaviruses, group A β-haemolytic streptococci, and *Toxoplasma gondii*. The true pathogenesis of JDM in relation to infection remains unclear.
- HLA associations include B8, DRB1, DPR1, and DQA1.
- TNF-α promoter polymorphisms have also been implicated in pathogenesis, and associated with calcinosos and ulceration.

Table 14.8 Bohan and Peter's criteria for the diagnosis of juvenile DM/PM

Feature	DM	PM
Characteristic rash	Yes	No
Symmetrical proximal muscle weakness in the absence of other rheumatic/endocrine disease	Yes	Yes
Elevated muscle enzymes	Yes	Yes
Muscle histopathology	Yes	Yes
Electromyographic changes of inflammation	Yes	Yes

Additional assessment tools
- Potential markers of disease activity on 'the horizon' and that may be more sensitive than serum muscle enzymes include:
  - phenotypic flow cytometry of peripheral blood mononuclear cells;
  - IL-17;
  - interferon alfa;
  - endothelial and macrophage activation markers, e.g. quinolinic acid and neopterin.

Drug treatment
- Regimens are similar to those in adult disease:
  - *initial:* corticosteroids and MTX, with adjuvant therapies such as HCQ, vit D, and calcium, topical therapies for ulceration, pain control, and physical and psychosocial management;
  - *second-line:* IVIG, AZA, ciclosporin;
  - *severe/non-responsive:* cyclophosphamide, MMF, tacrolimus, anti-TNF-α, rituximab.
- Rapid disease control is important to help prevent damage. iv or oral corticosteroids are first line, followed by MTX.
- JDM in particular benefits from early and aggressive therapy, which may prevent calcinosis and other complications:
  - methylprednisolone 30 mg/kg/dose (up to a maximum of 2 g) twice weekly for 1 month;
  - prednisone 2 mg/kg/day;
  - intravenous immunoglobulin 2 g/kg administered in divided doses over 5 days.
- Other treatments that have been used include iv immunoglobulin and ciclosporin. Cyclophosphamide is used for severe multisystem disease.
- Infliximab and iv bisphosphonates have shown some effect on muscle disease and calcinosis. Rituximab and autologous stem cell transplantation have been used in a small number of cases.
- Early physiotherapy and muscle strengthening is vital, and evidence suggests that this does not affect the inflammatory process.

Primary vasculitides

Introduction

- The vasculitides are a heterogeneous group of relatively uncommon diseases that can arise as primary conditions or secondary to an established disease such as rheumatoid arthritis (RA) (📖 Chapter 5, p 233) or systemic lupus erythematosus (SLE) (📖 Chapter 10, p 321).
- The vasculitides are linked by the presence of vascular inflammation, which can lead to one of two common outcomes:
  - *vessel wall destruction*, leading to aneurysm or rupture;
  - *stenosis*, leading to tissue ischaemia and necrosis.
- In 1990, the American College of Rheumatology developed a classification system based on vessel size, with the inclusion of a division between primary and secondary vasculitis (Table 15.1).
- In 1994, the Chapel Hill Consensus Conference (CHCC) developed a standard nomenclature for the primary systemic vasculitides based on clinical and laboratory features, and categorized by vessel size:
  - *large vessel:* aorta and its major branches ('great vessels');
  - *medium vessel:* main visceral arteries (e.g. renal, mesenteric);
  - *small vessel:* capillaries, arterioles, and venules.
- antineutrophil cytoplasmic antibody (ANCA; see next section) is helpful to define a subset of the small vessel vasculitides that have a predilection for the respiratory tract and kidneys. These 'ANCA-associated vasculitides' include Wegener's granulomatosis, microscopic polyangiitis, and the Churg–Strauss syndrome.
- This classification system is not perfect: patients with 'large vessel vasculitis' and 'small vessel vasculitis' can have disease that affects some medium-sized vessels. Moreover, not all patients with 'ANCA-associated vasculitis' have detectable levels of ANCA. However, this is a useful framework for the clinician, since categorizing the patient into one of these groups can narrow the differential diagnosis considerably.

Antineutrophil cytoplasmic antibody

- ANCA exist in 2 forms:
  - *cytoplasmic (C-ANCA):* caused by antibodies against proteinase-3 (PR3);
  - *perinuclear (P-ANCA):* caused by antibodies against myeloperoxidase (MPO).
- Other ANCA-staining patterns (i.e. non-cytoplasmic, non-perinuclear) can occur; moreover, the P-ANCA pattern may be caused by antibodies against antigens other than myeloperoxidase. These are sometimes referred to as 'atypical ANCA', and do not predict the presence of vasculitis, although they can be found in Crohn's disease, immune-mediated neutropenia, and other autoimmune diseases.
- C-ANCA is found in patients with Wegener's granulomatosis; patients with microscopic polyangiitis and the Churg–Strauss syndrome tend to be P-ANCA positive.
- Counter intuitively, patients with 'ANCA-associated vasculitis' can be ANCA-negative in up to 50% of cases; patients with active, untreated disease are more likely to be ANCA-positive.
- The exact role that ANCA may play in the pathogenesis of vasculitis is still controversial.

Table 15.1 A classification of systemic vasculitis

Dominant vessel	Disorders	Disorders
Large arteries	Giant cell arteritis. Takayasu's. Isolated central nervous system angitis	Aortitis in rheumatoid arthritis. Infection, e.g. syphilis
Medium arteries	Classical polyarteritis nodosa. Kawasaki disease	Infection, e.g. hepatitis B. Hairy cell leukaemia
Medium arteries/small Vessel	Wegener's granulomatosis. Churg–Strauss syndrome. Microscopic polyangiitis	Vasculitis secondary to autoimmune disease. Malignancy. Drugs. Infection, e.g; HIV
Small vessels (leucocytoclastic)	Henoch-Schönlein purpura. Essential mixed cryoglobulinaemia. Cutaneous leucocytoclastic angitis	Drugs. Malignancy. Infection, e.g; hepatitis B/C

Disease and damage assessment

- To be complete, any description of a chronic disease (such as primary systemic vasculitis) must include both a description of disease activity and a description of disease damage.
- The concept of damage denotes the aspects of disease that are unlikely to reverse with immunosuppression (such as pulmonary fibrosis or renal insufficiency).
- Clinical trials of vasculitis commonly use the Birmingham Vasculitis Activity Score (BVAS) and Vasculitis Damage Index (VDI) to assess activity and damage, respectively.
- Other clinical indices exist. The French Vasculitis Study Group (FVSG) has developed a prognostic Five Factor Score (FFS). This index provides another useful method of classifying patients with vasculitis. Patients with polyarteritis nodosa or ANCA-associated vasculitis who have a FFS>0 have substantially higher mortality than patients with a FFS = 0.
- The FFS was revised in 2008, and now includes the following: age >65, renal insufficiency, cardiac involvement, and gastrointestinal manifestations. The presence of ear, nose and throat signs was found to correlate with an improved outcome among patients with Wegener's granulomatosis.

Large-vessel vasculitis

- The 'large vessels' include the aorta and its main branches (i.e. the subclavian, carotid, and brachocephalic arteries). Primary and secondary forms of large vessel vasculitis are shown in Table 15.2.
- The classic forms of primary large vessel vasculitis are Takayasu's arteritis and giant cell arteritis. Because of the overlap in symptoms, polymyalgia rheumatica is sometimes considered to be a *forme fruste* of giant cell arteritis. Recent studies demonstrate that many patients with polymyalgia rheumatica have subclinical aortic inflammation, which seems to validate this classification scheme.
- The clinical manifestations of large-vessel vasculitis can be predicted by the pattern of vessel involvement. Arch aortitis leads to aneurysmal dilatation and aortic regurgitation. Subclavian involvement causes arm claudication and diminished pulses on examination. Carotid involvement may lead to visual loss, jaw claudication, and stroke. Involvement of any major blood vessel may cause bruits of physical examination.
- Unfortunately, it may be impossible to diagnose a large vessel vasculitis definitively until one of the above events has occurred.

Table 15.2 The causes of large-vessel vasculitis

Primary	Takayasu's arteritis
	Giant cell arteritis[*]
	Behçet's disease
	Cogan's syndrome
Secondary[†]	*Infection:* bacterial, fungal, mycobacterial, spirochaetal
	Rheumatoid arthritis
	Seronegative spondyloarthropathy
	Systemic lupus erythematosus
	Sarcoidosis
	Relapsing polychondritis
	Juvenile arthritis

[*] Giant cell arteritis is discussed in this chapter in the section on polymyalgia rheumatica.

[†] The secondary causes of large-vessel vasculitis are discussed in their respective sections.

Takayasu's arteritis

- Takayasu's arteritis (TA) is a chronic granulomatous arteritis that affects the aorta and the great vessels. The pulmonary arteries can also be involved, although this is relatively uncommon.
- It is most common in Japan, Southeast Asia, India, and Mexico. It is rare in the UK and in the United States its annual incidence is estimated at 2.6 per million.
- TA tends to affect women (90% of cases) with adolescents and young adults between 20 and 40 years at greatest risk. Classification criteria distinguish TA from giant cell arteritis (GCA) by age at onset (i.e. TA <40 years, GCA >50 years).
- Importantly, TA is not limited to patients of Asian descent; the majority of patients in the United States are white.
- The hallmark of the disease is arteritic inflammatory infiltrates that cause luminal narrowing or occlusion; clinically, this presents with bruits, claudication, and diminished (or asymmetric) pulses.
- Lightheadedness, visual disturbance, and strokes can occur. Subclavian steal can be an important cause of neurological symptoms.
- Hypertension may develop as a consequence of renal artery stenosis.
- Musculoskeletal symptoms, including arthralgias and myalgias, are not uncommon.
- Cardiovascular complications are an important cause of morbidity, and include aortic insufficiency, congestive heart failure, systemic hypertension, and ostial involvement of the coronary arteries.
- Traditionally, the diagnosis of TA has depended on angiography to demonstrate the characteristic changes of arterial dilatation, thrombosis, and aneurysm formation. Conventional angiography has the added benefit of allowing a comparison between central and peripheral blood pressures; because subclavian stenosis is a common consequence of this disease, a standard arm cuff blood pressure reading may underestimate central hypertension.
- Magnetic resonance imaging/angiography (MRI/MRA) has excellent resolution at the level of the large vessels, and may be the technique of choice for some patients. MR can also demonstrate evidence of vessel wall inflammation, which could support a diagnosis of TA.
- High-resolution ultrasonography is sensitive for detecting carotid lesions.
- Positron emission CT (PET) scanning is useful for identifying the presence of large vessel vasculitis, but it is not clear whether it can be used to monitor response to therapy.

Treatment

- Initial medical treatment is with corticosteroids (prednisolone 1 mg/kg/day). Most patients should also be treated with MTX 20–25 mg po per week; patients with severe forms of the disease should be treated with cyclophosphamide 2 mg/kg/day.
- An anti-TNF-α agent should be used for severe or resistant cases.
- Hypertension can be difficult to manage, and may require angioplasty or surgery to address renal artery stenosis.

- Surgical management ranges from angioplasty to bypass procedures. These are best performed during the inactive phase of disease. Angioplasty is often a temporizing measure, and lesions tend to restenose over time; when intervention is required, bypass is the treatment of choice. Overall operative mortality is 4%, associated mostly with aneurysm rupture.
- The prognosis depends mainly on the presence of hypertension and aortic incompetence. The majority of patients (75%) will have some impairment of daily living, and 50% are permanently disabled. Mortality is low, 5- and 10-year survival rates reported as 80 and 90%, respectively.
- TA is not a contraindication to pregnancy. Cytotoxic agents should be stopped and steroids kept to as low a dose as possible. Obstetric decisions can be made on their own merits and not because of co-existence of TA. The main complications are exacerbation of hypertension and congestive cardiac failure. The anaesthetist should be made aware of the diagnosis, as the patient may require invasive blood pressure monitoring during delivery.

Polymyalgia rheumatica and giant cell arteritis

Polymyalgia rheumatica

- The diagnosis of polymyalgia rheumatica (PMR) is based essentially on clinical symptoms and signs. The criteria of Jones and Hazleman (1981)[1] are succinct and practical (Table 15.3).
- There may be apparent muscle weakness on testing, which is due to pain rather than intrinsic muscle disease.
- PMR is rare in patients <50; the mean age of onset is 70. Prevalence among patients older than 50 years is 1 in 133, and women are affected more than men (ratio 2:1). There is also a higher frequency of diagnosis in northern latitudes.
- Parainfluenza, parvovirus B19, *Mycoplasma pneumonia*, and *Chlamydia pneumoniae* infections have been shown to have a temporal relation to incidence peaks of PMR, although other studies have found no relationship.
- HLA DRB1*04 and DRB*01 are associated with disease susceptibility.
- Symptoms may start asymmetrically, but soon become bilateral. Systemic features of malaise, weight loss, low-grade fever, and depression are common. Arthralgia and synovitis may occur. Up to 5% of patients with RA (📖 Chapter 5, p 233) have an initial PMR-like presentation.
- Pathological features of PMR are minor and include synovitis with a CD4+ T-cell infiltrate similar to that seen in giant cell arteritis (GCA) (see text below).
- The lack of specific clinical features, a specific laboratory test, and the presence of several conditions that can present with PMR-like symptoms, makes this a diagnosis of exclusion (see Table 15.4).
- PMR and GCA have a close clinical relationship. One-half of patients with GCA have symptoms of PMR and up to 20% of patients with PMR have histological or clinical evidence of GCA. The pathogenesis for both conditions is not known. It could be considered they are components of a single syndrome, the expression of which depends on currently unknown factors.

Giant cell arteritis (Table 15.5)

- GCA is a granulomatous arteritis of the aorta and larger vessels, with a predilection for the extracranial branches of the carotid artery. It is the most common form of primary systemic vasculitis. In the United States, for example, the annual incidence is estimated at 18 per 100 000.
- Like PMR, the female to male ratio is 2:1.
- Infectious and genetic associations are also similar to PMR with evidence of disease 'clustering'.
- GCA is rare among African-Americans.

---

1 Jones JG and Hazleman BL (1981). The prognosis and management of polymyalgia rheumatica. *Ann Rheum Dis* **40**: 1–5

- Severe headache and scalp tenderness localized to the occiput or temporal area are common initial symptoms, present in 70% of cases. The temporal artery can be swollen, tender, and pulseless. Scalp necrosis has also been reported.

Table 15.3 Criteria for the diagnosis of PMR

1	Shoulder and pelvic girdle pain which is primarily muscular in the absence of true muscle weakness
2	Morning stiffness
3	Duration of at least 2 months (unless treated)
4	ESR >30 mm/h or CRP >6 mg/mL
5	Absence of inflammatory arthritis or malignancy
6	Absence of muscle disease
7	Prompt and dramatic response to corticosteroids

Jones JG, Hazleman BL. The prognosis and management of polymyalgia rheumatica. *Ann Rheum Dis* 1981; **40**: 1–5.

Table 15.4 Conditions that can present with polymyalgic symptoms

1	Rheumatic disease in the elderly. Rheumatoid arthritis. Systemic lupus erythematosus
2	Inflammatory myopathy
3	Hypo/hyperthyroidism
4	Carcinoma, myeloma
5	Chronic sepsis
6	Bilateral shoulder capsulitis
7	Osteoarthritis
8	Depressive illness
9	Parkinsonism

- Large arteries are affected in 15% of cases, leading to claudication, bruits, absent neck and arm pulses, and thoracic aorta aneurysm and dissection.
- Visual disturbance is usually an early finding. Patients may complain of amarosus fugax, but visual loss due to retinal ischaemia may be irreversible within hours. Diplopia and ptosis may also be seen.
- Fundoscopy may show optic disc pallor, haemorrhages, and exudates. Optic atrophy is a late finding.
- Arteritic anterior ischaemic optic neuropathy is the most common finding, and must be differentiated from non-arteritic anterior

ischaemic optic neuropathy, an idiopathic cause of visual loss that does not respond to steroids.

- Jaw and tongue claudication are other common sinister features.
- Malaise, fatigue, weight loss, fever, and anaemia are common.
- The ESR and CRP are characteristically elevated, but can be normal in up to 3% cases.

Table 15.5 Diagnostic criteria for GCA

Diagnostic schme	Criteria
Jones and Hazleman (1981)	Positive temporal artery biopsy or cranial artery tenderness
	One or more of: visual disturbance, headache, jaw pain, cerebrovascular insufficiency
	ESR >30 mm/h or CRP >6 mg/ml
	Response to corticosteroids
American College of Rheumatology	Three or more of: • Age at onset >50 years • New headache • Temporal artery tenderness or decreased pulsation • ESR over 50 mm/h • Abnormal artery biopsies showing necrotizing arteritis with mononuclear infiltrate or granulomatous inflammation usually with multinucleated giant cells

Jones JG and Hazleman BL. The prognosis and management of polymyalgia rheumatica. *Ann Rheum Dis* 1981; **40**: 1–5.

- Patients suspected of having giant cell arteritis should be evaluated with bilateral temporal artery biopsies, taking segments of 1.5 cm each. Treatment should not be delayed; biopsies may be helpful to confirm the diagnosis after 2 weeks of treatment with steroids. Unlike most forms of vasculitis, GCA does not cause fibrinoid necrosis; the presence of fibrinoid necrosis on a temporal artery biopsy should prompt a search for another form of vasculitis, such as polymyalgia rheumatica, Wegener's granulomatosis or cryoglobulinaemia.
- Even following this protocol, temporal artery biopsies may be negative in 12% of patients with GCA. A negative temporal artery biopsy does not exclude this diagnosis.
- Doppler ultrasound and, more recently, MR have both been studied as possible substitutes for temporal artery biopsy, although this is not common practice. Ultrasound in particular is operator-dependent, and it may be difficult to find someone with the appropriate expertise to evaluate a patient for GCA.
- Similarly, PET is useful in showing abnormal metabolic activity in the aorta of many patients with GCA, but this is still an experimental modality.

Treatment of polymyalgia rheumatica and giant cell arteritis

- Both conditions require corticosteroid treatment; however, the amount and duration of treatment required are quite different.[1,2]
- PMR responds dramatically to low dose corticosteroids (i.e. prednisone ≤20 mg daily) within 24 h; many patients will report substantial relief within hours after their first dose. After treatment for 2–4 weeks, the prednisone dose may be decreased by 2.5 mg every 2 weeks until the patient reaches a maintenance dose of 10 mg/day. Prednisone may subsequently be tapered in 1-mg increments.
- GCA requires treatment with high-dose steroids (i.e. prednisone 60 mg daily), and the patient may take a week or longer to experience substantial relief. After treatment for 1 month, prednisone may be gradually tapered over 9–12 months.
- Some studies have demonstrated the efficacy of MTX as a steroid-sparing agent for both GCA and PMR. A recent meta-analysis of trials in GCA indicates that the use of adjunctive MTX lowers the risk of relapse. Although MTX for the treatment of GCA and PMR is not yet standard, it is worth considering for some patients.
- The treatment of GCA requires a few additional considerations:
  - patients with visual symptoms associated with GCA should be treated with intravenous pulse methylprednisolone therapy (1 g daily for 3 days) prior to initiating therapy with prednisone;
  - daily low-dose (e.g. 75 mg) aspirin may prevent cranial ischaemic events, such as stroke and blindness, and should be considered if there is no contraindication;
  - bone protection against steroid-induced osteoporosis.

1 Dasgupta B, Borg FA, Hassan N, et al. (2010). BSR and BHPR guidelines for the management of polymyalgia rheumatica. Rheumatol (Oxf) 49(1): 186–90.

2 Dasgupta B, Borg FA, Hassan N, et al. (2010). BSR and BHPR Guidelines for the management of giant cell arteritis. Rheumatol (Oxf) 2010 [Epub ahead of print]. Available at: http://www.rheumatology.org.uk/resources/guidelines/bsr_guidelines.aspx.

Polyarteritis nodosa

- Polyarteritis nodosa (PAN) was the first form of systemic vasculitis described in the literature. It is characterized by a necrotizing vasculitis of medium-sized arteries, leading to cutaneous ulcers, kidney infarction, gastrointestinal haemorrhage, and mononeuritis multiplex.
- Some cases of PAN have been linked to infection with hepatitis B. Patients with PAN should be screened for viral hepatitis, since these patients may require antiviral therapy in addition to immunosuppression.
- The Chapel Hill Consensus Conference created a distinction between 'classic' PAN (i.e. an ANCA-negative, medium-vessel vasculitis associated with renal infarcts) and microscopic polyarteritis nodosa (i.e. an ANCA-positive, medium- and small-vessel vasculitis characterized by glomerulonephritis). This re-classification (and the hepatitis B vaccine) have made PAN increasingly uncommon.
- The clinical features are shown in Table 15.7. Patients often present with non-specific features of systemic disease including myalgias, arthralgias, weight loss, and fever. About 50% of cases develop a vasculitic rash, often with 'punched out' ulcers in the lower extremities. Gastrointestinal (GI) and renal involvement is common—50% in both cases. Non-specific abdominal pain, gut/gallbladder infarction, and pancreatitis are all features. Renal disease usually appears in the form of renal infarct. Renal impairment is often mild and present in around 20% of cases. Isolated organ involvement is rare, but disease affecting the skin, testes, epididymis, breasts, uterus, appendix, and gallbladder has been reported.

Treatment and prognosis in all the small- and medium-vessel vasculitides is discussed at the end of this section.

Wegener's granulomatosis

- WG is the most prevalent of the so-called ANCA-associated vasculitides (AAV), a group of diagnoses that includes microscopic polyangiitis and the Churg–Strauss syndrome. Renal-limited vasculitis and drug-induced ANCA-associated vasculitis are less-common members of this group.
- WG is a worldwide disease with a variable incidence of 4–9 per million. WG is slightly more common in men than women, and most often appears in the fourth and fifth decades.
- Classically, WG is described as a clinical triad, with manifestations affecting the upper respiratory tract, lower respiratory tract, and kidneys. However, patients may present with a wide range of clinical manifestations. Some patients may have an indolent presentation characterized by respiratory tract involvement, such as sinusitis and pulmonary nodules. Others may have a more fulminant presentation, including rapidly progressive glomerulonephritis and pulmonary haemorrhage (Table 15.6). Different treatment strategies for these manifestations are discussed below.

Table 15.6 Modified American College of Rheumatology 1990 classification criteria of Wegener's granulomatosis—diagnosis requires 2 or more of the following:

1	*Nasal or oral inflammation:* development of painful or painless oral ulcers or purulent or bloody nasal discharge
2	*Abnormal chest radiograph:* the chest radiograph may show nodules, cavities, or infiltrate
3	*Urinary sediment:* microscopic hematuria or red cell casts
4	Histological changes of granulomatous inflammation on biopsy
5	PR3-ANCA (C-ANCA) positivity

The clinical features of WG

Ear, nose, and throat

- Up to 90% of patients have ear, nose, and throat involvement.
- Chronic sinusitis is a common initial presentation for WG, and many patients will have been treated with several courses of antibiotics before the correct diagnosis is reached.
- Other manifestations include nasal septal perforation, bloody nasal discharge ('crusts'), and nasal bridge collapse due to erosion of underlying cartilage ('saddle nose').
- Patients may also complain of diminished hearing, either due to sensorineural hearing loss or Eustachian tube dysfunction.
- Subglottic stenosis is a classic feature of WG, and may present with hoarseness and stridor. Subglottic stenosis may worsen even when a patient is otherwise in remission, and responds better to steroid injections than systemic therapy.

- In the oral cavity and oropharynx inflammation can lead to mucosal ulcers or gingivitis ('strawberry gums')
- It is thought that *Staphylococcus aureus* has a role in disease pathogenesis. Nasal carriage in WG patients is 3 times that of healthy populations. The exact mechanisms leading to disease are unclear, but trimethoprim/ sulfamethoxazole may benefit patients with WG by eliminating *S. aureus* colonization.

Pulmonary disease
- 80% of cases have pulmonary disease.
- The tracheobronchial tree may be locally involved before any signs of generalized disease. Subglottic pseudotumours and/or stenosis cause stridor or dyspnea. Lower bronchial stenosis may cause atelectasis and obstructive pneumonia. Multiple nodules with or without cavitation are found in the lungs of asymptomatic patients.
- Severe pulmonary disease is associated with alveolar capillaritis, haemorrhage, and haemoptysis, with infiltrates on the plain chest radiograph. The radiograph typically shows an alveolar or mixed alveolar–interstitial pattern; the distribution is often like that of pulmonary oedema and focal infection.

Renal disease
- Up to 90% of patients with generalized ('severe') WG have renal involvement.
- Renal involvement can range from milder focal and segmental glomerulonephritis (GN) to fulminant diffuse necrotizing (rapidly progressive) and crescentic GN, which may rapidly lead to end stage renal disease.
- The milder form of the condition is most common, manifesting in the asymptomatic patient as a nephritic picture of microscopic haematuria, active sediment, and mild renal impairment.

Skin disease
- 40% of cases have skin disease.
- Features include palpable purpura due to a leucocytoclastic vasculitis, necrotic papules ('Churg–Strauss nodules'), livedo reticularis, and pyoderma gangrenosum.

Rheumatic symptoms
- Rheumatic symptoms are observed in 60% of cases.
- Symptoms can range from mild myalgias (in 50% of the cases) and arthralgias to overt arthritis. 20–30% of rheumatic symptoms may be related to a non-erosive and non-deforming polyarthropathy.
- Migratory arthralgias are a classic presentation for WG.

Nervous system
- About one-third of patients with WG have involvement of the nervous system. Mononeuritis multiplex and distal sensorimotor polyneuropathy are the main lesions. Seizures and cerebritis are much less frequent events.
- Disseminated granulomatous lesions ('pachymeningitis') can spread to the retropharyngeal area and skull base with involvement of cranial nerves I, II, III, VI, VII, and VIII; pachymeningitis can also be associated with diabetes insipidus and meningitis.

Eye disease
- Granulomatous lesions may obstruct the nasolacrimal duct and cause orbital pseudotumour, with optic nerve compression from masses developing in the retrobulbar space. Rarely a purulent sinusitis may spread and cause secondary bacterial orbital infection.
- Manifestations in the generalized stage of WG include episcleritis (red eye), vasculitis of the optic nerve, and occlusion of retinal arteries, in addition to the granulomatous lesions described above.

Investigation of Wegener's granulomatosis
- Laboratory investigation should include ANCA, FBC with differential, routine chemistries, ESR, CRP, and urinalysis to look for an active sediment.
- Not all patients with WG will be ANCA-positive; a negative ANCA test does not necessarily exclude this diagnosis.
- When suspicion of kidney disease exists, renal biopsy may be useful to confirm a diagnosis of WG, and may provide prognostic information as well.
- Sinus biopsies confirm a diagnosis of WG in only 33% of cases; biopsy often shows non-specific evidence of inflammation, and is most useful to exclude concomitant infection or malignancy.
- Pulmonary nodules are often asymptomatic; a patient diagnosed with WG should undergo some form of chest imaging, regardless of symptoms.

Treatment and prognosis of WG is discussed with the other AAV, below.

Other forms of antineutrophil cytoplasmic antibody-associated vasculitides: microscopic polyangiitis and the Churg–Strauss syndrome

Microscopic polyangiitis

- Microscopic polyangiitis (MPA) is classified as a pulmonary-renal (haemorrhage) syndrome, a group that also includes Goodpasture's disease and systemic lupus erythematosus. WG may also occasionally present as a pulmonary-renal syndrome.
- MPA lacks the granulomatous manifestations characteristic of WG, such as sinus disease and pulmonary nodules.
- Unlike WG, MPA is characterized by MPO-ANCA antibodies, which are associated with a P-ANCA staining pattern. Up to 80% of patients with MPA will be ANCA-positive.
- Like PAN, the male: female ratio is 2:1, with the majority of patients being Caucasian. The mean age of presentation is 50 years.
- Most patients with MPA will present with renal involvement in the form of a necrotizing glomerulonephritis, similar to what can be seen with WG. Unlike most forms of vasculitis, glomerulonephritis from AAV is 'pauci-immune' (i.e. there is only minimal immunoglobulin deposition on immunofluorescence stains).
- Pulmonary hemorrhage presents as haemoptysis, and can be surprisingly subtle in some patients. Bronchoscopy with bronchoalveolar lavage will demonstrate hemosiderin-laden macrophages. Chronic pulmonary capillaritis may eventually lead to pulmonary fibrosis.
- Other clinical features of the disease are shown in Table 15.7.

Churg–Strauss syndrome

- This condition is often described as a clinical triad of adult-onset asthma, eosinophilia, and vasculitis.
- Typically, the asthma gradually worsens in intensity until the patient requires daily oral steroids for symptom control. Many of these patients will have been treated with a leucotriene inhibitor (although leucotriene inhibitors do not cause the disease).
- Peripheral blood hypereosinophilia is typically mild and resolves quickly upon treatment with oral steroids.
- Other manifestations of hypereosinophilia include 'fleeting' pulmonary infiltrates, myocarditis, and interstitial nephritis; frank glomerulonephritis is much less common in this diagnosis.
- Nerve involvement is a common manifestation of vasculitis among patients with the Churg–Strauss syndrome (CSS), and patients should be examined for evidence of a sensory neuropathy or mononeuritis multiplex.
- Classically, it is said that the asthmatic component improves dramatically after the onset of the vasculitis, although this is often not the case.

- Cutaneous granulomata that form along the elbows and fingers are called 'Churg–Strauss nodules'; ironically, they appear more commonly in association with WG.
- Treatment and prognosis in all the small- and medium-vessel vasculitides is discussed at the end of this section.

Table 15.7 Clinical features at presentation (as % of cases) in classical polyarteritis nodosa, microscopic polyangiitis, and Churg–Strauss syndrome

Clinical feature	Polyarteritis nodosa	Microscopic polyangiitis	Churg–Strauss syndrome
Renal impairment	25%	90%	50%
Pulmonary disease	40%	50%	General 50%, asthma 100%
Fever	60%	40%	
Skin vasculitis	40%	50%	50%
Gastrointestinal disease	45%	20%	60%
Cardiovascular disease	15%	20%	45%
Peripheral neuropathy	10%	10%	60%
Ear, nose, and throat	10%	20%	
Ocular disease	10%	20%	

ANCA-associated vasculitis: treatment and prognosis

The AAV are approached using the same treatment strategy, which consists of a *remission induction* phase and a *remission maintenance* phase.

Induction
- Regimens typically follow a modified National Institutes of Health protocol for the treatment of systemic vasculitis: oral cyclophosphamide (CYC) 2 mg/kg/day for 6 months, followed by an antimetabolite steroid sparing agent (MTX, AZA) for 1 year or longer.
- Prednisolone 1 mg/kg/day (up to 80 mg/day) for the first month is used in conjunction with CYC.
- Pulse iv CYC may be as effective as oral CYC, but this is controversial.
- Patients with mild disease may be treated with oral MTX 20–25 mg weekly and prednisone 0.5 mg/kg/day for remission induction.
- Patients receiving CYC should also receive trimethoprim/sulfamethoxazole for prophylaxis against *P. jiroveci* pneumonia (PCP). Patients receiving chronic steroids should receive osteoporosis prophylaxis.

Maintaining remission
- Once remission has been achieved with CYC, a less toxic drug may be used for remission maintenance. MTX and AZA are both standard remission-maintenance drugs, but mycophenolate mofetil and leflunomide may also have a role in the treatment of some patients.
- Patients should receive remission maintenance therapy for at least 1–2 years; the optimal duration of immunosuppression is not clear.

Other treatments
- Plasma exchange has been used with some effect in those with severe renal disease, although the benefit is transient.
- Intravenous immunoglobulin has been found to have short-lived benefit, but may be used in patients at high risk of systemic infection.
- Anecdotal reports have shown the benefit of infliximab, anti-TNF-α in combination with MTX or CYC for treatment of resistant vasculitis, although this is highly controversial in the United States. Studies demonstrate some efficacy, but in exchange for a high risk of infectious complications.
- Treatment of a vasculitis associated with an infectious disease (e.g. hepatitis B-associated PAN, hepatitis C-associated cryoglobulinaemic vasculitis) should always include treatment of the underlying pathogen whenever possible.
- There is evidence that respiratory tract infections may trigger a relapse of WG. Trimethoprim-sulfamethoxazole in patients with stable disease on maintenance therapy may decrease respiratory infection, and is also useful for prevention of PCP among patients treated with CYC.

Prognosis

Prior to the introduction of cyclophosphamide and steroids, mortality associated with generalized AAV approached 100%. Modern immunosuppressive regimens have transformed these diseases into chronic conditions, characterized by cycles of relapse and remission. For many patients, the consequences of treatment (such as steroid-associated complications) may lead to greater morbidity than the underlying disease itself. Mortality due to infection continues to be an important consideration for patients treated for AAV; indeed, patients with 'treatment resistant' AAV should be carefully evaluated for the presence of *Nocardia*, *Aspergillus*, and other infections that can mimic some of the manifestations of the AAV.

For a detailed analysis of the literature on induction of remission in ANCA positive disease the reader is referred to Jayne (2005)[1] and BSR guidelines.[2]

1 Jayne D (2005). How to induce remission in the primary vasculitides. *Best Pract Res Clin Rheum*, **19**: 293–305

2 Lapraik C, Watts R, Bacon P, *et al.* (2007). BSR and BHPR guidelines for the management of adults with ANCA associated vasculitis. *Rheumatol (Oxf)* **46**(10): 1615–6. Available at: http://www.rheumatology.org.uk/resources/guidelines/bsr_guidelines.aspx).

Small-vessel vasculitis

The definition of small vessel vasculitis is open to different interpretations. Small vessel disease can be one feature of WG, microscopic polyangiitis, and the Churg–Strauss syndrome. However, there are a range of clinical and pathological features that define a specific group of small-vessel vasculitides outlined in Table 15.8.

Leucocytoclastic vasculitis

- Histologically, leucocytoclastic vasculitis appears as a neutrophil infiltration in and around small vessels, with fragmentation of the neutrophils (leucocytoclasis), fibrin deposition, and endothelial cell necrosis. Immune complex deposition appears to be important in pathogenesis.
- Small-vessel vasculitis usually presents in the skin, although the microvasculature of any tissue may be affected, especially joints or kidneys.
- Some forms of cutaneous vasculitis are predominantly lymphocytic, without evidence of neutrophils or leucocytoclasis. However, the division into leucocytoclastic and non-leucocytoclastic (lymphocytic) vasculitis is not absolute. Likewise, the clinical presentation of cutaneous vasculitis can vary considerably.
- The finding of leucocytoclasis should prompt a thorough review of drug treatment (e.g. sulfonamides, penicillin, thiazides), a search for infection (hepatitis B, human immunodeficiency virus, β-haemolytic streptococcus), a screen for autoimmune rheumatic disease, malignancy (in particular myelo- and lymphoproliferative diseases), inflammatory bowel disease, chronic active hepatitis, and cryoglobulinaemia (see below).

Allergic (hypersensitivity) vasculitis

- Allergic vasculitis is the most common pattern of presentation in adults, both sexes being affected equally.
- Non-blanching haemorrhagic papules (palpable purpura), purpuric macules, plaques, pustules, bullae, and ulcers may occur, classically distributed maximally over the lower leg.
- A low-grade fever, arthralgias, and microscopic haematuria may accompany such presentation.
- Often the condition is self-limiting and identifiable causes should be managed as appropriate. Analgesia may be needed and systemic steroids may be required for acute organ disease, especially progressive renal impairment.
- AZA may be appropriate for refractory disease, but removal of the offending drug or exposure is the most effective treatment strategy.

Table 15.8 Conditions associated with small-vessel vasculitis

Leucocytoclastic vasculitis	Allergic vasculitis (hypersensitivity angiitis): drugs, infection, inflammation, autoimmune disease, malignancy, Henoch–Schönlein purpura
	Urticarial vasculitis (hypocomplementaemic vasculitis)
	Cryoglobulinaemia
	Hypergammaglobulinaemia
	Erythema elevatum diutinum and granuloma faciale
Non-leucocytoclastic vasculitis (lymphocytic vasculitis)	Drugs (penicillins, thiazides)
	Nodular vasculitis (see 'panniculitis')
	Livedo vasculitis
	Pityriasis lichenoides

Henoch–Schönlein purpura

- This tends to be regarded as a special form of allergic vasculitis. It occurs most often in children, but can affect adults of any age. IgA is usually detected in skin, gut, or renal biopsies.
- The classic presentation is with purpura, arthritis (50%), haemorrhagic GI disease (40%), and glomerulonephritis (50%). Corticosteroids given early may relieve joint and GI symptoms, but there is little evidence that they prevent progression of renal disease or influence overall outcome. If renal function is rapidly deteriorating, pulsed methylprednisolone and/or plasmapheresis may be of benefit.
- Patients who present with a nephritic or nephrotic syndrome have an increased lifetime prevalence of renal complications, including hypertension.
- Although most cases are self-limited, this can (rarely) become a chronic, relapsing disease. Such patients should be evaluated for the presence of a monoclonal IgA antibody, which may herald a pre-malignant lesion.

Urticarial vasculitis

- Urticarial lesions with arthralgias are the most common features of this condition, with men outnumbering women 2:1. The typical age of onset is 40–50 years.
- Morphologically the skin lesions resemble ordinary urticaria and sometimes may be mistaken for erythema multiforme. Unlike ordinary urticaria, the lesions of urticarial vasculitis tend to last for days (not hours) and tend to be burning and painful (not pruritic).
- Patients with hypocomplementemic urticarial vasculitis tend to develop more systemic features such as renal, GI, and pulmonary disease. Less common manifestations include lymphadenopathy, uveitis, and benign

intracranial hypertension. These patients are often ANA positive, and some may evolve into SLE.
- Systemic antihistamines are widely used, but tend to be disappointing.
- There are anecdotal reports of success with indometacin, hydroxychloroquine, colchicine, ciclosporin, and dapsone. AZA may be particularly effective.
- For the majority of patients, the condition is chronic and benign. For those with end-organ damage, chronic immunosuppression may be necessary.

Cryoglobulinaemia

- Cryoglobulins are immunoglobulins that precipitate when cold. They are divided into three types: type I (monoclonal), type II (mixed monoclonal and polyclonal), and type III (polyclonal).
- Mixed cryoglobulins are associated with autoimmune rheumatic diseases, infection, and lymphoproliferative disorders. Hepatitis B and C viral infection should always be excluded; the latter in particular is strongly associated with mixed essential cryoglobulinaemia.
- Mixed essential cryoglobulinaemia presents with purpuric skin lesions showing a leucocytoclastic vasculitis on biopsy; polyarthralgias (70%), weakness, progressive renal disease (55%), and transaminitis (70%) are common. Women are affected as twice as frequently as men.
- Less common problems include oedema, hypertension, leg ulcers, Raynaud's phenomenon, abdominal pain, neuropathy, and susceptibility to bacterial pneumonia.
- The prognosis is worse with renal disease; the main causes of death among patients with cryoglobulinaemia include renal failure and infection.
- Treatment requires management of the underlying cause; immunosuppression by itself is frequently unsatisfactory. Choice of immunosuppression should be dictated by the disease manifestations; the most severe forms may require treatment with CYC, pulse steroids, and plasmapheresis.

Hypergammaglobulinaemic purpura

- This is a rare, benign IgM condition presenting as long-standing leucocytoclastic purpura similar to the cutaneous features of Sjögren's syndrome (📖 Chapter 12, p 353).
- It should not be confused with Waldenström's macroglobulinaemia, a monoclonal IgM paraproteinaemia associated with lymphoma.

Erythema elevatum diutinum and granuloma faciale

- These are rare, but distinctive forms of chronic localized leucocytoclastic vasculitis. There is no systemic involvement and the aetiology is unknown.
- Erythema elevatum diutinum (EED) is characterized by slowly enlarging oedematous purplish-brown plaques or blisters over the backs of the hands, elbows, or knees. They heal very slowly (months to years) with fibrosis. It may respond to dapsone.
- Granuloma faciale (GF) presents as single or multiple pink-brown, well-defined, smooth papules and plaques on the face. They persist

for years. It is distinguished histologically from EED by the presence of eosinophils and a normal collagen beneath the epidermis. It may respond to intralesional steroids.

Non-leucocytoclastic (lymphocytic) vasculitis

- The differential diagnosis of nodular forms of cutaneous vasculitis embraces a wide range of disorders, including the panniculitides (📖 Chapter 18, p 489).
- Nodular vasculitis is regarded as a distinct group characterized by recurrent subcutaneous nodules usually found on the legs of young to middle-aged women. Patients are otherwise healthy. Streptococcal infection may be found; Bazin's disease is sometimes used to describe the nodular vasculitis that can occur in association with tuberculosis. The condition resolves spontaneously, but may take many years. Intralesional triamcinolone may help.
- Livedo vasculitis is characterized histologically by endothelial proliferation and intraluminal thrombosis leading to ischaemic damage. Livedo vasculitis has been attributed to defects in the tissue plasminogen activator (tPA) gene, although similar lesions can be seen in the antiphospholipid syndrome. The lesions heal with white atrophic scar ('atrophie blanche').
- Pityriasis lichenoides is an uncommon disorder of pink papules, which enlarge rapidly and may become haemorrhagic before becoming necrotic and heal with scarring. It is usually self-limiting and may respond to ultraviolet B irradiation.

Kawasaki disease

- This is a febrile, acute vasculitic illness of childhood. It is probably more common than rheumatic fever as the cause for rheumatic heart disease in children <5 years of age, and is associated with coronary artery aneurysms, myocarditis, and MI. Other organs involved include liver, pancreas, and kidney.
- It is seen most often in Japanese-Americans with a peak prevalence age of 18 months to 2 years, and is more common in males, ratio 5:1.
- Fever is usually present for >5 days and associated with conjunctivitis, erythema and oedema (skin, lips, and pharyngeal), and lymphadenopathy. Joint inflammation may also occur during the acute phase.
- Myocarditis may appear early, but arterial aneurysm formation appears later, its risk of occurring increases after longer periods of being febrile (14–16 days).
- There are no specific blood tests. Acute phase markers are usually high and cultures negative.
- An ECG and echocardiogram may show conduction defects and myocardial inflammation, respectively.
- Treatment should start with IVIG (2 g/kg) administered over 8-12 hours and aspirin (80–100 mg/kg/d, divided into 4 doses). Patients who fail to respond may benefit from re-treatment with IVIG, or pulse methylprednisolone therapy. The role of plasmapheresis and anti-TNF-α therapy is less clear.
- For further information, the reader is referred to the 2004 Scientific Statement from the American Heart Association on the diagnosis and management of Kawasaki's disease.[1]

1 Newburger JW, Takahasi M, Gerber MA, et al. (2004). Diagnosis, treatment, and long term management of Kawasaki disease. *Circulation* **110**: 2747–71.

Metabolic bone diseases and disorders of collagen

Osteoporosis

- Osteoporosis can be defined as a decrease in bone mass and strength resulting in an increased risk of fracture. Unlike osteomalacia, the ratio of matrix to mineral deposit in bone is normal in osteoporosis.
- The World Health Organization defines osteoporosis on the basis of bone density compared with the mean bone density for a young adult; this is known as a T-score. *Osteopenia* refers to bone mineral density (BMD) that falls 1.0-2.5 standard deviations (SD) below the BMD of a young adult. *Osteoporosis* is used if the BMD falls more than 2.5 SD below the BMD of a young adult.
- The risk of osteoporotic fracture is greater in women than in men; in both sexes, risk of fracture varies with site (Table 16.1).
- The age-adjusted incidence of hip fractures has been increasing steadily.

Table 16.1 Risk of osteoporotic fracture with site

Fracture site	Overall lifetime risk of fracture (%)	
	Men	Women
Hip	6.0	17.5
Vertebral	5.0	15.6
Distal forearm	2.5	16.0
Any of above	13.1	39.7

Pathogenesis and classification

- During childhood and adolescence, growth and modelling lead to an increase in the size, shape, strength, and composition of bone. Growth ceases with the closure of the growth plates (epiphyseal cartilage). However, remodelling and mineral homeostasis continue throughout life with bone resorption and deposition coupled by the interaction between osteoclasts and osteoblasts, respectively.
- Peak bone mass or maximal bone density, is usually achieved in the third decade. Peak bone mass is determined by both genetic (e.g. vitamin D receptor gene polymorphism, oestrogen receptor–cytokine interaction), and environmental factors. Changing lifestyle and behaviour patterns have been suggested as an effective way of increasing peak bone mass.
- After the age of 35 (presumably due to declining osteoblast activity), the amount of bone laid down is less than that resorbed during each remodelling cycle sequence. The net effect is an age-related decrease in bone mass. Trabecular and cortical bone mass decline by approximately 6 and 3% per decade, in women and men, respectively.
- Further bone loss occurs at the time of menopause with declining ovarian function and levels of oestrogens. Up to 15% of bone mass can be lost over the 5-year period immediately after menopause. A further 15% of bone mass can be lost if vitamin D deficiency co-exists.

- The mechanism of age-related bone loss is unknown. Several possibilities exist:
  - decreased intestinal calcium absorption;
  - decreased synthesis of vitamin D;
  - hyperparathyroidism (caused by the above);
  - increased osteoclast function;
  - fatty infiltration of the bone marrow, leading to loss of precursor cells and locally generated growth factors.
- Risk factors for osteoporosis include (Table 16.2):
  - race (White or Asian > African American);
  - age and gender (as above);
  - positive family history (maternal hip fracture);
  - previous 'fragility' fracture;
  - corticosteriod therapy;
  - malabsorption disorders;
  - endocrinopathies;
  - low body mass index (BMI <16);
  - short fertile period (late menarche, early menopause including early ovarian failure, hysterectomy and oophorectomy);
  - nulliparity;
  - sedentary lifestyle;
  - low intake of calcium (<240 mg daily);
  - excessive alcohol intake;
  - smoking;
  - malignancy (e.g. multiple myeloma).
- The World Health Organization has developed a Fracture Assessment Tool (FRAX) to identify patients at highest risk. Bone mineral density measurement alone may miss up to 50% of those at risk of fracture. The FRAX tool takes account of the following risk factors [with or without a bone mineral density (BMD) reading] in calculating a 10-year risk of fragility fracture:
  - age;
  - sex;
  - prior fragility fracture;
  - corticosteroid use;
  - parental history of hip fracture;
  - rheumatoid arthritis;
  - secondary osteoporosis;
  - current smoker;
  - alcohol >2 units per day;
  - low BMI.

The FRAX tool is available at www.shef.ac.uk/FRAX.

Table 16.2 Classification of osteoporosis

Major type	Causative factor(s)	Details
Primary (physiological)	Post-menopausal Age-related	
Idiopathic		
Juvenile onset		
Secondary	Endocrine	Hyperparathyroidism
		Hypopituitarism
		Thyrotoxicosis
		Hypogonadism
		Cushing's syndrome
		Insulin-dependent diabetes
	Drugs	Corticosteroids
		Excess thyroxine replacement
		Heparin
		Anticonvulsants
		Ciclosporin A
	Haemopoietic	Multiple myeloma
		Lymphoma
		Leukaemia
		Mastocytosis
		Gaucher's disease
	Inflammatory diseases	Rheumatoid arthritis
		Ankylosing spondylitis
	Congenital	Osteogenesis imperfecta
	Immobilization	
	Idiopathic hypercalciuria	
	Osteoporosis of pregnancy	

Idiopathic osteoporosis

- Idiopathic osteoporosis defines occurrence of the condition in pre-menopausal women or men under the age of 60 years, with no apparent cause. The female: male ratio is 10:1. Most cases are found to have 'low bone turnover' with low rates of bone formation. Some cases have 'high bone turnover' with hypercalciuria; these cases may respond to antiresorption drugs such as calcitonin and bisphosphonates.
- It is not clear if the majority of patients in this group will benefit from therapy. For most patients with idiopathic osteoporosis, in the absence of other risk factors, the absolute risk of fracture remains low. Anti-catabolic (anti-resorptive) agents are unlikely to shift the risk of fracture significantly.

Juvenile idiopathic osteoporosis

- Juvenile osteoporosis (JIO) is an uncommon disorder that occurs before, or at onset of puberty. It affects the sexes equally. The cause is unknown and there are no consistent biochemical abnormalities (Table 16.3).
- The child presents with pain, non-traumatic fractures around the weight-bearing joints, and collapsed vertebrae. No specific treatment is available and for most, bone mass increases to normal values as puberty progresses; however, in some cases fractures may lead to deformity. Supportive physical therapy should be made available.
- In the same way that height and weight charts are used to assess childhood development, there may be a role for serial bone density measurement in children with known low bone mass, as a surrogate assessment of appropriate development.

Corticosteroid-induced osteoporosis

- Corticosteroid-induced osteoporosis (CIO) is as a major concern. Treatment should be offered to all patients taking prednisone for a period likely to be 3 months or more. The risk is present at doses as low as 2.5 mg daily, although data would suggest it increases considerably for doses >5 mg daily.
- There is conflicting evidence as to the effect of inhaled corticosteroid on fracture risk. Patients on maximal doses of inhaled corticosteroids should be assessed for additional risk factors for osteoporosis and may require prophylaxis.
- The pathogenesis of CIO is controversial. Corticosteroids can affect calcium and phosphate metabolism both directly and indirectly in bone, kidney, and the intestine. Possible mechanisms are shown in Table 16.4.

Table 16.3 The causes of juvenile idiopathic osteoporosis

Type	Causative factor(s)
Primary	Calcium deficiency
	Idiopathic
	Osteogenesis imperfecta
Secondary	Endocrine (see Table 16.2)
	Intestinal: • malabsorption • biliary atresia • type I glycogen storage disease
	Inborn errors of metabolism—homocystinuria
	Leukaemia
	Congenital cyanotic heart disease

Primary hyperparathyroidism

Primary hyperparathyroidism is a relatively common disorder with an adult prevalence of about 0.2% in the fifth to seventh decades of life. It is 3 times more common in women than men, due to an increased incidence after the menopause. Mild hyperparathyroidism is often diagnosed after an incidental finding of hypercalcaemia on routine blood tests. The management of this condition will be discussed, later in this chapter.

Hypogonadism

• Hypogonadism due to any cause may lead to an increased risk of osteoporotic fracture.
• Causes of amenorrhoea include primary ovarian failure, use of oestrogen antagonists (e.g. in the management of endometriosis), hyperprolactinaemia, anorexia nervosa, and low body mass index (e.g. elite sportswomen).
• Causes of decreased testosterone levels include Klinefelter's syndrome, hypogonadotrophic hypogonadism, hyperprolactinaemia, anorexia nervosa, and testicular dysfunction following mumps orchitis.

Hyperthyroidism

Hyperthyroidism leads to osteoporosis as a consequence of high bone turnover, enhanced osteoclast recruitment, and increased bone resorption.

Table 16.4 Possible pathogenesis of corticosteroid-induced osteoporosis

Mechanism	Site	Effect
Reduced bone formation	Osteoblasts	Reduced activity
		Reduced recruitment
		Reduced collagen synthesis
		Reduced growth hormone
		Reduced cytokine levels
	Adrenal–testis	Reduced gonadal hormones
Increased bone resorption	Adrenal–testis	Reduced gonadal hormones
	Parathyroid	Increased PTH
	Intestinal	Reduced calcium absorption
		Reduced sensitivity to vitamin D
	Renal	Reduced calcium resorption
	Muscle	Decreased muscle mass

Malignancy

Malignant infiltration and replacement of marrow tissue occurs in multiple myeloma, lymphoma, leukaemia, systemic mastocytosis, and diffuse bone metastases. Mechanisms differ, for example:

- Over production of osteoclast-activating cytokines (such as IL-1 and TNF) in myeloma.
- Local synthesis of 1,25-hydroxyvitamin D by malignant cells in lymphoma.
- Over production of heparin, histamine, and prostaglandins that stimulate osteoclasts in mastocytosis.

Other factors

Potential factors that may cause generalized osteoporosis in inflammatory disorders, such as RA (🕮 Chapter 5, p 233) and ankylosing spondylitis (AS) (🕮 Chapter 8, p 281), include the systemic effects of inflammatory products, alterations in sex hormones, altered calcium metabolism, changes in load bearing, and the effect of drugs used in treatment. Immobilization per se leads to a net loss of bone (rates as high as 5% per month in the first 6 months).

Investigation of osteoporosis and low-trauma fracture

- Low-trauma fracture in those aged 50–75 years should be investigated to exclude the possibility of osteoporosis. The three most common sites of fracture are the wrist, vertebrae, and hip.
- Many now consider a low-trauma fracture in a person >75 years of age as strongly suggestive of osteoporosis and would treat without

measuring bone mass. Assessment and investigation for possible underlying disease is still required.

- Plain radiographs are an insensitive method of assessing bone mass. The high correlation between bone mineral density (BMD) and bone strength and, therefore, bone fragility has led to the development of several techniques for assessing BMD.
- The standard technique for measuring BMD is dual energy X-ray absorptiometry (DEXA). It is quick, has high resolution, precision, and accuracy, and can assess the lumbar spine, femoral neck, wrist, and whole body. DEXA gives two readings, the 'T' and 'Z' scores. The T score is the individual's bone mineral density compared with the mean bone density achieved at peak bone mass for the same sex (and, more recently, race). The Z score is the individual's bone mineral density compared with the mean bone density for someone of the same age and sex (and, more recently, race). Most analyses and studies have focused on the T score. The score is recorded as a + or − figure above or below the mean. For every one standard deviation (SD) below the mean there is a two-fold increase in the risk of fracture, i.e. an individual three SD below the mean has an 8-fold risk of fracture compared with a 'normal' individual of the same age, bearing in mind also that base-line risk increases with age in the 'normal' population.
- Quantitative CT allows volume measurements and can distinguish between cortical and trabecular bone in vertebrae. It is, however, costly and entails a high radiation exposure.
- Ultrasonography is a non-invasive technique that is currently being correlated with DEXA. US can be performed at the heel (calcaneus) and patella. Correlation seems poor and its role in clinical diagnostics remains unclear.
- Since the advent of non-invasive techniques, transiliac bone biopsy is no longer essential unless there is the need to diagnose osteomalacia as the underlying cause. Bone biopsy may be used as a tool in research, in particular for the quantification of rates of bone turnover.
- Routine biochemical and haematological tests are usually normal in osteoporosis. Investigation of the newly diagnosed osteoporotic person should include a screen for malignancy and metabolic bone biochemical abnormalities. This at least would include an ESR, renal function, liver function test (LFT), serum immunoglobulins, calcium and phosphate. Measurement of the sex hormones should also be considered.
- Biochemical markers of bone turnover are available but their precise clinical role has not been established. These include:
  - bone formation: serum bone alkaline phosphatase, osteocalcin (bone Gla protein), type 1 procollagen peptides;
  - bone resorption: fasting urine calcium and hydroxyproline, urine collagen cross links (deoxy)pyridinoline, serum tartrate-resistant acid phosphatase.
- These markers may be helpful in comparing 'high bone turnover' with 'low bone turnover' cases in established osteoporosis, and in monitoring the effects of and compliance with treatments.

Management of osteoporosis and low-trauma fractures

Prevention

Bone mass at any one time will be determined by 'peak bone mass', rate of bone loss with ageing, and with women, the rate and duration of post-menopausal bone loss. Genetic factors cannot be manipulated, but nutritional and environmental factors may. Pharmacological intervention in 'at-risk' individuals is good prevention practice. Currently this would include those in the age group 50–65 with a T score of <–3.0, or with a T score <–2.5 with other risk factors (especially fragility fracture), and those >65 with a T score of <–2.5 regardless of presence of additional risk factors.

Calcium

- Calcium supplementation is sensible in those who have a low-calcium diet (poor in dairy products, green leafy vegetables, nuts, dried fruits, etc.). There is conflicting evidence about whether supplements have any effect on preventing bone loss and, therefore, risk of fracture per se in the young adult.
- Calcium supplementation in prepubertal children enhances the rate of change in bone mineral density, but whether this translates into higher peak bone mass is unknown.
- In post-menopausal women, calcium supplements can lead to a reduction in the rate of decline of total-body bone mineral density.
- There is a role for calcium and vitamin D supplementation in the elderly osteoporotic; it can help prevent cortical bone loss and subsequent vertebral fractures.
- At present the use of calcium supplements is recommended for:
  - definite osteoporosis;
  - poor calcium diet (<400 mg/day);
  - supplement to any anti-catabolic (anti-resorptive) treatment in the elderly.
- Calcium supplementation may be associated with increased risk of ischaemic heart disease.

Exercise

There is some evidence to suggest that physical activity decreases the rate of bone loss around the menopause, although the level and type of activity remains unclear. The activity must, however, be weight-bearing. There is little impact of exercise in improving bone mass once osteoporotic, although it may aid in preventing further loss.

Hormone replacement

- Oestrogen replacement therapy is an effective way of preventing post-menopausal bone loss. The addition of a progestogen allows endometrial shedding and minimizes the risk of hyperplasia and neoplasia. The minimum oral dose of oestrogen required is 2 μmg/day, and conjugated oestrogen 0.625 mg/day. Gels and transdermal/depot treatments should be started at around 3 mg/day or 50 μg/day, respectively.
- Evidence suggests that the use of HRT increases the risk of deep vein thrombosis, coronary artery disease, breast cancer, and stroke. These agents should therefore be used with caution.

Treating established disease (i.e. osteoporotic fractures)

- Virtually all the treatments listed below have demonstrated in the order of 40–50% reduction in risk of fragility fracture, either vertebral or at the hip in post-menopausal women with established osteoporosis. In subgroups over the age of 80 there is evidence for greater efficacy for agents such as strontium ranelate and denosumab.

- Bisphosphonates are the most commonly used of all agents available in the treatment of established osteoporosis. They are potent inhibitors of bone resorption (anti-catabolic). Cyclical disodium etidronate (400 mg daily for 2 weeks, every 3 months) is approved for use in the Canada and Europe, but not the United States. Alendronate (10 mg daily or 70 mg weekly) is the treatment of first choice in the UK currently (NICE Guidance 2010). Risedronate (5 mg daily or 35 mg weekly) and ibandronate (2.5 mg daily or 150 mg monthly) are other agents currently available.

- In the UK intravenous zoledronic acid (like teriparatide (below) is available if oral bisphosphonates or strontium ranelate are not tolerated.

- In general, bisphosphates are well tolerated, but should be used with caution in renal impairment, history of oesophageal reflux/hiatus hernia, or poor dentition requiring dental work (risk of bone necrosis). Symptoms of nausea and reflux can be lessened by taking these medications with plenty of water and avoid lying down for at least 30 min afterwards. These agents should also be taken on an empty stomach as absorption is poor. Compliance rates with therapy are variable with reports from the United States of <30%, but reports in the United Kingdom of >80% at 2–4 years' duration of therapy.

- Calcium supplements should be taken alongside bisphosphonate therapy unless otherwise contraindicated.

- Calcium (800–1000 mg) and vitamin D supplements (400–800 IU) are recommended in the elderly and those whose diet is poor in them.

- HRT may be used as described above. Selective oestrogen receptor modulaters (SERMs), such as raloxifene may become more popular in the future as alternatives to HRT.

- Calcitonin is useful for its analgesic effect early after osteoporotic fractures. It has only a modest effect on bone mineral density, and therefore is generally not used as a primary treatment for osteoporosis.

- Strontium ranelate (Protelos®) has been shown to both increase osteoblastic bone formation and reduce osteoclastic bone resorption. Given at 2-g daily orally, studies have shown 36–41% reduction in fracture risk (hip and vertebral) against placebo. It is contraindicated if there is risk of thrombo-embolic disease.

- Strontium, by its incorporation into bone structure, gives false high readings on DEXA scanning, making assessment of change in BMD following therapy difficult to interpret at present. In the UK its place is as a first line agent in patients likely to be intolerant of bisphosphonates or where a bisphosphonate is contra-indicated.

- Teriparatide (Forsteo®) is a parathyroid hormone analogue and an anabolic agent now available for use in severe osteoporosis. It is given as a subcutaneous injection daily for 2 years. Teriparatide should not be co-administered with bisphosphonates.

- Denosumab (Prolia®) is the first fully human monoclonal antibody that specifically inhibits RANK Ligand, an essential up-regulator of osteoclasts. Prolia® is now licensed in Europe for a range of bone loss conditions including post-menopausal osteoporosis and bone loss in patients undergoing hormone ablation for prostate and breast cancer. It is given by subcutaneous injection every 6 months. Its place in UK guidelines on treatment is to be determined; in the first instance it may be a viable alternative to zoledronic acid and teriparatide, however it may also become a first-line alternative to oral agents.
- Acute back pain due to vertebral collapse is discussed in 📖 Chapter 20, p 525.

The NICE 2010 guidelines for the management of osteoporotic fractures are complex. There are different BMD T-score cut-off criteria for treatment by age, number of independent risk factors, and class of drug used. The reader is advised to visit the following online site: http://guidance.nice.org.uk/TA161/QuickRefGuide/pdf.

Osteomalacia and rickets

- Osteomalacia and rickets are characterized by defective mineralization of bone and cartilage and the accumulation of unmineralized bone matrix (osteoid), i.e. there is, unlike osteoporosis, a decline in the ratio of mineralized bone to matrix.
- Rickets is the term used for this defect in growing children before the closure of the epiphyses.
- There are many causes of osteomalacia, but essentially they all occur due to either a deficiency or resistance to vitamin D, or a non-PTH related defect in renal handling of phosphate (Table 16.5).
- Both vitamin D_2 (ergocalciferol) from vegetables in the diet, and D_3 (cholecalciferol) from animal tissues and *de novo* synthesis in skin, are metabolized in the liver to 25-hydroxvitamin D and then in the kidney to 1,25-dihydroxyvitamin D_3. The latter affects calcium metabolism by acting on the parathyroid glands (negative-feedback loop on PTH stimulation of renal vitamin D hydroxylases), GI tract (decreased absorption of calcium and phosphate), and bone (both bone resorption and osteoblast activation with bone formation).

Clinical and laboratory findings

- Classical symptoms are bone pain and tenderness, bone deformity (depending on age of onset), and a proximal muscle weakness with a 'waddling gait'. Muscle enzymes and biopsy are normal. Proximal myopathy is not a feature of X-linked hypophosphataemic rickets.
- The hypocalcaemia of osteomalacia is usually silent, but some individuals develop paraesthesia and tetany. Rarely, it is severe enough to cause cardiac dysrhythmia, convulsions, or psychosis.
- Children may be hypotonic and apathetic with growth retardation and delayed walking. On weight-bearing, bones become bowed, and there is irregularity of the metaphyseal–epiphyseal junction, usually at the wrist and costochondral junctions. The latter gives rise to the feature 'rachitic rosary'. An indentation may also arise along the attachment of the diaphragm to the softened ribs (Harrison's groove). Rapid growth of the softened skull leads to cranio-tabes, parietal bone flattening, and frontal bossing. Dentition is also delayed and poor.
- Many bony deformities persist despite treatment (unless due to simple dietary deficiency and treated early) and may require surgery, e.g. tibial/fibial osteotomy to correct lower limb alignment.

Table 16.5 The classification of osteomalacia

Abnormal vitamin D metabolism	Reduced availability	Poor diet
		Inadequate exposure to sun
		Malabsorption
	Defective metabolism	Hepatobiliary disease
		Chronic renal failure
		Anticonvulsant drugs
		Vitamin D-dependent rickets type I
		X-linked hypophosphataemia
		Oncogenic hypophosphataemia
	Receptor defects	Vitamin D-dependent rickets type II
Altered phosphate homeostasis	Malabsorption	
	Renal phosphate loss	X-linked hypophosphataemia
		Fanconi syndrome
	Defective mineralization	Aluminium and fluoride toxicity
		Bisphosphonate toxicity
		Hypophosphatasia
		Fibrogenous imperfecta ossium

- The classical radiographic change of osteomalacia is the pseudo-fracture (Looser's zone), found most often at the following sites:
  - ribs and clavicles;
  - outer border of the scapulae;
  - pubic rami;
  - femoral neck;
  - metatarsals.

They appear as incomplete, radiolucent fracture lines perpendicular to the cortex, with poor callus formation:

- Laboratory investigations of vitamin D deficiency demonstrate a low serum calcium and phosphate, elevated serum alkaline phosphatase, low urinary phosphate and low urinary calcium excretion, low levels of 25-hydroxyvitamin D, and a mild secondary hyperparathyroidism. The latter may cause a mild hyperchloraemic acidosis due to renal bicarbonate loss. If this acidosis is severe then it suggests a renal tubular defect (see 📖 p 445).

- Levels of 1,25-dihydroxyvitamin D may be normal and are therefore not helpful. If the serum calcium and 25-hydroxyvitamin D levels are normal as well, then the defect is likely to be renal handling of phosphate or end-organ resistance. If doubt remains as to the diagnosis of osteomalacia, a transiliac bone biopsy can be taken.

Features and treatment of abnormal vitamin D metabolism

- Vitamin D deficiency through poor diet intake is rare unless combined with exposure to sunlight. It is a phenomenon seen most often in the housebound elderly, and in immigrant Asian populations.
- Bone pain and muscle weakness respond quickly to replacement therapy though laboratory and radiological features may take longer to return to normal. Limb deformity can be prevented if simple vitamin D deficiency is treated early.
- Vitamin D_2 (ergocalciferol) at physiological doses of 200–400 IU/ day (5–10 micrograms) daily can prevent disease. In severe disease, a loading dose of ergocalciferol 50 000 IU can be administered weekly for 4–8 weeks.
- Intestinal disorders that lead to fat malabsorption can cause vitamin D deficiency, as vitamin D is fat-soluble. Cortical bone loss is usually irreversible in this group. Prevention of further damage is best achieved by annually monitoring levels of serum 25-hydroxyvitamin D and, if levels are low-to-normal or less, replacement with ergocalciferol or calcitriol and calcium. Calcium should be supplemented at doses of 800–1000 mg/day for adults.
- Chronic renal failure and renal osteodystrophy are discussed in the section on parathyroid disease and related disorders later in this chapter ([] p 448). Essentially, two problems arise as a consequence of renal failure: first a decline in production of 1,25-dihydroxyvitamin D, and secondly poor phosphate excretion and subsequent hyperphosphataemia. The latter worsens hypocalcaemia that, in turn, leads to parathyroid hyperplasia and secondary hyperparathyroidism.
- Type I vitamin D-dependent rickets is a rare autosomal recessive disease. Defective 25-hydroxyvitamin D 1 hydroxylase enzyme activity leads to low levels of 1,25-vitamin D. Children are often affected with rickets before the age of 2 years, and fail to respond to normal levels of vitamin D replacement. Treatment is most effective with physiological doses of calcitriol.
- Type II vitamin D-dependent rickets is a rare receptor defect disorder. About 70% of patients will have alopecia and this is an important prognostic feature when discussing likely outcome of treatment. In patients with normal hair, a remission can be achieved with high doses of vitamin D (as above). In patients with alopecia a 10-fold increase in vitamin D dosing is often required and about 50% will not respond.

Features and treatment of altered phosphate homeostasis

- Osteomalacia from phosphate depletion is rare and usually occurs as a consequence of abuse of phosphate-binding antacids over many years. Histologically it appears the same as vitamin D deficiency disease, although biochemically serum calcium is usually normal and vitamin D is high. Treatment is with phosphate supplements and avoidance of antacids.

- X-linked hypophosphataemic rickets (also known as 'familial hypophosphataemic rickets') is a disorder of vitamin D resistance. It is important to diagnose early as treatment can prevent deformity. It manifests itself as short stature and rickets in the homozygous men, with variable growth and expression of bone deformity in women. Dental delay occurs, but dentition is usually normal. Proximal myopathy is not a feature of this condition. Laboratory tests show a low serum phosphate, normal serum calcium and PTH, and a low/normal 1,25-dihydroxyvitamin D. Urine phosphate excretion is increased in the absence of abnormal acidification, glycosuria, or aminoaciduria. A combination of calcitriol (0.125–1.5 µg/day) and phosphate (25 mg/kg/day in infants, and 1–3 g elemental phosphorus in adults) is the most effective therapy. The induction of hypercalcaemia is a risk and the serum calcium should be monitored regularly every 2 weeks for a couple of months on induction of therapy and thereafter approximately every 3 months.
- Renal tubular acidosis (RTA) and Fanconi syndrome may be associated with osteomalacia and rickets. In RTA there is a disorder of bicarbonate handling leading to low plasma bicarbonate, metabolic acidosis, and an inappropriate urine pH. Type I, distal tubular RTA occurs as a result of failure to secrete hydrogen ions (Table 16.6).
- Type II, proximal RTA is a consequence of bicarbonate wasting. Type II RTA is often associated with Fanconi syndrome. The development of rickets in both forms of RTA is due to hypophosphataemia. The acidosis should be treated and vitamin D supplements given.
- Fanconi syndrome is associated with a number of acquired and inherited disorders. These include multiple myeloma, amyloidosis, heavy metal toxicity and disorders of carbohydrate metabolism. The net effect of the proximal renal tubular defects is glycosuria, aminoaciduria, phosphaturia, and hypophosphataemia. Treatment of the bone disease is with phosphate and calcitriol supplements.
- Oncogenic hypophosphataemic osteomalacia is a phenomenon seen with some tumours (usually mesenchymal). The proposed mechanism is the production of a humoral factor that affects proximal renal tubular handling of phosphate. The bone disease regresses after removal of the tumor. A similar condition occurs in fibrous dysplasia and neurofibromatosis. Treatment involves phosphate and calcitriol supplements.

Table 16.6 Some causes of type I, distal RTA

Hereditary	Primary	
	Renal	Medullary sponge, polycystic kidney
	Fructose intolerance	
	Ehlers–Danlos syndrome	
Acquired	Rheumatic	SLE, Sjögren's syndrome, sarcoidosis
	Renal	Obstruction, pyelonephritis, transplantation
	Endocrine	Hyper/hypothyroidism, hyperparathyroidism hyperprolactinaemia
	Hepatic	Chronic active hepatitis Liver cirrhosis
	Tuberculosis	
	Lithium toxicity	
	Cryoglobulinaemia	

Parathyroid disease and related disorders

This section will discuss hypercalcaemia in adults and children, and its relation to musculoskeletal disorders. Hyper- and hypoparathyroidism, and renal osteodystrophy are considered. For further information on vitamin D and phosphate imbalance the reader is referred to the previous section on osteomalacia and rickets.

Hypercalcaemia

- The clinical picture of hypercalcaemia can range from the asymptomatic to an acute medical emergency.
- Calcium plasma concentrations are normally balanced between the homeostatic mechanisms operating in the gut, skeleton, kidneys, and extracellular fluids. Hypercalcaemia arises most often as a result of excessive loss of calcium from bone, but may also occur due to excessive gut absorption. The excessive bone loss combined with a failure of the kidneys to handle high loads of calcium, and a failure of bone to reclaim minerals quickly enough, leads to the imbalance. Accelerated bone loss (osteoclast stimulation) may be driven by several causes including parathyroid hormone (PTH) and cytokines interleukin-1 (IL-1), TNF, and transforming growth factor (TGF). PTH also induces calcium reabsortion from the kidneys.
- The clinical presentation of moderate to severe hypercalcaemia includes:
  - joint, bone, muscle pain;
  - muscle weakness;
  - dehydration and polyuria;
  - lethargy;
  - fatigue;
  - acute confusional state—unconsciousness;
  - abdominal pains and vomiting;
  - renal colic pains;
  - electrocardiogram findings—short QT interval, etc.
- Hyperparathyroidism and malignancy are the most common causes of hypercalcaemia, accounting for 90% of all cases. A thorough history and examination is required when considering the cause of serum calcium (Table 16.7).

Table 16.7 Some cause of hypercalcaemia

Common	Primary hyper-parathyroidism	
	Malignancy	Lytic metastases: TNF, IL-1
		Ectopic PTH and TGF-α
		Ectopic 1,25 vitamin D
Uncommon/rare	Drugs	Thiazide diuretics
		Lithium
		Aminophylline
	Granuloma	Sarcoidosis
		Tuberculosis
		Histoplasmosis
	Endocrine/metabolic	Thyrotoxicosis
		Pheochromocytoma
		Excess vitamin A or D
		Renal failure
	Immobilization	

- Treatment options depend on the level of serum calcium, the presence of symptoms, renal impairment, and the underlying cause. For example, borderline high serum calcium in an asymptomatic individual with a mildly elevated PTH may simply warrant observation in the absence of renal impairment or vitamin D deficiency. On the other hand, an individual with severe hypercalcaemia, dehydration, and renal impairment due to a treatable malignancy would require urgent aggressive management.
- Dehydration is very common. Early rehydration is very important and often given for 24–48 h prior to review of serum calcium levels and the instigation of further therapies such as bisphosphonates and loop diuretics (Table 16.8).

Hypercalcaemia in infancy and childhood

- Chronic hypercalcaemia of infancy may not be associated with the more common clinical features mentioned above. More often there is a failure to thrive, abdominal pain, and irritability. Acute hypercalcaemia is very rare in children.
- Conditions to consider are listed in Table 16.9.

Table 16.8 Treatment of hypercalcaemia

General principles	Rehydrate with normal saline 4 L in 24 h if needed
	Correct hypokalaemia and hypomagnesaemia
	Mild metabolic acidosis need not be treated
Specific treatment	Loop diuretics when hydrated
	Bisphosphophates
	Calcitonin
	Corticosteroids (haematological malignancies and granulomatous diseases)

Table 16.9 Conditions that may be responsible for hypercalcaemia in infancy and childhood

Williams' syndrome	A spectrum of aortic valve stenosis and facial dysmorphism ('elfin' facies)
	Radioulnar synostosis impedes growth in 25% of cases. There is a deletion of the elastin gene on chromosome 7; pathogenesis is otherwise unknown
Idiopathic infantile hypercalcaemia	Similar milder appearance to Williams' syndrome can be seen. There are also features of inguinal hernias, hypertension, strabismus, and kyphosis
Familial hypocalciuric hypercalcaemia	See later in this section
Neonatal primary hyperparathyroidism	
Other	Fat necrosis
	Sarcoidosis
	Jansen syndrome (metaphyseal dysplasia)
	Overdosing of milk/vitamin D

Parathyroid disorders

Primary hyperparathyroidism

- Primary hyperparathyroidism (HPT) is a relatively common condition with an incidence of 1 in 1000. It occurs at all ages, although is much more common after the age of 60 with a female to male ratio of 3:1. It is unusual in childhood and should raise the possibility of familial multiple endocrine neoplasia (MEN) type I or type II.
- A single benign adenoma accounts for 80% of cases of primary HPT.
- Generalized gland hyperplasia accounts for 15–20% of cases.

- Parathyroid carcinoma is very rare.
- The condition is associated with bone, renal, GI, and neuromuscular complications. Bony problems can be seen on plain radiographs and range from mild subperiosteal bone resorption to full 'osteitis fibrosa cystica' with bone cysts, 'brown tumours', bone resorption of the distal phalanges and clavicles, patchy osteosclerosis (classic 'rugger jersey' spine), and multiple lytic lesions of the skull. These changes may often, however, be non-specific.
- Renal stones are a common complication. GI manifestations include peptic ulceration and pancreatitis. The myopathy of primary HPT is rare and more often a syndrome of fatigue and weakness is seen.
- Primary HPT is diagnosed by assaying PTH levels. The assays are sensitive and able to distinguish between non-parathyroid tumour secreting PTH and parathyroid hormone.

Treatment
- Medical management includes adequate rehydration and avoidance of high calcium intake. Clinical trials with calcimimetic agents (stimulate calcium receptors with consequent inhibition of PTH secretion) and in particular cinacalcet hydrochloride are ongoing and may be effective in primary HPT. At the time of writing, cinacalcet has received FDA and NICE approval for the treatment of secondary HPT in patients with chronic kidney disease.
- Some individuals (especially the elderly) have physiological mild elevation of PTH due to vitamin D deficiency with normal calcium levels. Vitamin D should be replaced and the serum calcium and PTH levels monitored after 8–10 weeks.
- Parathyroidectomy should be offered to individuals with moderate-to-high serum calcium and/or symptoms and complications of the condition, the latter regardless of whether serum calcium levels are 'borderline' raised or not. US imaging, thallium/technetium scans, MR, and CT are all useful ways of establishing the position of an adenoma. However, exploration by an experienced surgeon is equally effective.

Secondary and tertiary hyperparathyroidism
Secondary HPT occurs as a consequence of abnormalities in serum calcium and homeostatic 'sensing' of calcium levels. With time, PTH secretion becomes autonomous and the abnormality is then called tertiary HPT. This is most often seen in conditions such as end-organ renal disease and vitamin D resistance. Calcimimetics may have an important role to play in controlling secondary HPT but at present parathyroidectomy is the best treatment option. Vitamin D replacement to lower PTH secretion does not appear to be effective in patients with otherwise normal vitamin D levels.

Familial hypocalciuric hypercalcaemia or familial benign hypercalcaemia
- This condition is common, but most often asymptomatic. It is inherited as an autosomal dominant with high penetrance. Radiographs, PTH, and renal function are usually normal. Although parathyroid gland hyperplasia occurs, parathyroidectomy is invariably unsuccessful at lowering serum calcium levels.

- The two indications for parathyroidectomy are neonatal severe HPT and adult relapsing pancreatitis. Use of diuretics, oestrogens, or phosphate to regulate serum calcium has been unsuccessful. Patients should therefore be followed without intervention unless complications arise.
- In pregnancy the three situations to be aware of are:
  - asymptomatic hypercalcaemia in the affected offspring of a carrier;
  - severe neonatal hypercalcaemia in affected offspring of an unaffected mother (intrauterine secondary HPT, which usually resolves spontaneously);
  - hypocalcaemia in the unaffected offspring of an affected mother (foetal parathyroid suppression).

Familial hyperparathyroid syndromes

Up to 10% of cases of HPT may have a hereditary syndrome. The most common of these is multiple endocrine neoplasia (MEN). Type I, autosomal dominant and equal in both sexes, is associated with pancreatic and pituitary adenomas, and adrenal hyperplasia. Type IIA, autosomal dominant Sipple's disease, is characterized by pheochromocytomas and medullary carcinoma of the thyroid.

Parathyroid hormone resistant syndromes

- Pseudohypoparathyroidism (PHP) occurs as a result of resistance to PTH by target tissues. The biochemical consequences are hypocalcaemia, hyperphosphataemia, and elevated PTH.
- Cyclic AMP (cAMP) mediates many actions of PTH. Administration of bioactive PTH to normal individuals leads to increased urinary excretion of cAMP. The abnormal response to this test in individuals with PHP classifies them either type I—no increase in urine cAMP with bioactive PTH—or type II—normal increase in urine cAMP, but abnormal phosphate handling.
- The net effect is features similar to those of hypoparathyroidism of any cause (such as congenital parathyroid absence, or surgical removal).
- Common symptoms include:
  - neuromuscular irritability (due to associated hypocalcaemia);
  - muscle cramps;
  - pseudopapilloedema;
  - extrapyramidal signs;
  - mental retardation;
  - cataracts;
  - coarse hair/alopecia;
  - abnormal dentition;
  - personality disturbance.
- PHP type Ia [Albright's hereditary osteodystrophy (AHO)] manifests as short stature, round facies, obesity, brachydactyly, and SC(J) ossification. Albright observed that some individuals have these features without PHP. The term pseudopseudohypoparathyroidism was coined. This group have a normal serum calcium and PTH/cAMP test.
- Cases with PHP type, I but who lack features of AHO are classified type Ib. They often have the skeletal abnormalities seen in cases of hypoparathyroidism.

- In type II PHP there is a normal cAMP response, but an abnormal phosphate response in the kidney.
- The mainstay of therapy is the maintenance of serum calcium and phosphate levels. The complication of calcium and vitamin D supplements is the increased risk of renal stones due to hypercalciuria. One gram a day of calcium is recommended and products rich in phosphate (e.g. dairy foods) should be avoided. Hydroxyvitamin D supplements are valuable, but serum calcium and phosphate levels should be checked weekly for 4–6 weeks up to steady state and then every 3–6 months.

Renal osteodystrophy

- The kidneys regulate calcium/phosphate balance, are a target organ for PTH, and produce 1,25 dihydroxy-vitamin D (calcitriol). Renal osteodystrophy is the net effect on bone that occurs due to derangement of calcium homeostasis in chronic renal failure. Renal bone disease is classified as 'high turnover' or 'low turnover' depending on whether serum PTH levels are high or low/normal respectively. Low turnover, adynamic osteodystrophy, is related to excess bone aluminium deposition in dialysis patients and is also seen in diabetes mellitus and corticosteroid therapy and as part of aging.
- Hyperphosphataemia, hypocalcaemia, impaired calcitriol production, and skeletal resistance to PTH all contribute to secondary HPT in chronic renal failure. Serum PTH varies too widely in the condition to be useful in assessing treatment. Serum alkaline phosphatase is increased and is a useful marker though it does not distinguish between 'high' and 'low' turnover states.
- The clinical manifestations of renal osteodystrophy are shown in Table 16.10.

The management of renal osteodystrophy

- Good dietary control of phosphate can maintain normal calcium levels, but low-phosphate diets are often unacceptable and normal phosphate levels are best achieved with binding agents, e.g. calcium carbonate or calcium acetate.
- Small doses of calcitriol (vitamin D) may help to lower serum PTH levels. Some individuals may be sensitive to calcitriol and serum calcium levels may increase. Most patients require doses of 0.25–0.5 μg daily; children may require higher doses.
- Parathyroidectomy is indicated in persistent symptomatic hypercalcaemia, ectopic calcification, and severe bone pain.

Ectopic calcification and ossification

- Ectopic calcification can arise from any one of a number of causes of hypercalcaemia or hyperphosphataemia. These include renal failure, hyperparathyroidism, and sarcoidosis. Dystrophic calcification is also a feature of SScl (📖 Chapter 13, p 363), DM (📖 Chapter 14, p 385), and primary calcinosis.
- Ectopic ossification can be seen post-trauma and following myositis. It is also a feature of several rare conditions including pseudo-hypoparathyroidism and myositis ossificans progressiva. Early signs of muscle ossification are best detected with MR scanning. Later ossification it easily visible on plain radiographs. Treatment is difficult, but includes physiotherapy to maintain suppleness and possibly heparins or bisphosphonates to halt bone formation.

Table 16.10 The clinical manifestations of renal osteodystrophy

Clinical feature	Comment
Bone pain	Common
Skeletal deformity	Common. Affects appendicular and axial skeleton
	Children: onset <3 years, rachitic; onset <10 years, bowing of long bones, widened metaphyses, pseudoclubbing, slipped epiphyses
	Adults: lumbar scoliosis, kyphosis, distorted thorax
Growth retardation	
Proximal muscle weakness	
Ectopic calcification	Soft-tissues. Visceral. Vascular—if severe, individuals may develop ischaemic necrosis

Paget's disease of bone

- Paget's disease is a chronic disorder of accelerated bone resorption and formation resulting in deformity in size and shape of bone, as well as fragility despite apparent 'thickening' of bone.
- The condition is common (about 5% of the population over the age of 55) in the United Kingdom, the United States, Australia, and New Zealand, with a male to female ratio of 3:2. It is uncommon in Asia and non-White races.
- Very little is known of the molecular basis of Paget's disease. There is evidence to suggest that it may be triggered by exposure to a slow virus. Paramyxovirus antigens found in bone cells, and compatible with measles, respiratory syncytial virus, and canine distemper have all been implicated.
- The clinical features of Paget's disease are shown in Table 16.11.

Investigation and treatment

- Serum alkaline phosphatase, a measure of bone formation, is the most useful marker and may be elevated as much as 30 times above normal. Occasionally, in limited Paget's, the enzyme is normal. This should not be a deterrent to treating painful lesions. The differential diagnosis of increased bone alkaline phosphatase includes metastatic bone disease, osteomalacia, hyperparathyroidism, and hyperphosphatasia.
- Urine hydroxyproline excretion is also increased. Hydroxyproline is a breakdown product of collagen and a marker of bone resorption.
- There is a wide variation in radiographic appearance of the condition but the main features are sclerosis, bone expansion, and coarse, disorganized, trabecular bone.
- Isotope bone scanning is a sensitive investigation for defining the extent of lesions.
- Many rare hereditary dysplastic conditions are associated with bone sclerosis. These include osteopetrosis, Engelmann's disease, and pycnodysostosis. These conditions are beyond the scope of this book.
- Sclerosis is also a feature of many other conditions including metabolic disease (fluorosis, hypervitaminosis D, parathyroid disease, renal osteodystrophy), malignancy (lymphoma, myeloma, skeletal metastases), infection, sarcoidosis, and tuberous sclerosis.
- Thermographic improvement and pain reduction are correlated with effective treatment of Paget's; thermographic observations probably demonstrate a decline in bone and peri-osseous blood flow after treatment.

Table 16.11 Clinical features of Paget's disease of bone

Clinical feature	Details
Pain	Deep, boring pain, possibly correlated to blood flow
Bone expansion and deformity	Hands or feet 10% of cases
	Pelvis 75% of cases
	Lumbar spine 50% of cases
	Femur 35% of cases
	Sacrum 35% of cases
	Skull 35% of cases
	Tibia 30% of cases
	Radius 15% of cases
Fractures	
Heat	
Neurological syndromes	Deafness (sensorineural or conductive)
	Tinnitus
	Headache
	Brainstem/cerebellar compression
	Spinal cord/root compression
	Cranial nerve entrapment
High-output cardiac Failure	Rare—occurs when >40% of the skeleton is involved
Malignant osteosarcoma	Seen in 0.1% of cases, esp. if disease present for >10 years
Immobilization hypercalcaemia	Serum calcium levels are nearly always normal
Gout	
Retinal angioid streaks	

- There are several indications for treatment of Paget's disease:
  - pain arising from Pagetic sites;
  - deforming disease;
  - skull disease;
  - *complications:* progressive neurological syndrome, fractures, hypercalcaemia, high-output cardiac failure, serum alkaline phosphatase (over twice upper normal).

- Pagetic and related osteoarthritic pain may be reduced by simple analgesics, but pure Pagetic bone pain responds poorly to this. In most cases now the choice of treatment falls between bisphosphonates and calcitonin. These drugs are discussed in the section on osteoporosis.
- Etidronate may be given for 6 months at a dose of 5 mg/kg/day. Vitamin D supplements may minimize the mineralization defects that can occur with even low doses of etidronate.
- Risedronate may also be given at 30 mg daily for 1–2 months.
- Oral tiludronate 400 mg daily for 3 months has been licensed for the treatment of Paget's disease in the United Kingdom.
- Pamidronate may also be used and many in current practice offer a single dose infusion of 30–90 mg iv (dependent on renal function) to symptomatic patients, with follow-up and measurement of serum alkaline phosphatase after 3 months. Transient 'flu-like' symptoms of fever, myalgia, and arthralgia often occur after the first dose of iv pamidronate.
- Calcitonin (sc or im) may also be used in Paget's disease. The disadvantages are common symptoms of nausea and diarrhoea, relapse on therapy, and expense. Nasal spray calcitonin may be useful, but the therapeutic effect is weaker than with bisphosphonates. Typical dosing for salmon calcitonin would be a 10 IU test dose followed by 50–100 IU daily, reducing to 50 IU 2 or 3 times per week once a symptomatic response is achieved (usually after 4–8 weeks). If there has been no symptomatic response after 3 months, calcitonin therapy should be stopped.
- There is no consensus on whether or when to treat Pagetic joints *per se* prior to joint replacement.

Miscellaneous diseases of bone

Osteochondritis and osteonecrosis

- The osteochondroses are a heterogeneous group of disorders, defined by their radiological appearances. In a few instances, radiological osteochondritis may be an incidental finding, not associated with symptoms and may represent a normal developmental variant. Usually, however, it is painful, occurs in the growing skeleton between the ages of 3–16 years, and is more frequent in men and in the peripheral skeleton. Some cases are due to infarction (osteonecrosis) of subchondral bone. For others the aetiology is unknown.

- Osteonecrosis (synonyms: avascular necrosis, ischemic necrosis, aseptic necrosis) can occur at several sites and is associated with as many eponyms (Table 16.12). Bone infarction and subsequent pain occurs in susceptible areas because of limited collateral circulation and low perfusion pressure, e.g. in the femoral head. First, bone, and adjacent marrow becomes necrotic. Granulation tissue then advances into the dead bone, which is resorbed. Osteoblasts then lay down new osteoid. Advanced osteonecrosis leads to secondary osteoarthritis, severe disability, and eventually the need for joint replacement. Whether or not core decompression surgery should be performed in the acute phase of the condition remains open to debate.

- Aetiological factors for osteonecrosis include trauma, sepsis, radiation, thermal, and electrical injury. Caisson's disease is an obliterative endarteritis of the femoral head caused by expanding nitrogen gas in divers who decompress too quickly. Haematological causes include haemophilia, coagulopathies, and haemoglobinopathies. Endocrine causes include Cushing's syndrome and glucocorticoid use (high dose >60 mg/day over a period of months). There is an increased susceptibility to the condition in several rheumatic conditions including RA (📖 Chapter 5, p 233), SLE (📖 Chapter 10, p 321), SScl (📖 Chapter 13, p 363), and vasculitis (📖 Chapter 15, p 405). Finally, a miscellaneous group of associations with osteonecrosis include alcohol abuse, organ transplantation, dialysis, HIV infection, pancreatitis, chronic liver disease, hypertriglyceridaemia, and pregnancy.

- Osteonecrosis complicates 20% of cases of intracapsular hip fracture.

- Fat embolism may account for some cases, e.g. in alcoholism and Cushing's disease.

- Asymptomatic osteonecrosis in SLE may be as high as 35%.

Table 16.12 The osteochondroses

Skeletal area		Disease eponym	Mechanism
Upper limb	Basal phalanges	Thiemann	Trauma
	Second metacarpal head	Mauclaire	Trauma
	Lunate	Kienbock	Osteonecrosis
	Carpal navicular	Prieser	Trauma
	Humeral capitellum	Panner	Trauma/ osteonecrosis
Lower limb	Second metatarsal base	Freiberg	Osteonecrosis
	Fifth metatarsal base	Iselin	Trauma
	Tarsal navicular	Köhler	?Trauma/normal variant
	Talus	Diaz	Trauma-related
	Calcaneal	Sever	Traction apophysitis*
	Apophysis of tibial tubercle	Osgood– Schlatter	Traction apophysitis*
	Proximal tibia	Blount	–
	Inferior patella pole	Sinding–Larsen-Johansson	Traction apophysitis*
	Femoral epiphysis	Legg–Calvé–Perthes	Osteonecrosis
Axial skeleton	Vertebral epiphysis	Scheuermann	Repeated trauma

*Due to repetitive overloading of tendons, usually from sports.

- Osteonecrosis is diagnosed and classified radiologically (Arlet and Ficat classification): I = normal; II = osteoporosis, cysts, sclerosis giving mottled appearance; III = subchondral bone collapse; IV = abnormal bone contour and joint space loss. Isotope Bone Scan, CT, and MR are more sensitive. MR can identify early changes in bone marrow before bone necrosis and has greatest specificity once bone changes occur.
- Scheuermann's disease, although not consistently defined, is thought to be a vertebral epiphyseal osteochondritis that occurs in adolescence. Although an incidental radiographic finding, it is also associated with diffuse spinal pain which is more likely to be present if the osteochondritis is thoracolumbar (25%), rather than thoracic (75%) and the child is an athlete or very active. It can present with painless dorsal kyphosis with compensatory lumbar lordosis and lateral spine radiographs show irregularity of vertebral end-plates, anterior vertebral wedging, and kyphosis.

- Legg–Calvé–Perthes' disease is osteonecrosis of the femoral epiphysis and occurs in the age range 3–8 years, most frequently in boys (ratio 4:1). It is bilateral in 10–20% of cases. Symptoms include an insidious onset of limp and pain in the groin or referred to the knee/thigh that is relieved by rest. Limitation of hip internal rotation and abduction (due to adductor spasm) is typical. Leg length inequality suggests bone collapse. There may be spontaneous resolution, especially in younger patients, in whom conservative management is indicated.
- Osgood–Schlatter's disease is probably due to repetitive trauma at the site of patellar tendon insertion into the tibial tubercle, typically in athletic adolescents, especially young males aged 14–16 years. Pain on exercise usually eases with rest. The diagnosis is made clinically and on demonstrating an enlarged fragmented tibial tubercle on a lateral view radiograph. Bilateral knee views helps to distinguish normal from abnormal.
- Sinding–Larsen–Johansson's disease occurs as a consequence of over-loading of the patella at its secondary centre of ossification producing a traction apophysitis at the patella lower pole. Although not exclusive to the group, it is a typical sports-related injury in adolescent athletes who jump, e.g. high-jump, basketball. Treatment is with simple analgesia or NSAIDs, and rest.
- Köhler's disease is osteonecrosis of the tarsal navicular. Changes may represent a developmental variation in ossification and it presents with a painful limp. Weight bearing is more comfortable on the outside of the foot and the navicular is tender.
- Freiberg's disease, osteonecrosis of the metatarsal (usually the second) head following trauma, is most common in adolescent females. Pain is localized and worse on weight bearing with swelling sometimes detectable.

Osteochondritis dissecans

- This is usually a solitary lesion of the medial femoral condyle. A fragment of articular cartilage and subchondral bone becomes demarcated and may form an intra-articular loose body. The cause is unknown, but may be due to abnormal ossification or trauma. Similar features may occasionally be seen at the elbow, hip, and talus.
- The condition is seen most often in male adolescents. Symptoms are mainly acute onset pain, an effusion, and limited movement of the joint.
- Plain radiographs will show a well-circumscribed, sclerotic lesion.
- In young patients before skeletal maturity there is a good chance of healing. After the epiphyses have closed, however, there is more risk of a loose body and secondary osteoarthritis. Arthroscopy can assist in assessing the degree of damage and removing loose bodies. Surgery ranges from drilling the lesion *in situ* to encourage healing, to bone osteochondral allografts.

Osteoid osteoma

- This is a benign osteoid-forming tumor that can be an elusive cause of bone pain, radiculopathy, or arthritis in children and adults. It is uncommon and accounts for 10% of benign bone neoplasia. It is 2–3 times more common in men than women and the incidence is highest in the second and third decades of life. More than two-thirds of lesions occur in long bones and especially the femur and tibia.

- Pain is the primary symptom and may be referred.
- The typical lesion is seen on plain radiography as an isolated, well-defined area of sclerosis with a radiolucent nidus often containing speckles of calcium. Isotope bone scanning is a sensitive method of isolating a lesion and CT is valuable for localizing the nidus before surgical resection.
- Most individuals will respond, in part, to aspirin or NSAIDs. Provided the nidus is completely resected, surgery is curative.

Fibrous dysplasia

- This condition manifests as sporadic isolated or multifocal fibrous bone cysts and occurs most often in the second to third decade of life in isolated (mono-ostotic) disease, and before the age of 10 years in multifocal (polyostotic) disease.
- McCune–Albright syndrome is a triad of fibrous dysplasia, hyper pigmented 'café-au-lait' patches, and endocrine abnormalities.
- Laboratory tests are usually normal.
- There is no specific treatment. Some lesions regress. Fractures heal in the normal way. Girls with McCune–Albright-associated precocious puberty may respond to the aromatase inhibitor testolactone.

Molecular abnormalities of collagen and fibrillin

Collagen and fibrillin are major connective tissue proteins with important mechanical functions. This section will deal briefly with osteogenesis imperfecta (OI), Marfan syndrome (MFS), Ehlers–Danlos syndrome (EDS) and Joint Hypermobility Syndrome (JHS); the Hereditary Disorders of Connective Tissue (HDCT).

Genetics
- There are a number of types of collagen and a number of gene mutations leading to subtypes of collagen diseases. In this respect, we will focus only on common aspects of these uncommon conditions, although the reader should be aware that joint hypermobility syndrome (JHS), also considered to be the same as Ehlers-Danlos hypermobility type, is far more common than most clinicians realize and therefore under-diagnosed.
- The Villefranche nosology for EDS recognizes nine subtypes based on the severity of the clinical features, the underlying biochemical and genetic defect, and the pattern of inheritance (Table 16.15). Mutations in genes encoding collagens I, III, and V, and collagen-modifying enzymes have been identified in most forms of EDS.
- Procollagen Type I contains 2 α-1 and an α-2 polypeptide chain, encoded by single genes COL1A1 and COL1A2 on chromosome 17 and 7 respectively. Type V collagen contains 3 different polypeptides, the genes for pro-α 1 (V) and 2 (V), namely COL5A1 and COL5A2 being found on chromosomes 9 and 2.
- EDS Classical type is an autosomal dominant disorder caused by mutations in COL5A1 and COL5A2. Mutations of COL1A1 and COL1A2 are associated with EDS kyphoscoliotic type, and those of COL3A1 with EDS Vascular type. There are, however, many rare unclassified variants of EDS, the molecular basis of which is unknown.
- The defect underlying the most common EDS hypermobility subtype is unknown. The genetics of JHS also remains poorly understood with only a few family case reports in the literature. Some of the EDS hypermobility type/JHS phenotype may be accounted for by haplotype insufficiency in the expression of tenascin X, a large extra-cellular matrix glycoprotein.
- Molecular research has shown OI result from mutations in one of the two genes COL1A1 and COL1A2 that encode for type I collagen on chromosome 4.
- The Marfan syndrome is autosomal dominant in inheritance and associated with mutation of fibrillin 1 and 2. The causative gene for fibrillin 1 defects has been localized to chromosome 15q21. Many additional mutations have also been identified in *FBN1* and a related gene *FBN2*.
- If an HDCT is suspected additional morphological, biochemical and/or molecular analyses are available to confirm the diagnosis. A skin biopsy is required in order to perform biochemical analysis of collagen subtypes, and additional DNA analysis can be performed from the cultured fibroblasts. Molecular analysis of the fibrillin-1 gene can be performed on DNA extracted from leucocytes.

Table 16.13 Clinical and biochemical abnormalities in OI

Type	Clinical features	Inheritance	Defect
I	Normal bone growth. Normal dentition. Hearing loss in 50%. Blue sclera	Autosomal dominant	Decreased production of type I procollagen
II	Lethal. Stillbirths	Autosomal dominant. Autosomal recessive (rare)	Rearrangement of collagen IA/2A genes
III	Often deformed growth at birth and worsens. Poor dentition common. Hearing loss common. May have blue sclera	Autosomal dominant or recessive	Mutations in α-1 and α-2 collagen chains
IV	Often bone deformity and short stature. Poor dentition common. Hearing loss uncommon. Normal sclera.	Autosomal dominant	Mutations in the α-2 chains

Osteogenesis imperfecta

- OI (also known as brittle bone disease) is a spectrum of conditions ranging from stillbirth to asymptomatic signs. The pathogenesis centres around abnormalities of type I collagen that is found not only in bone but also ligaments, teeth, sclerae, and skin.
- Ligament laxity, joint hypermobility, easy bruising, and poor dentition are common features. The differences between the four types of OI are shown in Table 16.13.
- Generalized osteopenia, deformity, and fractures are common bone and radiographic findings. The differential diagnosis in children includes juvenile osteoporosis, Cushing's disease, and homocystinuria.
- There is no effective medical therapy for OI. Patients may need surgery in late childhood/adulthood for deformities, and good dental hygiene.
- Children may present with multiple injuries that lead the clinician to consider child-abuse as a source for these—absolute care must be taken in ensuring neither OI nor any other collagen disorder is present before considering further action.

Marfan syndrome

- The Marfanoid habitus is characterized by long extremities (span/height ratio >1.03), long fingers and feet (arachnodactyly) with a hand/height ratio >11% and foot/height ratio >15%, tall stature (with upper segment/lower segment ratio <0.89), pectus deformity of the chest wall (increasing risk of chest infections), high-arched palate, mandibular hypoplasia, lens dislocations and myopia, and joint laxity.
- There is a predisposition to mitral valve prolapse and acute aortic root rupture. All patients should have an echocardiogram and thoracic CT/MR to assess the aortic valve and arch.
- Beta-blockade has long been used to decrease the rate of aortic dilatation and improve long-term survival. However, there are little data to support this approach.
- In mouse models, losartan has been demonstrated to be an effective therapy through transforming growth factor-β antagonism, and may be an important advance in the treatment of this disease.
- It is an autosomal dominant condition with complete penetrance and prevalence of 1 in 25 000.
- The criteria for diagnosis are shown in Table 16.14.
- A subgroup similar to Marfan syndrome, but without vascular fragility exists. The condition is called congenital contractural arachnodactyly.
- Numerous gene mutations have been found for both conditions, both linked to abnormalities of the protein fibrillin type I and II.

The main aim of follow-up and assessment of these individuals is the early detection and referral of cardiac valve and aortic disease. Musculoskeletal symptoms should be managed in much the same way as outlined in the section below on joint hypermobility syndrome.

Table 16.14 The Ghent 1996 criteria for Marfan Syndrome

Major Criteria:	
1 Skeletal 4 or more of:	Pectus carinatum
	Pectus excavatum (requiring surgery)
	Marfanoid habitus
	Arachnodactyly
	Scoliosis >20°
	Reduced extension at the elbow (to <170°)
	Pes planus
	Protrusio acetabulae
2 Cardiovascular:	
Dilation of the ascending aorta involving at least the sinuses of valsalva *or* dissection of the ascending aorta	
3 Occular	Ectopia lentis
4 Dura	Lumbosacral dural ectasia on CT or MRI
5 Genetic	Parent, child, or sibling meeting the criteria *or* Presence of a mutation in fibrillin known to cause MFS
Minor Criteria:	
1 Skeletal	Mild–moderate pectus excavatum
	Joint hypermobility
	High-arched palate
	Facies: dolichocephaly, malar hypoplasia, enophthalmos, retrognathia
2 Cardiovascular	Mitral valve prolapse
	Dilatation of pulmonary artery below age 40 years
	Dilatation or dissection of the descending thoracic or abdominal aorta below age 50 years
	Calcification of the mitral annulus below age 40 years
3 Occular	Flat cornea, myopia
4 Skin	Striae, recurrent incisional hernia
5 Pulmonary	Spontaneous pneumothorax
	Apical blebs

In the absence of genetic confirmation, 2 major criteria and 1 other system involvement are required for the diagnosis. In a case where genetic mutations are known in the family, 1 other major criterion is required with involvement of one other organ system.

Ehlers–Danlos syndrome

- This is a clinically heterogeneous condition characterized by skin fragility, ligament laxity, short stature, spinal deformity, vascular fragility, and (rarely) retinal detachment. Retinal detachment and a history of early onset OA should lead the clinician to consider the diagnosis of Stickler's syndrome, a Collagen 1 abnormality.
- There are at least 9 genetic subtypes of Ehlers–Danlos syndrome (EDS), of which at least 5 have defined biochemical abnormalities. The classification, genetic abnormalities and clinical features of EDS are shown in Table 16.15. Various inheritance patterns are found dependent on the subtype of EDS. Hypermobility type EDS is the most common of these conditions and probably synonymous with JHS (see below).
- The clinician should be very sure they have confidently excluded vascular (type IV) EDS as this is associated with significant mortality.
- Therapy for these conditions centres on graded exercise and joint and skin protection. Some individuals require joint splints. Spinal deformity may need bracing or surgery, and retinal disease requires ophthalmic expertise.
- Vascular rupture is a major concern in vascular type (type IV). This may occur even in the absence of documented aneurysms. This risk should always be taken into account during surgery or pregnancy, indeed as should tissue fragility in general for all subtypes.
- Tissue vulnerability should always be at the forefront of planning any surgical intervention.
- Patients are often also resistant to local anaesthetics—the cause unclear. Failing to recognize this phenomenon can lead the clinician to inadvertently accuse the patient of being 'sensitive' or anxious without realizing that they truly do not get a full effect from the anaesthetic.
- Difficulties may arise during pregnancy—patients may get additional joint pain from increased body weight, early rupture of membranes and premature birth, cervical incompetence and spontaneous abortion, excessive tissue trauma during delivery, and musculoskeletal complications in the post-natal period due to lifting and caring for the newborn.
- The diagnosis is primarily clinical. Genetic testing can be done by looking for abnormalities of collagen types I, III, and V, although these tests may not be widely available. A skin biopsy is required.

(Benign) joint hypermobility syndrome

- Joint hypermobility can be totally benign and an asset (e.g. dancing, athletics) or, in the presence of other signs of an HDCT (especially skin and dislocations) be associated with a multitude of pathologies including:
  - chronic widespread pain;
  - fatigue;
  - cardiovascular autonomic dysfunction;
  - bowel dysfunction.

Table 16.15 Clinical features and genetics of EDS

Type	Inheritance	Genetic defect	Common clinical picture
Classical (type I and II)	AD	Abnormal pro-α 1 and 2 encoded by COL5A1 and A2 gene	Hyper-lax skin. Profound bruisig and scarring
Hypermobility (Type III)	AD	Not known. ? Tenascin X insufficiency	See BJHS, Table 16.16
Vascular (Type IV)	AD	Abnormal pro-α 1 encoded by *COL3A1* gene	Characteristic facies—wide spaced eyes, lobeless ears. Vascular rupture
Kyphoscoliosis (Type VI)	AR	Deficiency of lysyl hydroxylase	Severe hypotonia. Scoliosis. Scleral fragility
Atherochalasia (Type VII subtype)	AD	Abnormal pro-α 1 and 2 encoded by COL1A1 and A2	Severe dislocations. Skin laxity. Bruising. Hypotonia
Dermatospraxis (Type VII subtype)	AR	Deficiency of procollagen 1 peptidase	Severe, sagging skin. Bruising. Hernias
Rare forms:			
X-linked (Type V)	X-linked	Unknown	Milder version of Classical type
Periodontal (Type VIII)	AD	Unknown	Classical with gum fragility
Type X	?AR	Unknown	Milder version of classical type with platelet aggregation

AD—autosomal dominant; AR—autosomal recessive

- Hypermobility is usually considered present if a person satisfies four or more manoeuvres in the nine-point Beighton hyper-mobility score (Table 16.16).
- JHS is excluded in the presence of Marfan syndrome or Ehlers–Danlos syndrome (excluding hypermobility (Type III)). It may be synonymous with EDS hypermobility type.
- The revised (Brighton 1998) criteria for JHS are shown in Table 16.17. JHS is diagnosed in the presence of two major, one major and two minor, or four minor criteria. Two minor criteria will suffice where there is an unequivocally affected first-degree relative. The criteria serve to demonstrate the range of clinical findings in the condition.

Table 16.16 Beighton hypermobility rating

	Subject has the ability to:	Right	Left
1	Passively dorsiflex the fifth metacarpophalangeal joint to ≥90°	1	1
2	Oppose the thumb to the volar aspect of the ipsilateral forearm	1	1
3	Hyperextend the elbow ≥10°	1	1
4	Hyperextend the knee ≥10°	1	1
5	Place hands flat on the floor without bending the knees	1	
Possible total score		9	

Table 16.17 The Brighton (1998) criteria for (benign) joint hypermobility syndrome

Major criteria	A Beighton score of 4 out of 9 or greater (current or historical)
	Arthralgia for >3 months in four or more joints
Minor criteria	A Beighton score of 1, 2, or 3 out of 9
	Arthralgia in one to three joints or back pain, either for longer than 3 months, spondylosis/spondylolisthesis
	Dislocation/subluxation in > one joint, or one joint on > one occasion
	Soft tissue rheumatism in three or more sites
	Marfanoid habitus
	Abnormal skin: striae, hyperextensibility, papyraceous scars
	Eye signs: drooping eyelids, myopia,
	Varicose veins, hernias, uterine/rectal prolapse

Treatment of joint hypermobility syndrome
• Although hypermobility diminishes with age, the symptoms tend to continue and may worsen.
• It is important to remember that older patients may have been previously more mobile and that the Beighton score may not be an appropriate measure. A history of joint laxity should be sought.
• Hypermobility extends beyond the joints highlighted in the Beighton scale. The clinician should look at the fingers, shoulders, neck, hips, patello-femoral joint, ankles, feet, and skin laxity.
• Analgesics are often unhelpful for chronic pain, but have their place in acute symptoms. Pain and fatigue cause significant morbidity.

- Joint stabilizing exercises with particular reference to core stability, posture and proprioception are beneficial, as may be advice on avoiding overuse injuries and practical ways of managing day-to-day activities. A global approach to joint stability and function, as opposed to just treating regional symptoms, is effective.
- 'Pain management' should be considered in chronic pain cases. This might include for example, cognitive behavioral therapy and the processes similar to that used in fibromyalgia (📖 Chapter 18, p 489).
- The role of serotonergic/noradrenergic agents in these patients is unclear. In part there may be effective control of depression, however, there may also be direct analgesic properties to these agents.
- Neuroleptic agents for neuropathic pain have not been studied in this group of patients. However, gabapentin or pregabalin and other similar agents may have a role.
- Cardiovascular autonomic dysfunction requires specialist assessment and advice.
- Pregnancy is often a concern. Unlike the rarer forms of EDS, JHS is not associated with any major vascular hazard during pregnancy and labour. However, there are a number of considerations:
  - joint pain/dislocation may increase during pregnancy;
  - positioning during delivery should be careful to avoid excessive strain on joints;
  - labour may be rapid;
  - membranes may rupture prematurely;
  - there is an apparent resistance to the effects of local anaesthetics;
  - healing may be impaired and surgical technique may need to be modified accordingly;
  - there is no absolute indication for Caesarean section;
  - severe pelvic floor problems (uterine prolapse, etc.) may occur than otherwise anticipated.

Rare chondrodysplasias and storage disorders

There are >150 distinctive chondrodysplasias representing autosomal dominant, recessive, and X-linked patterns of inheritance. The first identified mutations were found in the collagen *2A1* gene, and are associated with premature osteoarthrosis. Such conditions include achondrogenesis, Kniest syndrome, spondyloepiphyseal dysplasia, and the Stickler syndrome. Clinical features in the latter three conditions include premature joint destruction, joint/bone deformity, short stature, and progressive myopia (with or without retinal detachment). Stickler syndrome patients are also prone to hernias, and cardiac valvular and conduction disorders.

Storage diseases associated with progessive skeletal dysplasia include:
- Mucopolysaccharidoses, e.g. Hurler, Hunter, Scheie.
- Mucolipidoses.
- Sphingolipidoses.
- Gaucher's disease.
- Fabry's disease.

The detail and complexities of these conditions is beyond the scope of this book.

Chapter 17

Infection and rheumatic disease

Introduction

Infectious agents have been linked directly and indirectly (through organism-specific and autoimmune responses) to a number of acute and chronic inflammatory rheumatic diseases. This chapter will introduce some examples of inflammatory mechanisms (Table 17.1) and infectious agents (Table 17.2) linked to rheumatic disease, and then discuss septic arthritis, osteomyelitis, Lyme disease, and rheumatic fever.

Table 17.1 Pathogenesis of rheumatic disease associated with infection

Inflammatory process	Basic process	Example	Susceptibility
Local infection at musculoskeletal sites	Infection. Tissue inflammation and direct damage	Pyogenic septic arthritis	Structural damage to joint replacement Diabetes, complement and immunoglobulin deficiencies
Pathogen and pathogen-specific immune response	Infection and organism-specific response. Immune response to intact organism or fragments, probable immune complex-mediated tissue injury	Syndromes associated with viral hepatitis, e.g. Sjögren's syndrome	Not generally established
Pathogens, immune response, and autoimmunity	i. Cross-reactive immune response ii. Infection inferred, but not established autoreactivity	Rheumatic fever Rheumatoid arthritis Juvenile idiopathic arthritis Systemic lupus erythematosus	Certain MHC class I and II genes Receptor genes MHC class I and II genes T-cell receptor genes

Table 17.2 Selected pathogens associated with arthritis

Class	Examples	Disorder
Bacteria	*Staphylococcus* and *Streptococcus*	Non-gonococcal arthritis
		Septic monoarthritis
		Osteomyelitis
	Neisseria spp.	Gonococcal arthritis
	Brucella	Septic monoarthritis
		Spondylarthropathy
	Chlamydia	Reactive/Reiter's
Mycobacteria	*M. tuberculosis*	Osteomyelitis
		Spinal disease
		Monoarthropathy
Atypical mycobacteria	*M. avium* complex *M. malmoense*	Septic arthritis in immunosuppressed patients
Spirochaete	*Borrelia burgdorferi*	Lyme disease
Viruses	Parvovirus B19	Fifth disease
	Rubella	Polyarthropathy
	Hepatitis B	Polyarteritis nodosa
	Hepatitis C	Cryoglobulinaemia
		Sjögren's syndrome
	HIV	Polyarthralgia and myopathy
		Vasculitis
		Sicca syndrome
Protozoa	Toxoplasma	Polyarthritis
	Giardia	Oligoarthritis
		Small-vessel vasculitis
	Trypanosoa	Myopathy
Helminths	Toxocara	All cause myositis and arthritis
	Dracunculus	
	Schistosoma	
Fungi	Histoplasma	Cause monoarthropathy
	Cryptococcus	

Pyogenic non-gonococcal and gonococcal arthritides

- Septic arthritis caused by a pyogenic bacterium is a medical emergency. Incidence in the general population is 2–10 per 100 000, rising to 30–70 per 100 000 in those with autoimmune rheumatic disease or prosthetic joint replacements.
- Most cases are due to haematogenous seeding during transient bacteraemia, but septic arthritis can also be caused by direct penetration through the skin, or by local spread from a contiguous infected site.
- Joints damaged by chronic arthritis [e.g. rheumatoid arthritis (RA), osteoarthritis (OA)] and prosthetic joints are at increased risk of infection. Immunodeficiency states and diabetes are added risk factors.
- Transient synovitis, particularly of the hip, is not uncommon in children, and generally occurs in the setting after upper respiratory tract infection. The presence of three of the following favours the diagnosis of septic arthritis: an elevated serum white blood cell count, inability to bear weight, recent history of fever, and erythrocyte sedimentation rate (ESR).
- The most common pathogens are *Staphylococcus aureus, Streptococcus* spp., and *Neisseria gonorrhoeae* in adults. The clinical features and natural history of gonococcal and non-gonococcal arthritis are sufficiently distinct to discuss them separately (Table 17.3).
- Unusual organisms may be involved in patients with a current history of iv drug abuse, or those who are immunosuppressed.
- Salmonella is a common cause of septic arthritis among patients with sickle cell disease.

Management of pyogenic joint infection

Three principles determine outcome—prompt diagnosis, immediate institution of appropriate antibiotics, and adequate drainage of joint.

- Specific tests for infection should include joint aspiration, Gram stain, and culture of synovial fluid; blood cultures, and (if relevant) skin/rash swabs, and oral and urethral swabs.
- Surgical drainage and washout or daily arthrocentesis may be required for non-gonococcal septic arthritis.
- Plain X-rays in early disease are unhelpful, since they show only soft tissue swelling. In later untreated disease, joint space narrowing and erosion will be seen. Ultrasound may show a joint effusion.
- An affected joint should be rested and non-weight-bearing until the inflammation and pain have subsided enough to allow passive mobilization. Mobilization should be encouraged as soon as possible.
- Empiric therapy with a third-generation cephalosporin should be started while awaiting culture data. Consider vancomycin in areas where community acquired MRSA is prevalent. *Pseudomonas* spp. should be suspected in intravenous drug users.
- In general, iv antibiotics are continued for 7 days until the swelling subsides and blood cultures become negative. Thereafter, uncomplicated cases will complete a 4-week course with oral

antibiotics. Prolonged courses of up to 6 weeks may be required in severe cases until swelling subsides, inflammatory markers normalize, and cultures become negative.

- There are no studies comparing long and short courses of antibiotics.
- Septic arthritis involving a prosthetic joint should be treated in a stepwise fashion. First, the prosthetic should be removed and replaced with an antibiotic-impregnated spacer; the patient should receive intravenous antibiotics for 6 weeks. Two to four weeks after antibiotics are finished, the joint should be aspirated; if there continues to be evidence of infection, intravenous antibiotics should be administered for another 6 weeks. When the aspirate shows no evidence of infection, the joint can be replaced, using antibiotic-impregnated cement.
- Under no circumstances should a joint be injected with corticosteroid if intra-articular infection is suspected, or if there is superficial infection over the skin covering a joint, e.g. cellulitis/psoriasis. Likewise, there is no benefit from intra-articular antibiotics; indeed, these drugs may cause a chemical synovitis.

Management of septic bursitis

- The two most common sites of bursal infection are the olecranon and prepatellar bursae. These are usually managed with serial aspiration and oral antibiotics. Those who do not respond will need iv antibiotics, and surgical incision and drainage.
- Osteomyelitis is a potential complication of chronic infected bursitis.

Table 17.3 Clinical features of gonococcal and non-gonococcal arthritis

Gonococcal arthritis	Non-gonococcal arthritis
Causative agents:	Causative agents:
Neisseria gonorrhoeae	*Staphylococcus aureus* (50% of cases)
Neisseria meningitidis	*Staphylococcus epidermis* (15% of cases)
	Streptococcus pyogenes/pneumonia (20% of cases)
	Gram-negative bacteria (10% of cases)
	Anaerobes (5% of cases)
Most often in young, healthy adults	Most often in the elderly, or underlying joint or medical condition
Women > men	Men > women
Hip disease uncommon	Hip disease common (20% of cases)
Migratory polyarthritis common	Polyarthritis uncommon
	Monoarthritis very common
Rash, skin blisters/pustules, tenosynovitis common	Extra-articular manifestations common
Synovial fluid analysis:	Synovial fluid analysis:
Gram's stain is positive in 25% culture positive, 50% lactate normal	Gram's stain is positive in 60% culture positive, 90% lactate raised
Rapid response to therapy	Often slow response, may require surgery
Full recovery in most cases	10% mortality; one-third residual damage

Mycobacterium tuberculosis

- Until 1985 the USA and Europe saw a decline in the number of tuberculosis (TB) cases. More recently, the recurrence of TB has become an important complication of new biologic disease modifying anti-rheumatic therapies.
- It is estimated that one-third of the world's population is infected with TB. In industrialized countries <5% of cases of TB develop infection of bone or joints.
- Tuberculosis of bone is usually a low grade and slow progressive infection associated with a variable degree of local and systemic symptoms, such as fatigue, weight loss, or night sweats. The onset is insidious and usually mono-articular or mono-osseous. Predisposing factors include pre-existing arthritis, alcoholism, prolonged use of corticosteroids, and immunosuppression.
- TB can affect any part of the musculoskeletal system. The spine is a common site, whether within a vertebral body, disc, or a paravertebral abscess. Spinal cord compression due to vertebral destruction and/or soft tissue swelling due to an abscess is a serious complication and must be treated urgently, with review by a neurosurgeon. Spinal stabilization procedures carry a good prognosis in preventing neurological sequelae. Monoarticular disease is seen most often in the weight-bearing joints of the hip, knee, ankle, or sacroiliac joint, in that order. The wrist and shoulder are less commonly affected. Osteomyelitis may affect any long bone, and is associated with either solitary or multifocal cysts.
- The diagnosis of TB is made by identifying acid-fast bacilli from a lesion or by histopathological changes in excised tissue. Occasionally, a high level of clinical suspicion, in the absence of other identified pathology, will lead the physician to treat empirically. Standard anti-TB regimes should be used for prophylaxis or treatment, and surveillance for 1 year after the end of treatment is recommended. Surgical intervention may be necessary; this may take the form, for example, of tissue-biopsy, debridement of necrotic tissue, or stabilization of a joint or long bone.
- Because of the association between TNF-α inhibitors and disseminated tuberculosis, the identification of latent TB has become increasingly important. This is accomplished using a tuberculin skin test (PPD). Induration of greater than 5 mm should be considered positive in patients who are immunosuppressed. QuantiFERON-TB GOLD, a blood-based interferon-gamma release assay, was recently FDA-approved, and is also useful for the diagnosis of latent TB. It has also recently been licensed in the UK.

Atypical mycobacterial infection

- Patients with autoimmune rheumatic diseases on immunosuppressant medication are at risk of developing atypical infections.
- These infections are usually chronic in nature and can mimic an inflammatory flare of rheumatic disease, which can make diagnosis difficult. *M. malmoense* has been described causing tensoynovitis and septic arthritis of the knee. *M. avium* complex and *M. chelonae* osteo-articular infections have also been described.
- Atypical infections should be considered in patients with autoimmune rheumatic disease who present with musculoskeletal symptoms that do not respond to conservative treatment.

Osteomyelitis

- This term is used to describe any infection involving bone or marrow.
- A number of general, local, and systemic factors need to be taken into account when managing osteomyelitis (Table 17.4).
- *Staphylococcus aureus* is the most common cause of osteomyelitis. Other important pathogens to consider, particularly in the immunosuppressed patient are tuberculosis, pseudomonas, and salmonella.

Investigations

- No single laboratory investigation is reliable enough to be used routinely for the diagnosis of osteomyelitis. An elevated white cell count and ESR may not be seen despite infection. Imaging plays an important part in establishing the diagnosis. Whether a particular imaging technique is successful at picking up osteomyelitis depends partly on the stage of the infective process.
- Once the pathogen has reached bone, a suppurative reaction and marrow oedema occurs. This can be seen using magnetic resonance (MR) imaging. The next stage, vascular congestion, ischaemia, thrombosis, and soft tissue swelling, is readily detected by computes tomography (CT). After 2–3 weeks, bone reactions including new periosteal bone formation and decalcification can be seen on plain films.
- Plain films should always be taken if the clinical setting is appropriate, even in assumed early disease, as they may be highly informative.
- Vertebral osteomyelitis is often seen early on plain films. There may be erosion of the vertebral body or disc, and paravertebral abscesses and vertebral collapse are common complications.
- Isotope bone scanning may be helpful in localizing an area of abnormality. $^{99}Tc^m$-labelled scans, however, are not specific and the negative predictive value is often greater than the positive predictive value in this scenario. ^{67}Ga- or ^{111}I-labelled leukocyte scans are often helpful in localizing infection.

Treatment

- Initial treatment in the acute phase is the same as that for septic monoarthritis (see 📖 Mycobacterium tuberculosis, p 480). In general, antibiotics are needed for 6 weeks, although chronic infection may require long-term (in excess of 3 months) low-dose treatment. In addition to the common iv antibiotics discussed above, a beta-lactimase-resistant penicillin (such as flucloxacillin) should be considered. Clindamycin and fluoroquinlolones are also used to treat osteomyelitits. Clindamycin should be used cautiously in the elderly because of the association with development of *Clostridium difficile* colitis.
- Surgery is required early in the acute phase especially if there is an abscess or spinal involvement. Chronic osteomyelitis implies that dead bone is present and this will require surgical debridement.
- Hyperbaric oxygen has also been used successfully in the treatment of air embolism, osteonecrosis, myonecrosis, and burn patients with infection.

Table 17.4 Factors relevant to the management of osteomyelitis

Factors	Examples
General	*Age:* neonates tend to harbour *S. aureus*, enterobacteriaceae, and β-haemolytic streptococci. In children > 4 years, *H. influenzae* is common, and in adults *S. aureus*
	Bone: long bones (especially lower limb) are more susceptible than short bones. Pelvic and cranial bones are infrequently involved
Local	Chronic lymphoedema
	Venous stasis
	Arterial disease with poor flow
	Scars
	Sensory neuropathy
	Prosthetic material
Systemic	Malnutrition
	Renal and liver failure
	Immunodeficiency
	Diabetes
	Malignancy
	Extremes of age
	Chronic hypoxia
	Parenteral drug use

Lyme disease

- Lyme disease is a tick-borne infection caused by the spirochaete *Borrelia burgdorferi*.
- Cases of Lyme disease have been reported from most states in the USA, as well as throughout Europe, the former USSR, China, and Japan.
- The highest incidence is in children under the age of 15 years and middle-aged adults, with seasonal variation, being most common in the summer months of June and July.
- The tick vector, *Ixodes*, is found on rodents mainly and in wooded, brush, or grassy areas. A history of potential exposure in an endemic country within the last 30 days is an important fact to establish in considering the diagnosis. A clear history of a tick bite is not necessary to make the diagnosis.
- The diagnosis is approached clinically, partly based on epidemiological history as well as classical clinical features (Table 17.5), and confirmed with laboratory tests.

Laboratory investigations

- Confirmation of Lyme disease may be by:
  - isolation of the spirochaete from tissue or body fluid;
  - detection of diagnostic levels of IgM or IgG antibodies in the serum or cerebrospinal fluid (CSF);
  - detection of changes in antibody levels between acute phase and convalescent paired sera.
- False-positive results occur in other infections, such as syphillis and treponema, as well as in RA and systemic lupus erythematosus (SLE). Western blotting is available as a confirming test, distinguishing between true seroreactivity and false positivity.
- If the serological status is negative then the diagnosis is unlikely and an alternative should be sought.

Treatment

Treatment of Lyme disease is summarized in Table 17.6.

Table 17.5 The clinical features of Lyme disease

System affected	Symptoms
Skin	*Erythema migrans (EM)*: begins as a red macule/papule expanding over days or weeks to a large round lesion often with partial central clearing. The lesion should measure 5 cm or more. There may be smaller secondary lesions[*]
	An expanding lesion is often accompanied by general symptoms: fever, fatigue, arthralgia, myalgia, headache
	Months later a chronic lesion, acrodermatitis chronicum atrophicans (AChA), can appear (violaceous infiltrared plaques or nodules)
Musculoskeletal system	Recurrent, brief attacks of joint swelling in one or a few joints (may become chronic—60% of untreated cases weeks to years after infection).
	A post-Lyme syndrome of fatigue, arthralgia and myalgia has been reported. Ongoing infection has been difficult to prove and this may represent a fibromyalgia/chronic pain syndrome.
Nervous system	Lymphocytic meningitis
	Cranial neuritis (especially facial nerve palsy)
	Radiculoneuropathy (differential Guillain–Barré)
	Encephalomyelitis
Cardiovascular	Acute second- or third-degree atrioventricular conduction defects often associated with myocarditis. Resolve in days to weeks
	Carditis—rare and remits spontaneously

[*] A similar lesion occurring within hours of a tick bite is usually a hypersensitivity reaction and does not qualify as EM.

Table 17.6 The treatment of Lyme disease

Clinical feature	Treatment
Skin disease	Doxycycline 100 mg twice daily for 3 weeks *or* cefuroxime 500 mg twice daily for 3 weeks
Septic arthritis	As above except may require treatment for up to 30 days
Neurological disease	Meningitis—iv penicillin, cefotaxime, ceftriaxone/imipenem
Carditis	As oral/iv doses above

Rheumatic fever

- Rheumatic fever is a delayed, non-suppurative sequel to a pharyngeal infection with Lancefield group A β-haemolytic streptococci.
- There is a latent period of 2–3 weeks before the appearance of the illness. A symptomatic pharyngitis is seen in 60% cases, migratory arthritis (typically of the large joints), myocarditis and valvulitis, and central nervous system disease (chorea).
- While the infection is often self-limiting, chronic, and progressive damage to cardiac valves occurs leading to cardiac decompensation and death.
- Although there has been a dramatic decline in the United States and Europe, the disease still occurs in these areas, and is common in developing countries. There are an estimated 10–20 million cases per year in these areas, with an annual incidence of 100–200 per 100 000.
- Associations have been described with HLA DR2, 3, and 4.

The clinical features are summarized in the revised 'Jones' criteria (Table 17.7).

Clinical manifestations and treatment of rheumatic fever

Arthritis

- Joint involvement is more common and often more severe in teenagers and young adults. It tends to start in the large joints of the lower limbs and migrate. Arthropathy tends to occur early and the pain can be severe in the absence of objective signs of inflammation. It lasts 2–3 weeks and is self-limiting.
- NSAIDs are the main treatment for the condition.
- Where one draws the line between the phenomenon of post-streptococcal reactive arthritis (seen in the absence of carditis) and rheumatic fever is difficult. Most patients will fulfill the Jones criteria and, therefore, should be considered as having rheumatic fever.

Cardiac disease

- Rheumatic heart disease is the most severe outcome of acute rheumatic fever. It remains the major cause of acquired valvular heart disease in the world. The mitral valve (stenosis) is involved more frequently than the aortic valve. When left unchecked, cardiomegaly, and cardiac failure secondary to valvular disease develops.
- Carditis may also occur and is associated with cardiomyopathy and conduction defects including second- or third-degree heart block.

Table 17.7 The revised Jones criteria for the diagnosis of acute rheumatic fever (diagnosis requires 2 major, or 1 major and 2 minor criteria)

Major manifestations	Carditis
	Polyarthritis
	Chorea
	Erythema marginatum
	Subcutaneous nodules
Minor manifestations	Fever
	Arthralgia
	Previous rheumatic fever or rheumatic heart disease
Laboratory tests	Raised ESR or CRP
	Normochromic normocytic anaemia
	Prolonged PR interval on ECG
Supporting evidence	Raised ASO titre*
	Positive throat cultures for group A streptococci
	Recent scarlet fever

*ASO = antistreptolysin O antibodies (titres peak at about 4 weeks, which is about 2 weeks into the clinical onset of rheumatic fever; they fall off rapidly over the following 2–3 months).

Chorea
- Sydenham's chorea (St Vitus dance) is a neurological disorder consisting of abrupt, purposeless movements, muscle weakness, and emotional disturbance. The hands and face are usually the most obviously affected parts. The movements are not present during sleep, but do occur at rest and may be more marked on one side of the body.
- Chorea may be the sole feature suggesting rheumatic fever (beyond observing new cardiac murmurs) and may occur weeks to months after onset of an arthropathy.

Skin
- The subcutaneous nodules of rheumatic fever are firm and painless. They are located over bony surfaces or near tendons, and are present for 2–4 weeks only, and more often in patients with carditis.
- Erythema marginatum is an evanescent, non-purpuric rash, usually affecting the trunk and proximal part of the limbs, but sparing the face. Because the rash often appears to make a ring, it is also called 'erythema annulare'. The lesions come and go in a matter of hours, and heat may make them appear or become worse. Again, it is more common in association with carditis. They resolve spontaneously.
- Erythema nodosum is rare.

Investigations
- There is no diagnostic investigation.
- Raised inflammatory markers and mild anaemia are often seen.
- Serial rises in anti-streptolysin O titres may be seen if measured every 14 days.
- Chest radiograph and electrocardiogram (ECG) to look for conduction defects/cardiomegaly.

Treatment of rheumatic fever
- The mainstay of treatment is an anti-inflammatory agent.
- If carditis is present, steroids should be started (2 mg/kg/day oral prednisone for 1–2 weeks followed by steroid taper over 2 weeks).
- Penicillin should be taken for 10 days, even in the absence of ongoing pharyngitis.
- Chorea can be treated with haloperidol 1–2 mg/kg/day, often given with prednisone, although there is little evidence that this gives added benefit.
- Recurrence is most common within the first 2 years; however, recurrence rates seem to be low, and the risk of recurrence declines with age at first attack.
- Prophylaxis in those who have had rheumatic fever should probably continue for life, although some clinicians would recommend up to 10 years, and antibiotic therapy to cover any dental or invasive procedure. Prophylaxis can be given either as oral phenoxymethylpenicillin or as benzylpenicillin, 1.2 million units im once every 3–4 weeks. Erythromycin at 250 mg daily may be used if there is an allergy to penicillins. The future may bring new streptococcal vaccines.

Miscellaneous conditions

Behçet's disease

- Behçet's disease is a systemic inflammatory disorder of unknown aetiology. It is most common in the Mediterranean basin, the Middle East, and Asia.
- The usual onset of the disorder is in the third or fourth decade.
- Onset is rare in children and after the age of 45 years.
- The male: female ratio is approximately equal, but the syndrome tends to run a more severe course in men and the young.
- Based on registries, the prevalence is about 1 in 300 000 in Northern Europe, 1 in 10 000 in Japan, and 40 in 10 000 in Turkey.
- The disorder is classically associated with HLA B5—its presence associated with greater disease severity. However, there are geographical variations. Patients from Mediterranean countries and Japan show this association with B5, but patients in the United States do not. In patients of Israeli origin there is an association with HLA B51.
- The full-blown disease might be easy to identify, but there are conditions that mimic the incomplete picture, including reactive arthritis and inflammatory bowel disease.
- There are no laboratory findings specific to the condition. The erythrocyte sedimentation rate (ESR) and C-reactive protein (CRP) are often only moderately raised.

Clinical features and their management

Skin and mucosa involvement (Table 18.1)

- Oral aphthous ulcers are always present, and may precede other features by several years. Idiopathic oral aphthous ulcers are common, and by themselves do not imply the presence of Behçet's. The ulcers associated with Behçet's are indistinguishable from ordinary ulcers, but tend to be multiple, more frequent, and may heal with scarring.
- Genital ulceration in men is most prominent over the scrotum (90%). Urethritis is not seen unless there is a meatal ulcer. In women, the labia are commonly affected. Cervical ulcers are rare.
- Skin lesions may be nodular (resembling erythema nodosum), acneiform, or vasculitic.
- The pathergy reaction, a hyper-reactivity of the skin to a needle prick, is peculiar to this syndrome and pyoderma gangrenosum. After skin puncture with a needle, a papule or pustule forms in 24–48 h. The reaction is seldom found in patients from Northern Europe or the United States, but is positive in 60 and 70% of patients from Japan and Turkey, respectively.
- Mild oral and genital ulceration may respond to topical colchicine 1.5 mg/day. More severe disease may require azathioprine (AZA) 2.5 mg/kg/day. Non-steroidal anti-inflammatory drugs (NSAIDs) can help pain control.

Eye disease

- This is a serious complication and a negative prognostic factor. Eye disease is more common in men and patients <25 years of age.
- Disease is bilateral in 90% of cases and is usually a chronic relapsing panuveitis. The presence of a hypopyon (cells in the anterior chamber)

is almost always associated with severe retinal vasculitis, after which there is almost always some structural damage despite treatment. The extent of this damage determines the course of eye disease in Behçet's disease.

- Topical steroids and mydriatics with close supervision may be sufficient in mild disease, but severe disease requires the addition of AZA 2.5 mg/kg/day, ciclosporin 5 mg/kg/day, or anti-TNF-α therapy.

Musculoskeletal involvement

- Joint involvement is seen in about 50% of patients. It is usually mono- or oligoarticular, but can be symmetric, mimicking RA.
- Chronic synovitis is rare, non-erosive, and non-deforming.
- In general, knees, ankles, wrists, and elbows are involved (in descending order of frequency).
- Back pain is rare.
- Pain may respond to NSAIDs. Inflammatory disease often requires the introduction of AZA 2.5 mg/kg/day or sulfasalazine 2–3 g/day

Table 18.1 The clinical findings in Behçet's disease

Lesion	Prevalence (%)
Aphthous ulcers	97–100
Genital ulcers	80–90
Skin lesions	80
Eye lesions	50
Arthritis	40–50
Thrombophlebitis	25
Neurological disease	1–15
Gastrointestinal disease	0–25

Cardiovascular and pulmonary involvement

- Endocarditis, myocarditis, pericarditis, coronary vasculitis, and ventricular aneurysms can all occur, but are rare.
- Venous involvement is one of the main features of Behçet's disease. Thrombophlebitis occurs in 25% of all patients. Limb venous thrombosis is often observed. Occlusion of the suprahepatic veins—Budd–Chiari syndrome—carries a high mortality.
- Pulmonary embolism is rare despite high rates of thrombophlebitis. It might be explained by the difference in architecture of thromboses seen in Behçet's disease and normal (e.g. post-operative) thromboses. The former tends to adhere throughout its length to the vein wall; the latter tends to have a long, non-adherent and potentially embolic tail.
- Arterial lesions can occur anywhere. Aneurysms may develop and rupture. This is frequently fatal.

- The pulmonary pathology of Behçet's disease is related to arterial vasculitis. Aneurysms, thromboses, and infarcts are found.
- Aspirin and NSAIDs can be used to relieve the symptoms of phlebitis. Aneurysms and arterial occlusion require cytotoxic therapy with cyclophosphamide 2.5 mg/kg/day and prednisolone 1 mg/kg/day; surgery may also be indicated. There remains debate as to whether to use heparin or oral anticoagulants for the thrombophlebitis; most physicians will choose to treat with anticoagulation in addition to immunosuppression.

Neurological involvement

- Prospective surveys suggest a prevalence rate of 5% for neurological disease in the condition.
- Pyramidal signs are the most common, followed by cerebellar and sensory symptoms and signs. The most common site is the brainstem. Meningeal irritation and dementia may also occur. As is the case with eye disease, central nervous involvement is often more severe in men.
- In contrast to other vasculitides, peripheral neuropathy is unusual.
- Central nervous system (CNS) disease should be treated with iv methylprednisolone, and cyclophosphamide should be considered.

Gastrointestinal involvement

- While seen in up to one-third of patients in Japan, gastrointestinal disease is rare in patients from the Mediterranean basin.
- The basic pathology is mucosal ulceration, seen most often in the ileum and caecum. The course is one of relapse and remission, with a distinct tendency to perforate.
- Ulceration may respond to prednisolone 0.5–1 mg/kg/day, sulfasalazine 2–6 g/day, or infliximab. Surgical evaluation may be necessary to manage severe sequelae.

Renal involvement

- This is seen much less than might be expected in a systemic vasculitis. There are occasional reports of glomerulonephritis. Amyloidosis usually presents with nephrotic syndrome.
- About 5% of men develop epididymitis. Treatment focuses on symptom control.

Treatment of Behçet's

- Colchicine 0.6 mg oral bd should be used to treat orogenital ulceration; dapsone, thalidomide, and anti-TNF-α therapy all have demonstrated efficacy.
- Azathioprine 2.5 mg/kg/day should be considered for the treatment of the systemic manifestations of Behçet's. Arteritis and other life-threatening manifestations should be treated with cyclophosphamide 2.5 mg/kg/day.
- Infliximab may be particularly effective for treating ocular manifestations of Behçet's that do not respond to topical therapy.
- Warfarin should be used in the usual way for thrombotic episodes. If thrombosis occurs in the setting of disease flare, immunosuppression may be required as well.

Sarcoidosis

- Sarcoidosis is a multisystem disease of unknown aetiology, characterized by the presence of multiple, non-caseating granulomas in involved tissue.
- It occurs worldwide, but the prevalence, clinical features, and outcome varies. It is seen more often in developed vs underdeveloped, Western vs Eastern, and in Northern vs Southern European countries. Sweden and Denmark have prevalence rates of 60 per 100 000: the United Kingdom 20 per 100 000. In the United States, sarcoidosis is 10–15 times more prevalent in the African American population than in Caucasians; African Americans may also present with a more severe form of this disease. There is also an increased incidence of sarcoidosis in families. Recently, studies have suggested a link between HLA B8, DR3, and acute sarcoidosis with arthritis.
- Acute sarcoidosis presents with rapid onset fever, erythema nodosum, and hilar lymphadenopathy. This condition has a high rate of remission and a good prognosis; the chest radiograph clears within 1 year in 60% of cases.
- Chronic sarcoidosis is less common and has a subtle, insidious, progressive, and highly variable clinical course (Table 18.2).
- Sarcoidosis is rare in childhood, and usually indolent. If arthritis occurs, it is usually before 5 years of age, and associated with eye and cutaneous disease.

Musculoskeletal manifestations of sarcoid

Joints

- Distinctive patterns of arthropathy are seen in both acute and chronic sarcoidosis. In acute disease, transient arthralgias may precede the emergence of other symptoms. Sarcoid arthritis is usually symmetric and persists for 1–4 months on average, and occurs in association with erythema nodosum (EN). Effusions are common at the knees and ankles. After recovery, acute sarcoidosis only occasionally recurs.
- Chronic arthritis is uncommon in sarcoidosis; when it does occur, it usually appears in the form of monoarthritis or involvement of the spine. Again, knees and ankles appear to be most often involved with inflammatory disease, characterized by acute exacerbation with synovial thickening and effusions. Unlike acute sarcoidosis, a history of EN is unusual. Chronic polyarthritis is also more frequent in women than men. It may cause joint deformity and destruction.

Bones

- Bone involvement occurs in 5% of all patients with sarcoidosis. Bone cysts are seen most often in the hands and feet and are most frequently seen in patients with persistent disease and/or lupus pernio (i.e. erythematous induration of the skin across the face). Cysts are often asymptomatic and found by chance on plain radiographs. Clinically, they can present in the phalanges with 'sausage-like' swollen digits.
- Other radiological features include thickening of cortical bone, acrosclerosis, and joint destruction.

Table 18.2 Clinical manifestations in chronic sarcoidosis

Organ/system	Clinical features
Lung	Parenchymal disease in >90% of cases
Skin	Lupus pernio, plaques, and nodules
Ocular	Uveitis, conjunctivitis, sicca
Lymphatics	Lymphadenopathy, splenomegaly
Bone marrow	Infiltration
Hepatic	Failure, granuloma, portal hypertension
Renal	Nephrocalcinosis, granuloma, glomerular disease
Cardiac	Arteritis, cardiomyopathy, conduction abnormalities
Nervous system	Central and peripheral neuropathy. Intracerebral lesions. Meningitis. Seizures
Granulomata	Endocrine and reproductive organs. Gastrointestinal tract. Salivary/lacrimal glands. Nose, tonsils, and larynx

- Occasionally, lytic lesions appear in vertebral bodies, leading to back pain and crush fractures. Lytic lesions may also be seen in the skull bones and long bones.

Muscles
- Often asymptomatic, in the early stages of acute sarcoidosis granulomatous muscle involvement is common (50–80%). It may present as proximal pain, tenderness, and weakness. Involvement may be focal with a granulomatous mass or diffuse and symmetrical myopathy, the latter leading to progressive weakness and atrophy.
- Electromyography looks similar to that of polymyositis.

Investigations and treatment of sarcoidosis

- A patient with a new diagnosis of sarcoidosis should receive an electrocardiogram, pulmonary function tests, computed tomography of the chest, and slit-lamp examination, in addition to a thorough physical examination and symptom-driven evaluation.
- The red cell count is usually normal. Leucopenia can be seen in up to one-third of cases, and eosinophilia in one-quarter. Thrombocytopenia is a relatively common problem.
- The ESR may be elevated in the acute phase, particularly if erythema nodosum (EN) is present; see later in chapter for EN/panniculitis.
- Reports of hypercalcaemia vary widely from 2–60%. The level tends to fluctuate and the reasons for such wide variation remain unclear.
- Liver function tests may be deranged.
- One-third of patients have significant proteinuria.

- Epithelial cells found in the granuloma produce angiotensin-converting enzyme (ACE). Serial measurements of this enzyme may be useful in monitoring the course of the disease.
- As sarcoidosis can resemble other diseases such as lymphoma and tuberculosis, the diagnosis should be confirmed by histology. Peripheral tissues such as skin or salivary glands may be helpful. Transbronchial lung biopsy is widely used and highly sensitive and specific.
- Acute, transient disease may resolve spontaneously, and require only supportive care. More severe disease may require treatment with corticosteroids, either alone or in combination with methotrexate.
- Addition of hydroxychloroquine may also help the skin and joint manifestations of sarcoidosis.
- Infliximab may be useful to treat refractory forms of this disease, including lupus pernio.
- Most patients with chronic disease will require steroid therapy, the decision to treat more often related to systemic involvement than articular disease.
- No therapy is required for asymptomatic osseous or cystic bone disease, or asymptomatic muscle disease. The place for steroids in chronic sarcoid myopathy remains uncertain.

Miscellaneous skin conditions associated with arthritis

Panniculitis

Panniculitis refers to inflammation within the subcutaneous fat. It is a dynamic inflammatory process involving neutrophils, leucocytes, and histiocytes that causes fibrosis, and sometimes granulomatous change.

There are four categories of panniculitis, based on histopathology:
• Septal panniculitis.
• Lobular panniculitis.
• Mixed type septal and lobular.
• Panniculitis with vasculitis.

Septal panniculitis

This includes EN and Vilanova's disease (subacute nodular migratory panniculitis). EN is a common, acute, and self-limiting condition found typically over the anterior tibial surface. It usually heals within 4–6 weeks without scarring, although a rare form can cause ulceration and a migratory form can occur for several years (more often in women around 45 years old). The causes and associations of EN are shown in Table 18.3.

Lobular panniculitis

Listed below are a number of conditions that cause lobular panniculitis:
• *Weber–Christian disease:* a relapsing, febrile, nodular non-suppurative disorder. There may be multiple recurrent nodules plus fever; arthralgia, myalgia, and abdominal pain are common. Any area of the body containing fat can become involved, e.g. mesentery, heart, lung, liver, kidney. There is a 10–15% mortality. Investigations may show:
  • typical histological features on biopsy;
  • elevated ESR;
  • anaemia;
  • leucopenia or leucocytosis.
• *Lipogranulomatosis:* this group of conditions tends to occur in children. Multiple lesions, often on the extremities, resolve with subcutaneous atrophy.
• *Post steroid use:* the pathogenesis of this rare condition is not understood. It seems to be limited to children, occurs on withdrawal of corticosteroids, and may clear up on steroid re-administration.
• *α1-antitrypsin deficiency:* may respond to doxycycline.
• *Acute pancreatitis.*
• *Calcifying panniculitis:* a feature of chronic renal failure. It is not the same as metastatic calcification. The prognosis is poor even with good calcium-phosphate balance. Parathyroidectomy may help.
• *Lipodermatosclerosis:* this condition may be a result of venous insufficiency and thrombophlebitis. It should be treated with compression stockings. Intralesional corticosteroids or low-dose aspirin may also help.

Table 18.3 Aetiological causes of EN

Cause	Examples
Infection	Streptococcal
	TB/leprosy
	Yersinia / Salmonella
	Histoplasmosis
	Blastomycoss
	Psitticosis
Drugs	Penicillin
	Sulfonamides
Pregnancy	
Diseases	Sarcoidosis
	Inflammatory bowel disease
	Collagen vascular disease (SLE, scleroderma, dermatomyositis)
	Malignancy (rare)
	Sweet's syndrome

- *Lupus profundus* is a rare manifestation of chronic cutaneous SLE, occurring in <3% of cases of SLE. The lesions are usually tender and may ulcerate and calcify. The lesions commonly occur on the face, upper arms, and buttocks, and may underly an area of discoid lupus. The lesions do not seem to follow the course of the systemic disease. It may respond to steroids.
- *Factitious.*

Panniculitis with vasculitis

This is seen in small-vessel and medium-vessel vasculitis. The reader is referred to 📖 Chapter 15, p 405.

Treatments include:
- Treatment of the underlying disease or agent.
- NSAIDs.
- Bed rest and limb elevation.
- HCQ
- Steroids.
- Dapsone.
- Colchicine.
- AZA
- Ciclosporin.

Neutrophilic dermatoses

The neutrophilic dermatoses are a group of non-infectious disorders characterized by the presence of an angiocentric, primary neutrophilic inflammatory cell infiltrate. The disorders can be divided into those that cause vessel wall destruction (vasculitis) and those that do not. Table 18.4 lists the causes of non-infectious neutrophilic dermatoses. The majority of diseases are discussed in detail in their own chapters in this book. This section will discuss Sweet's syndrome, and pyoderma gangrenosum.

Sweet's syndrome
- This condition is rare and occurs more often in women than men (ratio 3.7:1), between the ages of 30 and 70 years. It has occasionally been reported in children. The pathogenesis is unknown.
- The characteristic features are myalgia, fever, arthralgia, and painful erythematous plaques (occasionally nodules resembling EN). Untreated, the lesions resolve over 6–8 weeks, but new lesions will continue to appear. The condition is usually an acute, steroid-responsive, self-limiting disorder. If longer-term treatment is required, steroid dosage may be reduced by the addition of an NSAID, dapsone, colchicine, or possibly MTX.
- A secondary cause for the condition should be sought (Table 18.5).

Pyoderma gangrenosum
- This is an uncommon, ulcerative, cutaneous condition associated with several systemic diseases (Table 18.6).
- The lesion is characterized by an erythematous, violaceous border overhanging a central area of ulceration and necrosis. The lesions start as discrete pustules, most often on the legs, and are often extremely painful, healing with scars.
- There is no specific treatment. An underlying disease should be sought. Treatments include topical sodium cromoglycate or 5-amino salicylic acid, oral sulfonamides, dapsone, and corticosteroids.

Table 18.4 Non-infectious neutrophilic dermatoses

Group	Examples
Non-angiocentric	Psoriasis
	Reactive arthritis
	Acne fulminans
Angiocentric and vessel destruction	Leucocytoclastic vasculitis
	Polyarteritis nodosa
Angiocentric, no vessel destruction	Sweet's syndrome
	Pyoderma gangrenosum
	Bowel-associated dermatosis–arthritis
	Behçet's disease
	Rheumatoid arthritis
	Ulcerative colitis
	Familial Mediterranean fever

Table 18.5 The associations with Sweet's syndrome

Associations	Examples
Haematological malignancy	Leukaemia
	Lymphoma
	Myelodysplastic disorders
Solid tumours	Breast
	Gastric
	Genitourinary
	Colon
Infectious diseases	HIV
	Hepatitis
	Tuberculosis
	Salmonella
Inflammatory bowel disease	Ulcerative colitis
	Crohn's disease
Rheumatic diseases	Rheumatoid arthritis
	Systemic lupus erythematosus
	Sjögren's syndrome
	Behçet's disease

Multicentric reticulohistiocytosis

- This is a rare systemic disease, primarily a disorder of adults in their fifth decade. It is recognized clinically by the combination of papular and nodular skin lesions and a severe destructive polyarthritis.
- The disorder is distinct from the solitary nodule lesion of the reticulocytoma in that the latter is not associated with systemic disease. Multicentric reticulohistiocytosis may involve any organ system.
- The arthritis may mimic a RA pattern. Often the distal interphalangeal joints (DIPJ) are involved and the destruction may give a picture similar to arthritis mutilans.
- The skin lesions occur in approximately 90% of cases. Histologically, the infiltrate consists of multicentric giant cells and histiocytes from the monocyte-macrophage lineage. The lesions are usually numerous, non-pruritic, skin coloured (or yellow/brown), and range in size from a few millimeters to several centimeters in diameter. They occur most often on the dorsum of the hands and on the face (at the nose, corner of the mouth, and ears). Extensive facial involvement may lead to a 'leonine' facies.
- About 25% of cases have xanthelasma.

Table 18.6 Diseases associated with pyoderma gangrenosum

Association	Examples
Rheumatic diseases	Seronegative spondyloarthropathy
	Rheumatoid arthritis
	Osteoarthritis
	Psoriatic arthritis
	Systemic lupus erythematosus
	Wegener's granulomatosis
	Sarcoidosis
	Takayasu's arteritis
Haematological diseases	Leukaemia
	Myelofibrosis
	Gammaglobulinaemia
	Polycythaemia rubra vera
Gastrointestinal diseases	Inflammatory bowel disease
	Chronic active hepatitis
	Primary biliary cirrhosis
Other	Solid tumours
	Diabetes mellitus
	C7 complement deficiency

- One-third of cases have constitutional symptoms/signs, such as weight loss or fever.
- Approximately 25% of cases have been reported to have malignant (mostly solid tumour) disease. The investigation of the condition therefore requires a thorough screen for rheumatic and malignant disease.
- There are no specific laboratory markers. Histology is helpful. Biopsies may be taken from skin or inflamed synovium.
- The differential diagnosis includes:
  - rheumatoid or psoriatic arthritis;
  - sarcoid dactylitis;
  - xanthoma;
  - histiocytosis X—a disorder of children;
  - histiocytoma or tendon sheath giant-cell tumour—usually solitary.
- As a rule the condition 'waxes and wanes', and spontaneous remissions can occur.

- Multicentric reticulohistiocytosis has been associated with numerous forms of malignancy, and a new diagnosis should prompt a thorough investigation.
- Patients with multicentric reticulohistiocytosis may quickly develop a disabling arthritis, and should be treated aggressively. For patients with mild disease, MTX may be sufficient, but many patients may require treatment with cyclophosphamide or chlorambucil to prevent progressive damage.

Complex regional pain syndrome

This syndrome is characterized by variable dysfunction of the musculoskeletal, skin, neurological, and vascular systems. It may occur in a variety of situations with a number of clinical manifestations varying around central core features. As such several terms have evolved, describing the same phenomenon:

- Reflex sympathetic dystrophy.
- Sudeck's atrophy.
- Shoulder–hand syndrome.
- Transient osteoporosis.
- Regional migratory osteoporosis.
- Post-trauma painful osteoporosis.

Complex regional pain syndrome (CRPS) has 2 types; type 1 is symptoms in the absence of nerve injury, and type 2 ('causalgia') in the presence of nerve injury.

Epidemiology

- CRPS is a common disorder. It affects both sexes equally, and occurs at any age in all races and geographical regions. Typically, the syndrome involves the distal part of a limb, e.g. forearm or foot.
- The early clinical features of the condition include:
  - Pain;
  - soft tissue swelling (may be synovitis if over a joint);
  - reticular/livedo rash;
  - warmth over affected part occasionally there may be localized;
  - sweating and piloerection.
- The pain has several particular characteristics and is often described as 'burning'. The features include:
  - *allodynia*—an otherwise innocuous stimulus produces pain;
  - *hyperalgesia*—increased pain perception to a given stimulus;
  - *hyperpathia*—delayed over-reaction, often after repetitive cutaneous stimulus.
- Trauma (whether accident, burn, surgery, etc.) is the most common triggering event. The event may have even seemed trivial or minor at the time.
- Several neurological conditions may act as triggers, including, for example, hemiplegia and meningitis. Peripheral nerve root injury may also lead to the syndrome.
- Pregnancy, tumours, and prolonged immobilization have also been linked as possible triggering factors. However, 25% of cases have no clear trigger.
- It is important to try and identify psychosocial stresses.

Staging

- The signs and symptoms of pain, swelling, etc. (see above), are traditionally placed as 'stage I' of the condition. In most cases, the symptoms persist and fluctuate, though they may just gradually resolve. Stage II is a period of dystrophic change (Plate 9). This tends to occur several months after onset of the disorder. The affected region becomes cool, pale, and often cyanosed in colour with abnormal sensation (dysesthesia). There is a decrease in hair and nail growth, osteopenia develops, and eventually atrophy (stage III) of skin and subcutaneous tissue occurs; at this point the condition becomes difficult to treat and reverse. Most cases tend not to progress beyond stage I, or at most early stage II.

Investigations

- Laboratory values, including acute phase reactants and metabolic profiles, are normal. However, there may be evidence of bone demineralization, with elevated 24-h urine hydroxyproline excretion.
- Although essentially a clinical diagnosis, CRPS does have some radiological and nuclear medicine imaging characteristics. No technique is diagnostic. Plain radiographs, dual energy X-ray absorptiometry (DEXA), and MR may show features of osteoporosis.
- Thermography can demonstrate changes in cutaneous temperature.
- Perhaps of most value, and high specificity, is the triple-phase isotope bone scan, showing three phases of abnormal early regional blood flow, blood pool, and late bone uptake respectively.

Management

- Success in treatment of this condition probably hinges on focusing on the whole individual and not the regional symptoms, and making an early and accurate diagnosis. Attention to anxiety, psychosocial stressors, pain behaviour, and sleep disturbance is important. The patient often requires repeated reassurance and counselling. The aim should be to resume premorbid levels of activity if possible. In this respect, early intervention with physical therapy and hydrotherapy should be considered.
- Tricyclic antidepressants can help correct sleep disturbance and increase the pain threshold; neuropathic analgesics, such as gabapentin or pregabalin, may also be of value.
- Transcutaneous electrical nerve stimulation (TENS) may help pain control and allow entry into a physical activity program.
- In severe cases, regional sympathetic or ganglion blocks can control pain sufficiently to start more vigorous physical therapy or exercise programmes.
- Some clinicians have also had success with corticosteroids and with pamidronate. There are no controlled trials of this or any other therapy mentioned above.

Relapsing polychondritis

- This is an uncommon multisystem disorder of unknown aetiology, characterized by episodic and sometimes progressive inflammation of cartilage leading to destruction and fibrosis.
- Common sites of involvement include the ear, nose, larynx, joints, heart, and eyes (cornea and sclera; Table 18.7).
- Similar patterns of disease may be seen in Wegener's granulomatosis; also, some patients with relapsing polychondritis are antineutrophil cytoplasmic antibody (ANCA) positive.
- The disease predominantly affects Caucasians in the fourth to fifth decades of life.
- Approximately 30% of cases have an underlying systemic rheumatic or autoimmune disease, such as RA, systemic lupus, Sjögren's syndrome, thyroiditis, or ulcerative colitis.
- There are no specific laboratory tests. The diagnosis is made on clinical grounds.

Treatment of relapsing polychondritis

- There are no controlled trials and the condition is rare. Intervention is based on anecdotal experience.
- Mild symptoms may be controlled with NSAIDs alone. Dapsone may also be of value. Corticosteroids (high doses, 1 mg/kg daily) may control systemic disease, particularly respiratory complications. Persistent or severe cases may be treated with AZA, MTX, cyclophosphamide, or infliximab.
- Patients should be assessed for tracheal involvement (e.g. stridor). Some cases may require temporary or permanent tracheostomy if laryngeal involvement is severe.

Table 18.7 Extent of organ involvement in relapsing polychondritis

Organ	Clinical feature	Prevalence (%)
External ear		95
Arthritis	Non-deforming and non-erosive	85
Nose		48
Eye	Episcleritis, uveitis, retinal vasculitis	57
Respiratory tract	Dysphonia, dyspnoea, stridor	67
Inner ear		53
Skin	Erythema nodosum vasculitis, Behçet-like ulceration	38
Kidney	Glomerulonephritis (poor prognosis)	8
Heart	Pericarditis, aortic valve incompetence, heart block	8
Blood vessels	Aneurysms	12

Trentham DE, Le CH. Relapsing polychondritis. *Ann Intern Med* 1998; **129**: 114–122.

Miscellaneous disorders of synovium

Pigmented villonodular synovitis

- The term pigmented villonodular synovitis (PVNS) is used for a group of conditions that are characterized by the proliferation of synovial cells and supporting tissues of the joint, tendons, and bursa.
- The condition is rare (estimated 2 cases per million).
- As the name implies, there is a villous and nodular proliferation. This is non-malignant, and associated with iron and fat deposition. Repeated small haemorrhages and lipid deposits stain the synovium red-brown and yellow, respectively.
- The cause of the condition remains unknown, although some studies have proposed a link with chronic repetitive trauma or haemarthroses.
- Experimental models and clinical experience with patients with bleeding disorders have, however, not reproduced the condition.
- The classic presentation is with a monoarthritis. Any age may be affected, although it tends to occur more often in both sexes in the third or fourth decade. The knee is the most commonly affected joint and 'diffuse' disease is more aggressive and more likely to recur.
- Insidious onset of pain and swelling in the absence of trauma, with a sero-sanguinous synovial fluid aspirate and a characteristic synovial biopsy are the basis for a diagnosis of PVNS. There are some important conditions to consider in the differential diagnosis:
  - malignant synovioma;
  - synovial haemangioma;
  - synovial chondromatosis;
  - tuberculous arthritis;
  - amyloidosis;
  - haemophilia.
- Imaging may be helpful. Plain radiographs are often normal, but it may show soft tissue swelling that can be radiodense with hemosiderin deposition. Calcification, however, is not a feature of PVNS and would suggest a malignant lesion or perhaps chondromatosis (see below).
- Erosions and subchondral cysts (also on non-weight-bearing surfaces) can be seen. Loss of joint space can occur late in the condition. Typically, this is not associated with juxta-articular osteoporosis or osteophyte formation. MRI can be highly suggestive of PVNS if there is sufficient haemosiderin and fat deposition in the lesion.

Treatment of PVNS

- Localized forms of PVNS are treated by marginal excision of the lesion.
- The prognosis is good.
- Diffuse forms of PVNS tend to be progressive and recurrent.
- Treatment techniques have included synovectomy, radiation therapy, arthrodesis, and arthroplasty. No single technique has particularly good results; however, there is only limited experience and little long-term follow-up.
- The most commonly reported treatment is surgical synovectomy.

Synovial chondromatosis

- This condition is characterized by chondrometaplasia of the sub-synovial connective tissues. The joint is filled with a thickened white/blue nodular synovium.
- The cause is unknown, the disorder uncommon, and the process non-malignant. It tends to occur more often in middle-aged men and has never been reported in prepubertal childhood.
- Clinically the condition resembles PVNS (above), but tends to be slowly progressive and sometimes self-limiting with regression. Plain radiographs may show punctate calcification outlining the joint margin.
- The diagnosis should be confirmed on synovial biopsy. In rare cases, there may be transformation to a chondrosarcoma.
- Treatment is surgical and usually managed with arthroscopy, removing loose bodies and/or the synovial membrane.

Amyloidosis

- A number of disorders and clinical settings are associated with the extracellular deposition of amyloid, a proteinaceous, fibrillar material. The low solubility of amyloid and its relative resistance to proteolytic enzymes contributes to the irreversible and often progressive course of amyloidosis.
- Despite morphological similarities (including the formation of a beta pleated sheet), amyloid is a heterogeneous group of proteins. All types of amyloid fibrils have a carbohydrate moiety in the form of glycosaminoglycans and proteoglycans. Most forms of amyloid also contain the extrafibrillar protein, amyloid-P.
- The different amyloid proteins are often related to distinct clinical forms of amyloidosis. At present, at least 17 proteins have been characterized. The detail of these proteins is beyond the scope of this book. However, two types are important as manifestations of a response to chronic systemic inflammation; amyloid-L (AML) and amyloid-A (AMA).
- Protein AML consists of monoclonal immunoglobulin light chains and is seen in idiopathic and myeloma-associated amyloidosis. The clinical features of AML and AMA are shown in Table 18.8.
- Protein AMA (derived from serum amyloid A (SAMA), an acute phase apolipoprotein), is associated with conditions such as secondary 'reactive' amyloidosis and FMF (Table 18.9).
- The mechanisms by which the various precursor proteins are converted to insoluble amyloid fibrils, the reasons for the predilection of certain proteins for particular organs and tissues, and the reasons why not all cases of a particular chronic inflammatory disorder develop amyloid are not clear. The most studied mechanisms are those associated with the reactive AMA type amyloidosis.
- Reactive AMA amyloidosis is mainly associated with long-standing infectious or non-infectious inflammation, and less frequently with cancer. In the context of rheumatic disorders AMA amyloidosis is mainly seen in:
  - adult RA;
  - JIA;
  - AS.
- There are several rheumatic conditions that are rarely associated with AMA amyloidosis. In these conditions there is a relatively low level of the acute-phase protein SAMA. These conditions include:
  - SLE;
  - systemic sclerosis;
  - Sjögren's syndrome (SS).

Table 18.8 The clinical features of AL and AA amyloidosis

	Organ/condition	Comment
AL amyloidosis	Heart	Death occurs in 50% of cases from: restrictive cardiomyopathy, congestive heart failure, conduction disturbances
	Lungs	90% develop cough and dyspnoea
	Skin	40% of cases: papules, nodules, tumours
	Neuropathy	10% of cases develop carpal tunnel syndrome
	Macroglossia	
	Vasculopathy	
	Amyloid arthropathy	
	Autonomic disturbance	
Common to AL and AA	Weakness	
	Fatigue	
	Weight loss	
	Renal	Nephrotic syndrome/renal failure—major cause of death in AA*, cause of death in one-third of AL patients
	Gastrointestinal tract	Malabsorption, obstruction, diarrhoea, hepatosplenomegaly

*In AA amyloid the spleen, liver, and kidneys are often involved first.

Investigations

- The diagnosis of amyloidosis is made by tissue biopsy (usually abdominal subcutaneous fat), and alkaline Congo red stain showing the amyloid deposits as apple green/yellow under the polarizing microscope.
- The strong calcium-dependent affinity of protein AP for amyloid fibrils is also used diagnostically in radiolabeled serum amyloid protein (SAP) scintigraphy. This technique may localize amyloid and could be of value in assessing degrees of response to treatment.
- Other laboratory tests include DNA analysis to detect the genetic variants of proteins known to make up the hereditary amyloidoses.

Treatment of amyloidosis

- The condition is progressive and there is no cure. Marked heterogeneity of the hereditary amyloidoses makes counselling difficult as well. The processes by which the disorder may be controlled include liver transplantation for lysosomal amyloidosis and bone marrow transplantation.
- In the rheumatic diseases, cytotoxic drugs such as cyclophosphamide (often in combination with corticosteroids) have improved the prognosis in RA and JIA patients.

Familial Mediterranean fever

- This condition has been in the literature since the early 1900s and was more recently characterized in the 1960s.
- Most cases (80%) present before the age of 20 and it is very rare to present with a first attack after the age of 40.
- Abnormalities of the gene coding for the protein pyrin (on chromosome 16) have been identified and constitute the only test specific for the diagnosis of Familial Mediterranean Fever (FMF). This is an autosomal recessive disorder. It most frequently affects people of eastern Mediterranean descent, especially Armenians, Arabs, and Sephardic and Ashkenazi Jews.
- The most common symptoms of abdominal pain and pleuritis are related to serositis, present in up to 95% of cases. 75% of cases develop an arthritis that may be erosive and is most often isolated to a single joint. A rash with dermal neutrophil infiltration (rather than a vasculitis) is common and looks not unlike erysipelas.
- Amyloidosis can occur in up to 40% of cases and does not appear to be associated with severity or frequency of attacks of FMF. Patients may develop renal failure, proteinuria, or malabsorption.
- Treatment includes NSAIDs for pain and continuous colchicine (1–2 mg daily). Up to 65% of cases can achieve complete remission with this regimen. A further 30% can achieve partial remission. All remaining cases should stay on 2 mg colchicine daily to help prevent amyloidosis. Concern over long-term use of prophylactic colchicine in FMF has not been borne out, the benefits of controlling the condition outweighing any complication. It is, however, recommended that amniocentesis be a routine part of antenatal treatment to exclude colchicine-related chromosomal aberrations.
- Newer agents such as anakinra, etanercept, and infliximab may play a role in the management of patients who are refractory to colchicine.

Table 18.9 The clinical features of familial Mediterranean fever

Clinical feature	Comments
Short attacks of high fever (39–40°C)	Repeated and unpredictable
Painful inflammation	Abdomen—90% of cases (may develop adhesions)
	Chest—45% of cases. Often febrile pleurisy
	Joints—most often monoarthropathy, especially the knee with acute onset pain and swelling with resolution over 1–4 weeks. Aseptic necrosis
	Skin—erysipelas-like erythema, often below the knee to the dorsum of the foot
	Other—orchitis, mild splenomegaly
AMA amyloidosis	Renal—early, terminal renal failure, cardiac, hepatic, GI (Table 18.8)
Autosomal-recessive inheritance	Virtual ethnic restriction: Sephardi Jews, Ashkenazi Jews, Armenians, Anatolian Turks, Arabs

Tumour necrosis factor-associated periodic syndrome

- This term covers a group of conditions similar to FMF but occurring in non-Mediterranean areas and associated with mutations in the TNF receptor superfamily type 1A.
- The onset is in the second decade and presents with rash, fever, abdominal pain, disabling arthralgia, and myalgia.
- 20% of patients develop amyloid AMA.
- Colchicine is not efficacious. Corticosteroids may reduce the length and severity of attacks. Etanercept has been used successfully in some patients.
- Etanercept, infliximab, tacrolimus and anakinra have been studied in the treatment of TNF-associated periodic syndrome. Large cohort studies on comparative efficacy are lacking.

Fibromyalgia and chronic widespread pain

- Chronic widespread pain (CWP) is a common finding present in 5–10% of the general population. In the absence of diffuse degenerative or inflammatory rheumatic disease the two most common conditions found in association with CWP are fibromyalgia (FM) and joint hypermobility syndrome (JHS) (📖 Chapter 16, p 431).
- CWP affects women more than men with a ratio of 1.5:1, and is defined as pain for >6 months in 2 or more sites both above and below the pelvis.
- Treatment of CWP is similar to that for FM and JHS.
- Fibromyalgia is a subtype of CWP that has two cardinal features: sleep disturbance and diffuse tenderness at discrete anatomical sites (Table 18.10 and 📖 Chapter 2, p 19).
- Using the classification criteria for FM (Table 18.10), prevalence rates range from 0.5–4% with a female: male ratio of 10:1.
- FM cases tend to aggregate within families.
- FM is also found in up to 25% of patients with RA (📖 Chapter 5, p 233), AS (📖 Chapter 8, p 281), and SLE (📖 Chapter 10, p 321). It is also commonly found in association with JHS (📖 Chapter 16, p 431) and overlaps symptomatically with this condition and chronic fatigue syndrome in many ways. Care must be taken to avoid misdiagnosing CWP/FM as the only cause for pain when there is autoimmune rheumatic disease present.
- FM is a controversial condition and its existence as a distinct entity remains uncertain. Its aetiology is multifactorial, with neurological, psychological, and behavioural factors important in its development.
- Psychological stresses may precede the onset of FM and CWP.
- Both FM and CWP are often associated with other somatic symptoms, such as chronic fatigue, irritable bowel syndrome, multiple chemical sensitivities, and headache syndromes. Other causes of fatigue should always be excluded e.g. hypothyroidism, hypoadrenalism, and anaemia.
- Alterations in hypothalamic–pituitary axis function in response to stress have been explored, but no differences between FM and controls have been found.
- Both CWP and FM are associated with alterations in peripheral and central pain processing. Painful stimuli are detected at lower levels in affected patients. Allodynia (pain in response to non-painful stimuli) found in these conditions is thought to be due to central sensitization and an 'amplification' phenomenon.
- FM patients have been found to have increased levels of substance P in the CSF—this may be a marker for these conditions, but not a routine clinical test! CSF levels of noradrenaline and serotonin metabolites are decreased in FM. These transmitters are involved in descending spinal cord pain inhibitory pathways, and the observed reduction may be responsible in part for central sensitization.

Table 18.10 ACR 1990 criteria for diagnosis of fibromyalgia (FM)

History of widespread pain:

Pain is considered when all of the following are present
- Pain in the left and right side of the body
- Pain above and below the waist
- Axial skeletal pain
- Pain present for 3 months

Pain in at least 11/18 tender point sites on digital palpation with 4 kg pressure*. One point is given for each side of the body at the following 9 sites:

1	*Occiput:* at the suboccipital muscle insertions	
2	*Low cervical:* at the anterior aspects of the inter-transverse spaces at C5–C7	
3	*Trapezius:* at the midpoint of the upper border	
4	*Supraspinatus:* at origins above scapula spine near medial border	
5	*2nd rib:* at 2nd costochondral junction	
6	*Lateral humeral epicondyles:* 2 cm distal from epicondyles	
7	*Gluteal:* in upper outer quadrants	
8	*Greater trochanter:* posterior to trochanter	
9	*Knees:* at medial fat pad proximal to joint line	

*Positive tender point when subject says palpation was painful, 'tender' is not considered painful.

Fibromyalgia said to be present when both criteria are satisfied. FM is not excluded by the presence of another disorder.

Treatment (see 📖 Chapter 21, p 550–563)
- It is of paramount importance to consider carefully the way in which an explanation is given as to the nature of the condition. Many patients have suffered disappointment, and blows to self-esteem and confidence. It may take some time and may be best approached over several visits. Many will be seeking a physical cause for the pain and may misinterpret discussion about pain amplification and its treatment as 'labelling' their condition as psychological. The label 'psychological' is, in itself, also legitimate medically, but to the layperson it often stirs ideas of 'crazy', 'all in the head,' or 'malingering'.
- It is important to assess the effect of symptoms on the patient's life, and to develop a good rapport so that psychosocial issues can be discussed. Chronic fatigue can be very disabling.
- The emphasis in the explanation should be reassurance that there is no serious underlying inflammatory or systemic condition, or damage to the joints and muscles. Reassure that other conditions are absent and that no further investigations are needed.
- Although exercise may cause a short-term increase in pain, a prolonged exercise programme has been shown to be beneficial. Low impact exercise, such as Pilates may be helpful. The presence of JHS should be identified first before deciding on type of exercise; failure to do so could cause harm.

- Pacing of activities is also important, avoiding patterns of periods of over-activity when feeling well, followed by periods of inactivity due to pain and fatigue afterwards. Pacing is one key component of cognitive behavioural therapy, a chronic pain programme that, alongside aerobic rehabilitation, may be of significant benefit to patients with FM, CWP, and JHS. This multidisciplinary approach (psychologists, physiotherapists, occupational therapists, doctors) has been tried with some success, but remains incompletely studied.
- Education of family and partners is invariably helpful and often essential.
- NSAIDs and corticosteroids are not effective as the pain is not due to inflammation or tissue damage, and may cause increased morbidity due to side effects. Narcotics should be avoided. Many patients will have tried analgesics with little effect. This in itself can fuel anxiety as to the cause and severity of their underlying condition, as well as frustration and lack of confidence in their doctor.
- Tricyclic antidepressants such as amitriptyline (10–50 mg qds) are often helpful in improving quality of sleep, decreasing morning stiffness and alleviating pain. Patients should be warned of side-effects such as dry mouth and that they may take 3–4 weeks to take effect. Patients are often also wary of being given an antidepressant. An explanation that it is being used as an analgesic is important to improve adherence. Amitriptyline is one of a group of drugs that increase 5-hydroxytryptamine.
- Amitriptyline is often combined with tramadol successfully.
- The efficacy of selective serotonin reuptake inhibitors (SSRI) is controversial. The use of fluoxetine, sertraline, or citalopram improves mood, but are less effective than tricyclics in treating pain, fatigue, and sleep disturbance.
- Venlafaxine (serotonin and noradrenaline reuptake inhibitor) in high dose is effective in treating multiple symptoms in FM. Low dose treatment is ineffective.
- Sedative hypnotics may be used to improve sleep.
- Both CWP/FM are conditions with relapses and remissions. Most patients will have ongoing symptoms. Patients with appropriate coping strategies, improvements in psychosocial stressors, and good social support networks are more likely to have a better outcome.

Common upper limb musculoskeletal lesions

For a detailed view on the differential diagnosis of the entire range of upper limb lesions, see 📖 *Chapter 2, p 19*

Shoulder (subacromial) impingement syndrome

Shoulder impingement syndrome is caused by compression of the rotator cuff by the acromion. This results in shoulder pain, particularly when the patient reaches overhead or rolls over the shoulder at night. Weakness and loss of range of motion at the shoulder are also commonly reported:

- Shoulder impingement syndrome is the most common type of presentation of shoulder pain in adults.
- Pain is often referred to the upper arm.
- The causes include acute rotator cuff tendonitis (which may be calcific), subacromial bursitis, rotator cuff tear with cuff instability and impingement, and glenohumeral instability owing to a number of different lesions (e.g. labral tear, synovitis due to crystalline arthritis).
- Inferior acromial osteophytes/acromioclavicular joint (ACJ) osteoarthritis (OA) can accompany any subacromial lesion, and are risk factors for recurrent rotator cuff disease.
- Long-term rotator cuff disease can lead to 'cuff arthropathy', with OA of the glenohumeral (GH) joint and significant chronic morbidity.
- In children or young adults with shoulder impingement syndrome, consideration of an underlying glenohumeral (instability) lesion is mandatory.

Making a diagnosis

- Exclude alternate causes of shoulder pain, including rotator cuff tear, adhesive capsulitis, and referred pain from the neck or abdomen (e.g. cholecystitis with pain referred to the shoulder).
- Elicit evidence of shoulder impingement by testing passive range of motion at the shoulder while applying 5–10 lb of pressure down on the acromion (Table 19.1).
- An AP X-ray can show specific changes that identify underlying glenohumeral or bony pathology. Plain radiographs are also useful for identifying calcific tendonitis. Consider requesting an AP view with 30° external rotation at the arm, an outlet Y view, and an axillary view.
- MR may be necessary to rule out subtle glenohumoral pathology. MR characterizes sites of cuff inflammation and is more sensitive than US in identifying cuff tears.

Conservative management of cuff/subacromial bursal inflammation

- Avoid overhead arm activities.
- Trial a full-dose regular NSAID for 2 weeks.
- If the rotator cuff is intact, consider steroid injection (e.g. triamcinolone acetonide 40 mg; Plate 4) and local anaesthetic injection (e.g. 5 mL 1% lidocaine). Approach laterally or posteriorly.
- Consider physical therapy 1–2 weeks later if the cuff muscles are weak.
- Consider a second injection after 6 weeks (Fig. 19.1).

Table 19.1 The range of disorders presenting with a subacromial impingement pattern of pain. Clinical testing, though it can be elaborate, has been shown repeatedly in studies not to be as specific as the original literature appeared to suggest

Condition	Diagnosis made by
Supraspinatus/cuff tendonitis	MR or US
Subacromial bursitis (e.g. trauma, RA, gout, CPPD)	US/MR
Rotator cuff tear (partial or full)	MR
Long head of biceps tendonitis	Clinical, US/MR
OA ACJ (impingement of osteophytes on cuff)	Clinical, X-rays, MR
Glenohumeral instability due to labral trauma (e.g. SLAP lesion), arthritis GH joint	MR
Enthesitis (e.g. deltoid origin at acromion) in SpAs (📖 Chapter 8, p 281)	Clinical, US
Lesion at suprascapular notch (e.g. cyst, tophus)	MR

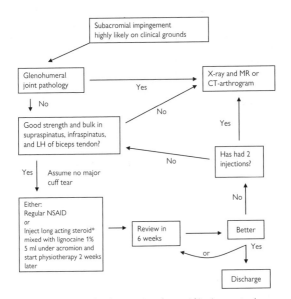

Fig. 19.1 Pragmatic algorithm for managing subacromial impingement pain
*Use 20–40 mg triaminolone acetonide or methylprednisolone acetate.
LH – Long head.

Adhesive capsulitis

Pain and diminished active and passive range of motion (in the absence of an intrinsic joint disorder) is highly suggestive of adhesive capsulitis (AC). The aetiology is unknown, but it involves capsular and coracohumeral ligament contractures. The condition is more common in women than men (typically affecting women age 40–60 years), and is four times more common in diabetics. AC occurs bilaterally in 15% of patients. Recurrence is unusual. If left alone, pain usually resolves within 2 years, but the patient may be left with long-term restriction of shoulder movement.

Making the diagnosis

- Do not confuse AC with shoulder impingement syndrome. With impingement, passive range of motion remains intact, and is less painful than active movements. With AC, passive and active range of motion are equally impaired.
- Clues to the diagnosis from examination include marked restriction of external rotation; also, with abduction, the scapula moves very early—normally it doesn't move until 30° of abduction has been completed.
- If the presentation is delayed (e.g. >6 months), a secondary impingement syndrome may have evolved and is exposed as some range of motion begins to return.

Principles of management

- Rule out associated conditions: diabetes, hypothyroidism, lung carcinoma, myocardial infarction, stroke, and protease inhibitor use for human immunodeficiency virus (HIV) infection.
- Control pain during the initial painful/stiff phase of the condition. Consider NSAIDs, intra-articular steroid injections (e.g. 40 mg triamcinolone acetonide +5–10 mL 1% lidocaine), suprascapular nerve block, or a short course of prednisone 30 mg/day for 3 weeks.[1]
- Mobilize with physical therapy early, but be aware this may be limited by poor pain control.
- Consider surgery if conservative management fails after 6 months. Surgical procedures focus on releasing contracted/fibrotic tissue of the antero-inferior capsular structures. Procedures associated with good results include arthroscopic or open release with manipulation under anaesthesia or arthroscopic release alone. The latter may be combined with steroid injections.

1 Buchbinder R, Hoving JL, Green S, et al. (2004). Short course prednisolone for adhesive capsulitis: a randomised, double blind, placebo controlled trial. *Ann Rheum Dis* **63**: 1460–9.

Lateral epicondylitis (tennis elbow)

This condition is common, affecting 1–3% of the adult population, typically in the age group 40–60 years. The dominant arm is most affected. It is rare in elite tennis players, but up to 40% of social players get it at some time. About 90% of all patients seen in clinical practice do not get this from playing tennis!

It is thought to be due to cumulative trauma overuse disorder from mechanical overloading. If chronic, it can lead to tendon degeneration and osseous changes. Poor prognosis is associated with manual work, high level physical strain at work, and high baseline pain and distress.

Making the diagnosis

- The main differential diagnoses are: elbow joint lesions, referred neck pain and enthesopathies (e.g. DISH or enthesitis linked to spondyloarthropathies—📖 Chapter 8, p 281).
- Pain is elicited by resisted force in pronation (e.g. handshakes, turning doorknobs, carrying bags).
- There is tenderness at the lateral humeral condyle with pain elicited by resisted finger and wrist extension. Pain often extends down the extensor side of the forearm.
- Enthesopathies, tendon tears, and joint lesions may be diagnosed by an experienced musculoskeletal ultrasonographer.
- MR may miss mild epicondylitis/enthesitis and appearances are not specific. MR is more useful for ruling out tendon tears and joint lesions. Do not use MR of the elbow to discriminate elbow lesions from referred neck pain.

Principles of management

- During the acute phase, lateral epicondylitis should be treated with activity restriction, pain control, and immobilization.
- Injection around the epicondyle with triamcinolone should be considered if conservative therapy is insufficient (Plate 5).
- In patients failing to respond to steroid injection or physical therapy, injection with autologous blood has demonstrated some efficacy.
- Isometric grip exercises may also help with recovery.
- Surgery is rarely indicated, and should be considered only in patients with persistent symptoms despite several months of therapy (Fig. 19.2).

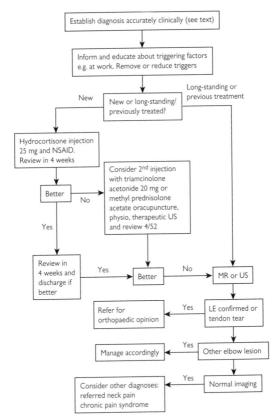

Fig. 19.2 Pragmatic algorithm for managing lateral epicondylitis (LE).

Back pain

Categorizing of back pain

Non-spinal back pain

It is important to remember that pain may radiate from other structures, e.g. renal, aneurismal, or pleuritic disorders and retroperitoneal fibrosis.

Acute non-specific back pain

- This accounts for 80–85% of all acute.
- Typically 90% of cases will recover within 6 weeks (the threshold for reassurance).
- Some will be neuropathic in nature.

Chronic back pain

- Describes pain that has been present for >12 weeks.
- Some will be neuropathic in nature.

Neuropathic pain

- This type of pain accounts for approximately one-third of acute and chronic low back pain.
- painDetect® is a useful assessment tool, as well as an *aide memoire* for the typical symptoms of neuropathic pain: burning, prickling, hot/cold dysaesthesia, sensitivity to touch and pressure, numbness, and sudden 'electric shock'-like symptoms.

'Red' and 'Yellow' flags

This terminology is used to identify potentially serious secondary physical (Red) and psychosocial (Yellow) pathologies (Table 20.1).

Table 20.1 Warning signs for sinister pathology in back pain

'Red flags':	'Yellow flags':
Age of onset <20 years & >55 years	Belief that pain and activity are harmful
Recent trauma	Abnormal 'sickness behaviour', e.g. extended rest
Pain constant, progressive, and no relief with rest	Low/negative mood
Thoracic pain	Work environment (low support/satisfaction conflicting evidence for high pace/demand)
Past history of malignancy	Seeking treatments that seem excessive/inappropriate
Osteoporosis risk	Inappropriate expectations
Infection risk (immunosuppressed)	Lack of social support in private life (moderate evidence)
Systemically unwell—weight loss/fever, etc.	Compensation claims
Progressive neurological signs/including bladder dysfunction	
Structural deformity	

Conditions causing acute or sub-acute back pain in adults

Acute mechanical back pain

- Most cases in a primary care setting are due to lumbar muscle strain or sprain; this presents with diffuse pain in the lower back to buttocks, and resolves spontaneously. If pain is related to posture or movement, especially of the thoracic cage, and local tenderness is felt at the lumbosacral junction then the pain is highly likely to be musculoskeletal.
- The clinician should be aware of 'Red flags' that may indicate more thorough investigation. Although far less common (<15% of all cases) the following should be considered (% of cases in back pain population):
  - compression fracture (4%);
  - symptomatic herniated disc (4%);
  - spinal stenosis (3%);
  - malignancy (0.7%);
  - ankylosing spondylitis (0.3%);
  - cauda equina syndrome (0.04%) (saddle anaesthesia, leg weakness, bilateral sciatica, and bladder dysfunction);
  - spinal infection or inflammatory radiculopathy (0.01%).
- Herniated discs account for 4% of lower back pain. Disc herniation presents with leg pain radiating past the knee, and is most common in patients between 20 and 50 years old.
- Degenerative causes of back pain, including degenerative disc disease, facet joint hypertrophy and spinal stenosis, are more common in older patients.
- The immediate management is adequate and regular analgesia, advising only minimal bed rest, encouraging mobilization and normalization of activities.
- Short courses of muscle relaxants such as diazepam should be considered; these agents decrease muscle spasm and aid sleep.
- The clinician should explore patient fears (Yellow flags) and, where appropriate, reassure that serious illness is unlikely, tests are not usually needed, severe pain is often short-lived, but milder pain may be present for longer, and that recurrences are common.
- Radiographs are likely to be unhelpful for planning management in most cases and radiologists often advise against getting them. MR of the lumbar spine, for example, frequently demonstrates abnormal findings in asymptomatic patients; the relationship between such findings and clinical symptoms is not always clear.
- A rehabilitation approach should be considered (Table 20.2). The strength of evidence for therapies is variable. Adherence may be a problem with rehabilitation programs, but adherence may be augmented by providing patient education literature.

Table 20.2 Therapies used in facilitating rehabilitation after acute mechanical low back pain

Manipulation	Either done by an osteopath, chiropractor, or physiotherapist. Some controversy as to the level of benefit owing to poor methodological studies. Avoid using in cases of intractable back pain (see 📖 Chapter 20, p 525, Management of chronic back pain).
McKenzie exercises	Passive extension exercises designed to improve pain and stiffness associated with disc and anterior spinal structure pathology. May aggravate pain from posterior spine structures, e.g. facet joints, spinous processes.
Hydrotherapy or balneotherapy	Poorly studied, but warmth can ease movement and augment land-based exercises. Might be considered after initial painful phase to regain normal movements and mobility. May only suit a few patients and resources may be limited.
Graded activity programs	Useful for patients who require guidance and would be unable to gain optimally from home exercise regime. A plan for rehabilitation with milestones is useful for some patients.
Behavioural programs	Focuses on psychological aspects of pain, involves moderate supervision and planned withdrawal of treatment. Differs from some other approaches in that the therapist takes over the 'control' of the back pain. Limited resources may restrict provision of this approach.

Back pain and nerve root lesions

See also 📖 Chapter 2, p 19.

- Root compression occurs most often because of acute or sub-acute disc prolapse or foraminal stenosis. The peak incidence is age 30–50 years. About 70% resolve within 3 months and 90% within 6 months.
- Root compression should be suspected if acute or sub-acute back pain is associated with segmental nerve or sciatic leg pain.
- Acute sciatic pain (affecting the outer and posterior leg) is often sharp or burning in nature, and most frequently arises from acute disc prolapse of either L4/5 or L5/S1 (>90% cases). Sciatica is characterized by leg pain projecting past the knee, which may be more severe than the associated back pain.
- A patient with a herniated disc may present with complaints of sciatica; evidence of disc herniation may be elicited of physical examination by straight leg raise or crossed straight leg raise (i.e. elevation of unaffected leg). These tests are positive if pain is felt in the buttock or back at a leg angle of 30–60°. Pain elicited at a leg angle <10° is consistent with musculoskeletal back pain.
- A neurological examination is essential: L5 root lesions give decreased strength of the foot and great toe dorsiflexion, standing on heel, and decreased ankle reflex and sensation over great toe. S1 root lesions give decreased strength in plantar foot flexion, difficulty in weight-bearing on toes, and decreased ankle reflex and sensation on the sole or outer part of foot.

Principles of management
- The natural history is such that 30–60% of patients recover in 1 week.
- Non-steroidal anti-inflammatory drugs (NSAIDs), paracetamol (acetaminophen), and muscle relaxants should be considered first. Some patients will require narcotics for pain control. Bed rest should be limited; prolonged bed rest leads to worse outcomes.
- An epidural steroid injection can improve pain in the short-term, but data from RCTs does not show better long-term outcome at 3 months or longer compared with controls. A meta-analysis showed that 1 in 7 patients having a steroid epidural experience >75% improvement in pain in the short-term, and 1 in 13 experience >50% symptom improvement in the long-term.
- Physical therapy and supervised rehabilitation using lumbar extensor exercise regimes may be of benefit.
- MR can characterize lesions, but 25% of asymptomatic people have frank disc protrusions; thus, MR gives poor specificity. MR should be used to confirm a diagnosis, not to reach for one.
- The absolute indications for surgery (Table 20.3) are cauda equina, progressive muscle weakness, and neuropathy causing functional disability.

Facet hypertrophy/facet joint syndromes
- Facet joint (FJ) osteoarthritis (OA) of the lumbar spine is common in middle aged/elderly adults, can be part of inflammatory generalized OA, and is associated with spondylolytic spondylolisthesis (i.e. forward slippage of a vertebrae, usually L5, in relationship to the vertebrae below).
- Psoriatic arthritis (📖 Chapter 8, p 281) can also affect FJs and is under-recognized as a cause of low back pain.
- Calcium pyrophosphate deposition (CPPD) arthritis (📖 Chapter 7, p 269) may also affect FJs.
- Typical symptoms include pain on hyperextension or rotation of the lower back; pain is referred to the upper buttocks, is worse while standing still, and eased by forward lumbar flexion.
- Facet hypertrophy itself cannot be felt, but FJ syndrome is accompanied by muscle spasm and superficial soft-tissue tenderness.
- Arthritic FJs may be seen on oblique spinal radiographs; however, imaging in general cannot reliably identify symptomatic FJ joints. FJ injection with anesthetic may confirm the diagnosis if this results in significant pain relief.

Management of FJ syndromes
- Patients can be treated according to principles applied for all patients with acute mechanical back pain except that extensor exercises are contraindicated as they will aggravate symptoms.
- Short courses of analgesics and/or NSAIDs as for OA (📖 Chapter 6, p 259).
- Generally advise minimal bed rest.
- Steroid injection of FJs is a frequently used treatment modality, although studies have failed to demonstrate benefit over placebo injection.

Table 20.3 Surgical approaches for lumbar disc prolapse

Discectomy	Essential for discs causing cauda equina syndrome and progressive neurological deficits. Excluding above indications, compared with conservative therapy, in a RCT 66% vs 33% patients were satisfied following surgery at 1 year, and 66% vs 51% were satisfied at 4 years; thus, benefit of surgery in the long term is small. Adverse events with surgery include: mortality (<0.2%), dural tears (4%), and permanent nerve root injuries (<1%). 70% success rate in short term. Risk of failure from surgery relates to hysteria or hypochondriasis scores on MMPI* and presence of litigation claims.
Microdiscectomy	Smaller surgical field results in earlier mobilization and less post-operative disability. Outcomes similar to those of conventional discectomy.
Percutaneous discectomy	Suctioning of central disc material causing disc decompression and relieving nerve root pressure. Associated with low complication rate and rapid rehabilitation. Non-RCT data suggest similar efficacy to discectomy.
Chemo-nucleolysis	Injection of proteolytic enzyme into disc. RCTs suggest standard discectomy is superior. Rare, but devastating neurological complications and risk of anaphylaxis (0.3%).
Laser lumbar discectomy	Vapourizing of part of disc by laser introduced through a needle probe. Efficacy possible similar to discectomy. No RCT data.
Prosthetic intervertebral disc replacement	Also indicated for degenerative disc disease, post-laminectomy syndrome and non-specific persistent low back pain. Artificial discs consist of 2 endplates separated by pliable inner core. Anterior approach needed. Good results reported in open series for pooled patient groups. Complication rate may be high (up to 45%).

*MMPI = Minnesota Multiphasic Personality Inventory.

RCT = Randomized Control Trial

- Radio frequency denervation of medial branches of dorsal rami supplying FJs can help, but the procedure should only be considered if local anesthetic block works first.

Spinal stenosis

- The diagnosis is frequently missed in the elderly.
- It presents mainly with achy, stiff pains in the legs increasing on walking and eases if the patient stops walking, sits, or leans forward (neurogenic or pseudo-claudication).
- Pain, numbness/tingling, and weakness are the most common symptoms. Neurological leg signs can be accentuated after exercise.
- The diagnosis is made using MR imaging the L-spine.

- Non-surgical management (including pain control and physical therapy) is often adequate.
- Decompressive laminectomy is required urgently to address rapidly progressive neurological symptoms, bladder dysfunction, or cauda equina syndrome.

Non-traumatic vertebral collapse: evaluation

- This is usually due to osteoporosis, collapse into an abnormal vertebra (e.g. vertebral haemangioma), or secondary to malignancy or infection.
- The history should therefore focus around identifying risk factors for these conditions. Post-menopausal status or hypogonadism, previous fracture history, steroid use, and alcoholism may all contribute to osteoporosis. Weight loss or B-type symptoms may indicate the presence of malignancy or infection.
- Kyphosis and loss of height can occur after vertebral collapse; a full examination should be performed to evaluate the possibility of cord compression or malignancy.
- Investigate with AP and lateral spinal X-rays, MR, bone biochemistry [intact parathyroid hormone (PTH)], morning luteinizing hormone (LH) and free testosterone, 25-OH vitamin D, thyroid function tests (TFTs), and serum/urine electrophoresis.
- MR is good at discriminating infection and tumours from osteoporosis, but biopsy for histology and culture is essential if tumour or infection has not been ruled out by MR.

Management of non-traumatic vertebral collapse

- The patient should be placed on bed rest and monitored for evolving neurological deficits.
- Pain control often requires long-acting narcotics, with short-acting narcotics for breakthrough pain.
- Calcitonin 100–200 IU bd sc or 200 IU/day by nasal spray has an analgesic effect and reduces bone turnover in osteoporosis. Paracetamol (Acetaminophen) and NSAIDs alone are unlikely to be sufficient.
- Osteoporosis should be treated aggressively (📖 Chapter 16, p 431), at minimum with calcium and vitamin D supplements. The use of bisphosphonates in women of childbearing years is controversial due to their long half-lives and unknown impact on the foetus.
- Discuss any pathological malignancy-related fracture with a radiation oncologist.
- Consider vertebroplasty or balloon kyphoplasty.

Post-surgical back pain

- There are numerous causes and no single entity (Table 20.4).
- Imaging with gadolinium-enhanced MR may be helpful to delineate inflammatory tissue around the surgical site.
- Persistent pain after surgery may be associated with adverse psychological and social factors, and outstanding litigation or insurance claims.
- Nerve root blocks, epidurals, and spinal stimulators may be used.

Sterile discitis

- This inflammation of the intervertebral disc is often associated with annulus enthesitis at the vertebral end-plates and vertebral osteitis.
- The causes include disc degeneration, CPPD disease, ankylosing spondylitis (AS; Romanus lesions) and other spondyloarthritis (SpAs) including SAPHO (📖 Chapter 8, p 281).
- The lesion should be identified with MR and treatment should include bed rest and aggressive analgesia. In RCTs, steroid disc injections have been shown to be little help overall. Bisphosphonates (iv, e.g. pamidronate 60–90 mg) has anecdotally been shown to help AS and SAPHO discitis.

Table 20.4 Implicated causes of post-surgical back pain

Recurrent disease	E.g. further disc protrusion and radicular features. If re-operation not appropriate consider nerve root block, steroid epidural, etc.
Operation for wrong lesion	MR appearances can highlight lesions, which may not be relevant to clinical features. More than 1 or 2 lesions can co-exist. Detailed clinical assessment *prior* to imaging is essential.
Misdiagnosis originally	A structural lesion treated when an inflammatory disease, typically SpA-related disease, was present and causing on-going symptoms.
Adverse rehabilitation conditions	Resolution of symptoms and regaining functional capacity if slow has been associated with significant psychological and social factors. Poor result of surgery also associated with an outstanding insurance claim or litigation.
Arachnoiditis	Thought to be a direct effect of surgery. Dural tissue becomes inflamed. In nerve root/disc surgery often associated with sensory root symptoms for some months afterwards. Diagnosis with gadolinium-enhanced MR. Where associated with sensory radicular symptoms, may respond to steroid root block, epidural. If radicular symptoms chronic and disabling consider spinal cord (implanted) stimulator.

Management of chronic back pain

Chronic back pain requires a special approach, with an emphasis on psychological and social management. Patients are likely to have set beliefs about their problem, the ability of healthcare systems to help them, and are more likely to have developed coping strategies than patients with acute or sub-acute back pain. However, those with chronic back pain who continually seek further and different healthcare options are likely to have less successful coping strategies.

Initial approach to the care of patients with chronic low back pain

See Table 20.5.

- Be confident that there is no undiagnosed condition affecting back pain [e.g. hypermobility (🕮 Chapter 16, p 431)] and that no new neurological lesions have evolved. If examination raises concern, use MR to rule out lesions.
- Establish empathy and trust, taking time to get information about the patient's:
  - social situation;
  - health and illness beliefs;
  - intra-family dynamics;
  - true role and perception of their role at work;
  - view on conventional and complementary therapies;
  - view on what does and doesn't work, and on their specific view of exercise therapy.
- Plan the management approach with the patient and establish short- to mid-term goals, including whether, and what type of, supervision is required (e.g. graded programme of exercise) and how often a review is needed.
- Consider 'domains' of therapy under the following headings:
  - physical therapy;
  - work/life commitments;
  - psychological and social support;
  - painkillers and medications;
  - education (insight and coping strategies).
- Plan to review progress at regular intervals.
- Evaluate patients carefully at baseline if considering long-term opiate use. There may be an increased risk of dependency if the patient currently or previously abused drugs, there is a high level of psychological distress, if short-acting opiates are used, or drugs are prescribed 'as needed'.
- Although many strategies, especially those that combine techniques, can be costly, these costs to healthcare are likely to be offset by the saving in lost wages.

Table 20.5 Management options for chronic low back pain

Exercises	RCT evidence supports use. Greater evidence of effect when combined with behavioural methods. Aerobic exercises augment effect of 'back school'. Should be essential part of outpatient physical retraining programme. Less evidence on how much should be supervised, by whom, and how often.
Manipulation	Trials show efficacy on pain in the long term.
Transcutaneous electric nerve stimulation (TENS)	Disappointing results from few RCTs in patients with chronic back pain, although efficacy for other specific diagnoses are unknown.
Posture training	May be more appropriate than corset use and easy to combine training with supervised exercise therapy.
Oral medications	NSAIDs best reserved for acute-on-chronic pain exacerbations. Low-dose tricyclics (e.g. amitriptyline, nortriptyline) are useful particularly if chronic neuropathic pain is present. Try to avoid long-term opiate drugs. Chronic opiate use for chronic low back pain has not been extensively studied. A mental health evaluation before long-term prescribing is essential to avoid triggering dependency (see text); short courses, initially for a trial period, are sensible. Best supervised by a specialist with experience in pain management.
Back school	Regular programme carrying an educational component. Programmes vary from one to many sessions. May be more effective in occupational setting. Long-term changes in behaviour have not been extensively studied. Non-compliance and relapse are problems.
Psychology-orientated rehabilitation programmes	Intensive courses often run by psychologists and 'hands-off' physical therapists can help (highly) selected patients. Focus is on learning to cope with pain and increased control of effects of pain on functioning and psyche. Not suitable for many patients. Courses few and far between. Cost-effectiveness of courses not proved.
Complementary therapies	Increasingly used (📖 Chapter 23, p 599). By consensus, chiropractic has been shown to be helpful for chronic low back pain. Acupuncture has yet to be proved successful in robust studies. Poor evidence base otherwise.
Intrathecal opiates	Conflicting results from (only) non-controlled studies. Generally results show overall short-term improvements regarding pain perception, but not function. Best reserved for patients where all else has failed.
Spinal cord stimulator (SCS)	A number of good studies show that SCS is effective for neuropathic including radicular pain. Technique is relatively safe. Careful patient selection is important. Studies show 50% reduction in pain long-term.

Additional sources of reference materials on the value of interventions

American College of Physicians/AmericanPain Society Guidelines.

Chou R, Qaseem A, Snow V, *et al.* (2007). *Ann Intern Med* **10**:492–504.

European Acute Low Back Pain Guidelines.

Van Tulder MW, Bedler A, Brekkering T, *et al, Eur Spine Journal* 2006, **3**:Suppl 2:192–300.

UK Beam: Various publications between 2004 and 2007.

Cochrane databases:

2003—Multidisciplinary Bio-psychosocial, Rehabilitation, Muscle relaxants.

2004—Back schools.

2005—Bed rest, Exercise therapy, Behavioural therapy, Acupuncture.

2007—Herbal medicine, Traction, Insoles, Opioids, Injection therapy, Prolotherapy, and Laser therapy.

Management of back pain in children and adolescents

Children with spinal problems present with deformity, back pain, limping, systemic features, neurological features, or a combination of effects. Back pain in children is common—up to 30%, but is rare in the those <10 years. If severe enough to warrant hospital admission there is frequently an underlying cause. Age determines the likelihood of cause, with infection and tumours being more common in young children compared with adolescents (Table 20.6).

The principles behind history and examination in children are discussed in 📖 Chapter 2, p 19.

Non-specific low back pain

- The annual incidence is 10–22% in schoolchildren.
- Adolescent back pain is linked with familial clustering, physical inactivity, sports injuries, and psychosocial factors.
- Most children have self-limiting symptoms.
- Management should focus on an explanation of the short natural history, reassurance, addressing predisposing factors (see above) that remain a trigger for recurrence and increasing general health/exercise to improve muscle strength.

Idiopathic scoliosis

- This is often vertebral malalignment in the coronal plane associated with spinal rotation accentuated on spinal flexion.
- It occurs in up to 3% of schoolchildren.
- Most (70%) are asymptomatic. Progression is more likely in the presence of pain or thoracic curve convex to the left—conditions that should be investigated for more serious underlying spinal pathology.
- Progressive scoliosis (Fig. 20.1) requires bracing or surgery. Usually curves of 25–45° are braced and those >45° are best considered for surgery.

Congenital (CS) and neuromuscular (NMS) scoliosis

- Congenital scoliosis (CS) is associated with genitourinary malformations (20%) and, rarely, congenital heart disease. CS is associated with spinal dysraphism (20%), myelodysplasia, and Klippel–Fiel syndrome.
- Neuromuscular scoliosis (NMS) is associated with cerebral palsy, muscular dystrophy, spinomuscular atrophy, and myelodysplasia.
- To avoid rapid progression and increased long-term morbidity and disability, refer for prompt correction of progressive curves. Orthotic treatment is an adjunct to, not a substitute for, surgery.

Table 20.6 Causes of back pain in children

Developmental
- Painful scoliosis
- Spondylolysis and spondylolisthesis
- Scheuermann disease

Infection
- Discitis
- Vertebral osteomyelitis
- Spinal epidural abscess

Inflammation
- Juvenile arthritis
- Osteoporosis

Mechanical
- Herniated disk
- Muscle strain
- Fractures

Neoplasms
- Benign (osteoid osteomas, osteoblastoma, aneurysmal bone cyst)
- Malignant (leukaemia, lymphoma, sacroma)

Visceral
- Pyelonephritis, appendicitis, retroperitoneal abscess

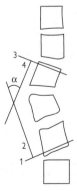

Fig. 20.1 Measurement of the degree of scoliosis by the Cobb method: 1, the lowest vertebra whose bottom tilts to the concavity of curve; 2, the erect perpendicular to line 1; 3, the highest vertebra whose top tilts to the concavity of curve; 4, the drop perpendicular to line 3; α, the intersecting angle. Curves less than 20° are considered to be mild, 20–40° are moderate, and above 40° are severe.

Scheuermann's osteochondritis

- This is perhaps the most common cause of spinal deformity and back pain in children and adolescents (3–5% of all adolescents usually 13–17 years). The aetiology is unknown.
- If severe it can form a kyphosis and then frequently becomes symptomatic. Compensatory lumbar lordosis evolves.
- The typical radiographic pattern is one of wedge deformities (<10°) of contiguous thoracic vertebrae with irregular vertebral end-plates.

Management

- Avoid repetitive stress-loading activities such as running.
- Extensor exercises for the back and abdominal muscle exercises may improve symptoms, but will not correct kyphosis.
- Brace treatment usually prevents progression of kyphosis.
- Surgery is reserved for severe persistent pain, if there are severe or progressive deformities (>70°) or there is great concern about the appearance.

Spondylolysis and spondylolisthesis

- Spondylolysis is a defect in the pars interarticularis, most commonly seen at L5. Alone as a lesion it is common (4% preschool children and 6% at age 18 years).
- Spondylolysis is a risk factor for asymptomatic and symptomatic spondylolisthesis [slippage of one vertebra on another (Fig. 20.2)].
- Progressive slippage is rare in children, but can occur during the adolescent growth spurt.

Management

- On serial radiographs if slippage is >25% (Grade II, III, or IV) then advise against contact sports or sports involving lumbar hyperextension.
- Advise should be given on regular abdominal muscle exercises, avoiding gaining abdominal obesity, and consider regular bracing.
- Surgery is considered for *progressive* vertebral slippage or Grade III/IV slip.

Herniated disc

- This is infrequent in children. Most occur in children older than 11 years and are often associated with scoliosis.
- Diagnose disc herniation by MR, but be cautious in interpreting normal developmental changes in the growing spine.

Management

- Without nerve root impingement management is conservative: short period of bed rest, adequate analgesics, and NSAIDs with early exercise-based rehabilitation regime.
- Over 50% improve with conservative treatment, but reported results from surgery for significant nerve root lesion (persistent severe pain or neurological deficit) are very good.

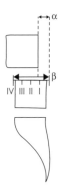

Fig. 20.2 Spondylolisthesis measured as a % slip of L4 on L5 (α/β). Grade I <25%, Grade II 25–50%, Grade III 50–75%, and Grade IV >75%.

Spinal tumours

- Although rare in children, spinal tumours frequently present with back pain (80% cases).
- It is important to recognize painful scoliosis, radicular pain, night pain, stiffness, and effectiveness of NSAIDs which are all (though not specific) features of spinal tumours.

Management

- Urgent radiographs (may be negative in early disease) and MRI are needed to delineate the nature of the problem and the clinician should consider isotope bone scan (with SPECT) or focal CT to identify posterior element tumours (e.g. osteoid osteoma).
- Adequate analgesia is required: NSAIDs—ibuprofen in recommended doses for weight may not be sufficient, consider naproxen 15 mg/kg/day for adolescents.
- Bed rest is not essential, although wise if scans show there is risk of vertebral collapse or cord compression. If the latter is a worry this should be discussed urgently with a paediatric spinal surgeon and radiation oncologist.
- Initiate a search for other tumours known to metastasize to spine (Table 20.7).
- Investigation within an adolescent unit is advisable given the specific multidisciplinary input often needed.

Table 20.7 Primary spinal tumours in children and adolescents (see also Table 2.17)

Osteoid osteomas

Benign. Not uncommon. Mainly adolescents. Posterior vertebral bone usually. Pain can be severe. Discriminated from osteoblastomas by size (osteomas are <1.5 cm, osteoblastomas >1.5 cm) as histology is often identical. Lesions are associated with scoliosis (63% cases). Surgical excision is treatment of choice.

Aneurysmal bone cyst

Benign. Symptoms often triggered by vertebral collapse. Take care when considering biopsy to discriminate from malignant lesions. Discuss in detail with musculoskeletal radiologist.

Eosinophilic granulomas

Benign—often occurs around age 10 years. Rare. Lytic lesion. May occasionally be multiple/disseminated—staging important. Symptoms often triggered by vertebral collapse. Cord and radicular compression can occur. Biopsy essential to discriminate from malignant lesions. Surgical excision or internal spine fixation not usually needed. Consider radiotherapy if cord compression threatened. Consider external brace fixation in all and monitor for spontaneous resolution. Disseminated lesions can be treated with chemotherapy.

Ewing sarcoma

Overall rarely affects spine (~10% cases). Can affect any part of spine including sacrum (latter cases often delayed diagnosis). Suspicion of it requires biopsy. Treat with combination chemotherapy and local radiotherapy. 5-year survival ~50%. Outcome better for tumour sizes < 8 cm or localized disease.

Leukaemia

Consider in all cases of spinal osteopaenia or single/multiple vertebral collapse. Notorious association with delayed diagnosis. Associated systemic symptoms may not necessarily be present, but normal FBC at presentation unlikely (~10% cases only). Also look for eosinophilia and hypercalcaemia, and consider bone marrow aspirate.

Lymphomas

Rarely presents with back pain; however, known cause of persistent back pain. MR is imaging of choice. MR can show vertebral collapse and/or soft tissue paraspinal mass. Biopsy is diagnostic. Case reports of plasmacytomas presenting similarly.

Secondary malignant tumours

Neuroblastoma, rhabdomyosarcoma, Wilms tumour, retinoblastoma, and teratoblastoma are known to present with back pain. Usually biopsy evidence for triggers a search for the underlying primary neoplasm.

Part III

Medicine management and emergencies

Drugs used in rheumatology

Drugs used in the management of hyperuricaemia, pulmonary hypertension, and osteoporosis are discussed in 📖 Chapter 7, p 269, 📖 Chapter 13, p 363 and 📖 Chapter 16, p 431, respectively.

Introduction

A variety of pharmacological agents are used across the breadth of rheumatic diseases. Therapeutic options are discussed in each of the disease-specific chapters in Part II of the book.

This chapter highlights common themes pertinent to prescribing for pain relief and control of auto-immune rheumatic disease. It is not the intention of this chapter to describe all of these in detail, although specific issues are discussed. Protocols for the use of certain agents such as iloprost and pooled-immunoglobulin will also be described.

For a detailed description of a specific drug it is recommended the reader use a National Formulary.

The chapter starts with a reminder that rehabilitation is an integral part of disease management and should complement pharmacological interventions whenever appropriate.

Table 21.1 lists the common classes of drug used in rheumatology and is the framework for the content of this chapter.

Table 21.1 Pharmacotherapy of rheumatological diseases

Drug type	Examples
Pain relief	Paracetamol and compound analgesic
	Opioid analgesics
	NSAIDs
	Antidepressants
	Anticonvulsants
	Hypnotics and muscle relaxants
	Topical agents
Disease-modifying drugs	Glucocorticoids (oral, im, intra-articular)
	Azathioprine
	Ciclosporin
	Cyclophosphamide
	Chlorambucil
	Gold
	Hydroxychloroquine
	Leflunomide
	Methotrexate
	Mycophenolate mofetil
	Penicillamine
	Sulfasalazine
Biological therapies	Anti-TNF-α; etanercept, infliximab, adalimumab, certolizumab
	Anti B-cell: rituximab
	IL-6 antagonists: tocilizumab
Other	Anaemia: iron, erythropoietin
	Hyperuricaemia (📖 Chapter 7, p 270)
	Osteoporosis: calcium and vitamin D, bisphosphonates, teriparatide, denosumab (📖 Chapter 16, p 432)
	Ischaemia—iloprost
	Vasculitis—iv immunoglobulin

Principles of rehabilitation

In addition to pharmacological interventions, consideration of the role of rehabilitation is also very important.

Adults

It is beyond the scope of this book to address the many techniques employed in rehabilitation. The reader should discuss and observe the management of patients with arthritis with the rehabilitation team:

- In the last decade the development of a multidisciplinary approach to rehabilitation has transformed the way most rheumatologists think about disability.
- Two main types of measurement exist for assessing outcome in rehabilitation (beyond the various scoring systems for particular diseases).
- 'Generic' measures take a global view of disability and afford later comparison. Generic measures also help in assessing different programs, populations, and practices. 'Specific' measures deal with the individual patient and their function in their own environment.
- No one single instrument will suffice and there are now many, some well-validated, disability scores:
  - Ritchie index—inflammation and response to NSAIDs;
  - Health Assessment Questionnaire—disability;
  - SF36;
  - Beck depression score—depression;
  - Spielberg score—anxiety;
  - Sickness Impact Profile (SIP);
  - multi-dimensional pain inventory—psychological response to pain and disability.
- Important components of rehabilitation for patients with arthritis include:
  - a co-ordinated team;
  - problem-solving approach;
  - functionally relevant programme;
  - education;
  - community orientated;
  - cognitive and psychological behavioural therapy;
  - addressing social factors, e.g. work, housing etc.;
  - access to support services;
  - commitment to long-term follow-up and reassessment.
- As such, the team will consist of doctors, specialist nurses, physical and occupational therapists, counsellors, psychologists, orthotists, chiropodists, dieticians, rehabilitation engineers, and social workers.

Childhood

There are important additional issues to consider in the management of children:

- A child's rheumatic disease always has an impact on their family. Many normal activities are impossible or time-consuming, and financial hardship is common.

- Siblings may feel neglected, and parents are often overburdened with tasks and worries to focus completely on the family. The 'team' aims to share out that burden and assist the whole family.
- The child should be integrated in school ('mainstream' preferably) and social life as much as possible. It is important to achieve the highest level of integration, hopefully ceasing a child's perception of sickness and difference, acquiring a sense of belonging and purpose.
- The therapist will spend as much time preventing deformity in early disease as dealing with chronic disability, the aim being to maintain or restore function.
- For a child with chronic progressive disease a regular, often daily, therapy programme is necessary. The best way to guarantee this is to involve the parents or care provider. With education on the role of splints/exercise and the impact of rehabilitation on disease progression, most parents are eager and capable participants.
- Joint protection training is important—proper positioning, use of several joints in a task, safe transfer of loads, avoidance of prolonged position, planning of rest breaks, and adapted aids and devices should all be addressed.
- Chronic diseases may elicit different emotions in different children—frustration with lack of mobility in the young, and peer group issues and psychosexual anxieties in the adolescent. Positive adjustment, focusing on strengths not weakness, is important, as is the constant awareness of such issues in those that make up the support structure. Competence comes in many forms, not simply physical ability, and should be praised at every level, building a child's self-esteem.
- Many children who have learned to cope with their disease develop a more mature personality earlier than others in their age group. As such the adolescent may be earlier and better qualified to bid for an independent life despite physical limitations and should be supported.

Adolescents

At some point in a patient's development from childhood to adulthood, the paediatric physician must start to relinquish care to the adult physician. This phase of patient management, the 'transition', should be handled carefully. Some important principles to consider are stated below.

- Transfer should only occur when a young person feels ready to function in an adult clinic.
- From an early stage adolescents should be encouraged to take responsibility for medications.
- The whole concept of independence should be introduced well ahead of an anticipated 'transfer time'. This could be introduced at about the age of 11 years and encouraged by trying to see the adolescent by themselves for part of their consultation by the time they are 13–14 years of age.
- A schedule of events leading to 'transition' and finally to transfer of care should be drawn up.
- Adolescents should be given information on health care rights and taught how to recognize changes in their disease (good or bad) and how to seek help from health professionals.

Pain relief

The descriptors of pain and assessment of impact are discussed in 📖 Chapter 1, p 3.

Many patients will seek non-pharmacological methods of pain relief, having experienced a lack of efficacy or intolerance with analgesic medications, or because of concerns over side-effects. Likewise, patients seek homeopathic remedies, including systemic and topical herbal products (📖 Chapter 23, p 599).

Patients will also use the term 'addiction' to express concerns over the long-term use of stronger analgesics. Rather than 'substance abuse' the patient is most likely reflecting on the possibility of 'tolerance,' i.e. 'becoming used to' the analgesic so that that stronger and stronger agents will be required over time to gain benefit. This often needs clarification during discussion.

That said, abuse of opiates, whether addiction or 'diversion' (recreational use), and deliberate self-harm by overdose with analgesics is a legitimate cause for concern for the prescribing clinician. The safety and suitability of these agents is very much based on assessment of the individual patient.

Non-pharmacological methods of pain relief include:

- Hot/cold/pressure compress.
- Physical therapies—land based and hydrotherapy.
- Transcutaneous electrical nerve stimulation (TENS).
- Acupuncture.
- Hypnosis.
- Cognitive and behavioural therapy (CBT).
- Biofeedback.
- Pulsed radiofrequency and nerve ablation therapies.
- Low level laser therapy (LLLT).
- Massage.
- Relaxation therapy.
- Meditation.
- Aromatherapy.
- Reflexology.
- Reiki.
- Pet relief.
- Cupping.

When assessing the efficacy of analgesic medications one must always ascertain:

- The frequency and maximum dose tried.
- Whether there was any relief that then wore off. Patients may say their painkiller did not work, but on further questioning one discovers that either:
  - they did not take enough, or did not take them frequently enough— here it is about the clinician being clear over dose 'escalation and combination'.
  - the drug actually worked for a few hours and then wore off. Here, it is about the clinician being familiar with 'analgesic half-life'.

Analgesic escalation and half-life

- A clear description of the options for increasing dosage according to tolerability and efficacy should be given, including the principle of starting at the lowest dose whenever possible (particularly in the elderly and infirm). Clear guidance puts the patient in control of their pain relief.
- If a single agent fails to relieve pain, either a compound analgesic or a second drug utilizing a different mechanism can be prescribed. The benefit of using two separate agents (e.g. codeine and paracetamol), rather than a compound is in flexibility of dosage according to fluctuations in need. Equally, a compound agent may be considered easier for the patient to manage albeit that this then restricts flexibility to the number of tablets as opposed to agents used.
- Most analgesics have a short half-life. This makes them suitable for use 'as required'. However, when being used on a daily basis, patients may experience the 'on-off' effect in pain control. This can lead the patient to think that the medication is ineffective; it is often most obvious after periods of sleep. Having identified that the analgesic does give relief, the clinician should look to prescribing a slow-release formulation, aiming to remove the peaks and troughs in systemic concentration of the agent, giving better coverage across longer periods of time, in particular over-night.

Paracetamol and compound analgesics

Paracetamol

Paracetamol (acetaminophen) is available over the counter in many countries. At 4.0 g/day (typical adult dose 1.0 g qds) it is effective in managing soft tissue injury, joint pain, dental pain, and headache. It is usually given orally, but is available in suppository and intravenous formulations also.

It is reasonable to try paracetamol first; most general practitioners will. In doing so, it is important to assure the patient of its efficacy; often the specialist will hear patients say 'my GP just gave me paracetamol'. Perhaps its availability over the counter makes it appear less 'powerful' as an analgesic, its prescription somehow belittling or ignoring the perceived severity of the pain? Common concerns and interactions are shown in Table 21.2.

Table 21.2 Cautions and side effects with paracetamol

Caution	Comment
Hepatic toxicity	Avoid in known significant liver disease, alcohol abuse
Renal toxicity	Note that the effervescent formulations contain sodium—avoid in moderate–severe renal impairment
Blood dyscrasia	E.g. thrombocytopenia, leucopenia can be induced or worsened
Pregnancy and breastfeeding	Not known to be harmful
Common interactions	
Coumarin (warfarin)	Paracetamol may enhance the anticoagulant effect
Absorption and metabolism	Metoclopromide increases absorption, carbamazepine accelerates metabolism of paracetamol

Paracetamol compounds

Paracetamol 500 mg is also available in compound analgesics, such as co-codamol (paracetamol and codeine), co-dydramol (paracetamol and dihydrocodeine), and paracetamol and tramadol. Care should always be taken [as with 'over the counter' aspirin products and other non-steroidal anti-inflammatory drugs (NSAIDs)] that patients ensure they do not take more than the maximum daily dose of paracetamol, irrespective of the combination of single and compound medications used together.

The codeine content varies in these formulations between 10, 15, and 30 mg per tablet to a maximum total daily dose of 240 mg divided in 8 tablets and taken as 2 tablets qds.

Codeine is discussed in 📖 Opioid analgesics, p 555.

Because of safety concerns (primarily related to toxicity in overdose) co-proxamol (paracetamol and dextropropoxyphene) is only available in the UK by special arrangement on a named-patient basis.

Opioid analgesics

For all opioid drugs there are general cautions. These are shown in Table 21.3

Table 21.3 Cautions and side effects of opioid analgesics

Caution	Comment
Hypotension	Particular care when also taking anti-hypertensives, anti-psychotics, or anti-depressants
Sedation and respiratory suppression	Avoid in chronic obstructive pulmonary disease, head injury, any situation of reduced level of consciousness; take particular care when also taking anti-psychotics, anti-depressants, or anti-histamines. Counsel caution over driving and use of machinery
Hepatic toxicity	Avoid in known significant liver disease, reduce dose in mild disease
Renal toxicity	Avoid in known significant renal disease, reduce dose in mild disease
Blood dyscrasia	E.g. thrombocytopenia; leucopenia can be induced or worsened
Porphyria	Avoid
Pregnancy	Avoid
Breastfeeding	Preferably avoid. Note codeine is not known to be harmful as concentration are very small; however, individuals vary in rate of metabolism and close observation should be made for signs of infant morphine overdose
Gastrointestinal	Opioids induce nausea, vomiting, constipation, pancreatitis, obstruction
Neuropsychiatric	Opioids induce head ache, confusion, dys/euphoria, hallucinations, mood change, seizures
Genito-urinary	Sexual dysfunction, urinary retention, avoid in significant obstructive prostatic hypertrophy
Age	Reduce dosage in the elderly, avoid in childhood

Commonly used weak opioids

Codeine

As well as use in compound agents with paracetamol as described above, codeine is often used as a single agent to maximum daily adult dosage of 240 mg as 2 × 30 mg tablets qds.

Codeine is marketed in various salt compounds including phosphate and sulphate (typical in the United States, Canada, and UK), hydrochloride (continental Europe), hydro-iodide and citrate.

Low dose codeine is available 'over the counter' in some countries and is also found in cough suppressants. In the majority of countries, however, it remains prescription only, with concern over dependency and misuse, and in some countries it remains classed as an illegal substance. Travellers with legitimate prescriptions are advised to carry documentation of their condition from their physician. Other common interactions:

- Cimetidine increases plasma concentration of codeine.
- Metoclopramide and domperidone are antagonized by codeine.

Tramadol and meptazinol

Tramadol is a weak opioid agonist. It inhibits the reuptake of both serotonin and norepinephrine at the dorsal horn. The maximum recommended adult dose is 400 mg/day in divided doses. It is available in modified release (200 mg bd) and in combination with paracetamol.

Meptazinol has a similar profile and is given at 800 mg/day in divided doses.

These agents are often tried after or instead of codeine compounds given the difference in mechanism, and before escalating to strong opioids. Although they too cause gastrointestinal (GI) side-effects, this may be one reason for trying them before codeine in those prone to constipation. In the authors experience this benefit may, however, be off-set by a greater risk of intolerance from neuropsychiatric effects.

Commonly used strong opioids

These include morphine sulphate, dihydrocodeine (also available as modified release), and oxycodone hydrochloride 5–10 mg, both 4–6-hourly (can be titrated up to 400 mg per day in severe cases); the latter also has compound of oxycodone/naloxone, which may be beneficial in those with severe constipation from opioids despite trials of different classes of laxative. Thereafter, escalation might move to morphine salts, but before any of these are utilized it is common to try patch formulations.

Patches

These are applied to the skin and, therefore, in addition to the cautions above, be aware of allergic reaction with localized sensitivity.

Buprenorphine (also available orally as Temgesic® 200 μg) is produced as BuTrans® and Transtec®; **fentanyl** as Durogesic DTrans®. Both have formulations that allow a wide variety of dosing; again, starting at the lowest dose, e.g. BuTrans 5, and gradually building up, perhaps every couple of weeks depending on tolerance and severity of symptoms.

Non-steroidal anti-inflammatory drugs

- Anti-inflammatory agents are commonly used in rheumatological disorders. Most have licensed indication for osteoarthritis (📖 Chapter 6, p 259) and rheumatoid arthritis (📖 Chapter 5, p 233); some have license for ankylosing spondylitis (📖 Chapter 8, p 281). In reality, most are prescribed in effect 'off licence' for a number of rheumatic conditions outside these diagnoses, but based on the fact that they are highly effective analgesics with the capacity to reduce inflammation such as occurs in soft-tissues, tendonitis, and synovitis.
- **Ibuprofen** and **aspirin** compounds are available over the counter in many countries. **Naproxen** (250–500 mg bd) and **Diclofenac** (150 mg daily in divided doses) probably represent the two most commonly prescribed NSAIDs worldwide.
- Oral preparations are most often prescribed, also utilizing the benefit of slow-release formulations (as discussed 📖 Chapter 21, p 545, Introduction).
- Although per-rectum agents are also available these do not appear to reduce side-effects (specifically gastric) enough to necessarily warrant their preference over oral in the majority of cases.
- Topical agents have variable efficacy, often with limited evidence of benefit. That said, they are popular with patients as part of their management. Many will also try homeopathic topical agents (📖 Chapter 23, p 599). Common proprietary agents include: **Feldene®**, **Ibugel®**, **Mobigel®**, **Traxam®**, and **Voltarol®**.
- NSAIDs are classified by their inhibitory action on cyclo-oxygenase I (COX-I) or COX-2, recognizing that some agents (e.g. oxicams) demonstrate inhibitory action against both enzyme pathways. It is reasonable to try a NSAID from a different class when another has failed.

Cautions

A number of adverse reactions are recognized; caution applies to all NSAIDs, particularly avoiding their use in hepatic and renal impairment, pregnancy, and GI ulceration. These are shown in Table 21.4. Using the lowest possible dose for the shortest period of time lessens the risk. It is inevitable, however, that those with long-term conditions for which remission is less than optimal will require long-term therapy.

Cardiovascular

Whilst cardio-vascular (CV) complications occur, many patients with cardiovascular disease and risk factors use NSAIDS, particularly if the benefit is considered to outweigh the risk (e.g. improved function/exercise tolerance encourages a healthier lifestyle). It is imperative that blood pressure and renal function are monitored regularly (preferably every 3 months).

The highest risk of CV complications is with diclofenac, COX-2s (see below), and high dose ibuprofen (2.4 g daily); the lowest risk is with naproxen (1 g daily) and ibuprofen (1.2 g or below daily). It is not uncommon for individuals to also be on aspirin for its platelet inhibitory function.

Gastrointestinal

The gastro-intestinal risks are documented in Table 21.3. The greatest risk is seen with **azapropazone**, medium risk with **diclofenac, etodolac, indometacin, ketoprofen, naproxen,** and oxicams, and the lowest risk with ibuprofen.

Renal

NSAIDs should be used with caution and avoided if possible. The 'rule of thumb' of lowest possible dose for shortest possible period of time applies. Note that NSAIDs can induce acute renal failure, as well as exacerbate chronic impairment.

Respiratory

The exacerbation of asthma is a recognized concern; however, it should not be an absolute contra-indication to prescribing. Many patients may well have inadvertently tried aspirin and ibuprofen over-the-counter compounds without complication. The clinician may therefore gain some sense of tolerability. The decision to prescribe should always be based on the severity and responsiveness/stability of asthma in each individual.

Disease-modifying anti-rheumatic drug

Concern is often expressed over the co-administration of disease-modifying antirheumatic drugs (DMARDs) and NSAIDs. Toxicity monitoring is a fundamental responsibility when managing DMARDs. The general principles of monitoring introduction of DMARDs are described in Table 21.7. Typically, this is intensive for 6–12 weeks, then settles to 3-monthly. This applies irrespective of concomitant use of NSAID. Perhaps more importantly, the early intensive monitoring regimen should also apply when an NSAID is introduced to the patient already on a stable dose of DMARD.

Pregnancy and breastfeeding

It is generally advised that NSAIDs should be avoided in pregnancy unless the benefits to well-being significantly outweigh the risk. Even then usage applies to the first and second trimester. In the third trimester added risk occurs including non-closure of the foetal ductus arteriosus, delay in onset and an increase in the duration of labour. In addition, pulmonary hypertension may affect the newborn infant.

In some cases, studies show concentrations of certain NSAIDs to be too low in breast milk to warrant concern. In general, manufacturers advise avoiding NSAIDs for the duration of breastfeeding. Aspirin is absolutely contra-indicated.

Table 21.4 Adverse reactions of NSAIDs

Organ/ complication	Occurrence	Comments
GI tract	Common	Gastritis, bleeding, and perforation. High risk in the elderly and those with a history of ulcers
Renal	Common	Fluid retention, papillary necrosis
Hypertension	Common	Interference with drugs such as thiazide diuretics
Myocardial infarction	Increased risk in those with cardiovascular risk factors	COX-1 and COX-2 drugs
Pulmonary	Not uncommon	Exacerbation of asthma, pneumonitis (naproxen)
Skin	Not uncommon	Hypersensitivity, erythema multiforme
Central nervous system (CNS)	Not uncommon	Tinnitus, fatigue, cognitive disturbance
	Rare	Aseptic meningitis
Hepatic	Uncommon	Drug-induced hepatitis
Haematological	Rare	Bone marrow dyscrasias

Aspirin

As the prototype NSAID, Aspirin is available in single and compound formulations over the counter. Whilst it is rarely prescribed as an NSAID it is important to acknowledge its availability, as well as its common use in lower dosage (75–150 mg od) as a cardio-protective agent, when prescribing other NSAIDs, and advising on side effects and drug interactions.

For analgesic effect aspirin is dosed at 300–900 mg qds (max. adult dose 4 g per day). It is available in oral and suppository formulations.

Aspirin should not be given to children under the age of 16 years given the risk of Reye's syndrome.

Oxicams

This group of NSAIDs was developed for their longer half-life. **Meloxicam** and **piroxicam** are the two most commonly used agents.

Coxibs/COX-2 inhibitors

These agents were introduced because of their efficacy and selective COX-2 inhibition, recognizing the value of preserving COX-1 'protective' enzyme activity, particularly in relation to gastro-intestinal tolerability.

However, large-scale phase III control trials, an integral part of modern pharmalogical practice and essential in seeking approval for license, demonstrated an appreciable cardiovascular risk. As a consequence, several COX-2 inhibitor drugs (rofecoxib, valdecoxib) have been withdrawn, and more is now understood from retro/prospective studies of NSAIDs in general, triggered by the concern that older agents have never had this rigorous assessment.

Celecoxib and **etoricoxib** are available in Europe. **Celecoxib** is available in the USA; in Dec 2007 the Food and Drug Administration (FDA) voted not to approve etoricoxib. Both require regular monitoring of blood pressure.

Antidepressants

- Several drugs in this group are used in the management of pain, usually as a single nocturnal agent, sometimes in combination using different mechanisms of action, and often at lower doses than typically used for controlling depression.
- There is often a need to explain to patients that these drugs are being used for pain control and not for depression, even if there is a degree of reactive-depression present as a consequence of chronic pain.
  The idea arises in some patients that the clinician just thinks they are depressed or that the pain is 'in the mind,' and that is the real reason why they have been prescribed an 'anti-depressant'. They initially fail to appreciate the potential value of these drugs as analgesics.
- Educating the patient and explaining the mechanisms of action (blocking pain messages from travelling up the spinal cord and modifying the response to pain in the midbrain), one can gain greater compliance and enhance the clinician–patient relationship. A detailed exploration of the mechanisms is beyond the scope of this book, but most agents are thought to have a dual effect by modifying responsiveness of spinal opioid receptors, and changing mood and perception centrally.
- These agents are perhaps most logically used when pain disturbs sleep. A mild sedative and relaxant effect may also be beneficial.

Serotonin and norepinephrine reuptake inhibitors

Tricyclics

Tricyclics are predominantly serotonin and/or norepinephrine re-uptake inhibitors. The 'typical' agents in this group include Amitriptyline, clomipramine, imipramine and dosulepin.

Amitriptyline is the agent most frequently used (although sometimes Nortriptyline is better tolerated). Given at doses up to 75 mg/day, it is often titrated from a baseline of 10–25 mg in 10 mg steps every 3–4 days until a balance between maximum efficacy and tolerability is reached. Common side effects and interactions are shown in Table 21.5.

Selective serotonin reuptake inhibitors

This group includes **fluoxetine** (20–40 mg), **sertraline** (50 mg), and **paroxetine** (20 mg). Randomized control trials in fibromyalgia demonstrate efficacy similar to that of 25 mg amitriptyline; however, the average impact on pain reduction and quality of life is only about 15–20% and, as such, these agents are probably not suitable candidates as analgesics when used in isolation. The side effect profile in Table 21.5 applies.

Mixed serotonin-norepinephrine reuptake inhibitors

Increasing interest in the complexities of central pain pathways and the action of serotonin-norepinephrine reuptake inhibitors (SNRIs) has led to several studies demonstrating efficacy in the chronic pain condition fibromyalgia (FM; 📖 Chapter 18, p 489).

Table 21.5 Cautions and side-effects of serotonin/norepinephrine re-uptake inhibitors

Caution	Comment
Sedative	Care needed when used with other potentially sedating agent. Note: CNS toxic effects of tramadol can be enhanced (serotonin syndrome). Also note caution with driving or using machinery.
Anti-muscarinic action	Caution in those with ocular (closed-angle glaucoma), genito-urinary (retention, prostatic hypertrophy), dry eyes/mouth, constipation
Cardiovascular	Risk of dysrhythmias especially ventricular (e.g. increased with concomitant use of sotalol and amiodarone)
Hypotension	Increased risk in patients on diuretics
Thyroid disease	Amitriptyline enhances effects of thyroid drugs
Epilepsy	Amitriptyline antagonizes anti-epileptics reducing the threshold for seizures
Sexual dysfunction	
Hyponatraemia	
Hepatic impairment	Try to avoid in severe liver disease—risk of sedation
Pregnancy and breastfeeding	Avoid unless being used for psychiatric reasons and in the best interests of well-being
Neuropsychiatric	Induction of hallucinations, delusions, (hypo)mania, neuroleptic malignant syndrome, and suicidal behaviour
Motor function	Tremor/extrapyramidal signs
Endocrine	Breast enlargement, galactorrhoea

The FDA (USA) approved **duloxetine** (in 2008) and **milnacipran** (in 2009) for treatment of FM in adults. Neither is approved for use in children.

Duloxetine is given as 60–120 mg daily; milnacipran at 100 mg bd. Side effects include nausea, headache, insomnia, dizziness, constipation, hepatic dysfunction, hyponatraemia, and orthostatic hypotension (duloxetine) and hypertension (milnacipran). Like all anti-depressants duloxetine carries a warning highlighting an increased risk of suicide, especially among children and young adults.

Tramadol should not be co-administered with duloxetine; there is a risk of developing serotonin syndrome. Through cytochrome P450 enzyme system interactions, duloxetine may prolong effects of opioids.

Hyponatraemia can be rapid in onset and profound, leading to serious cardiovascular and neuropsychiatric complications, and occasionally death.

Anticonvulsants

Carbamazepine (100–200 mg daily) is an analgesic option in the management of trigeminal neuralgia, glossopharyngeal neuralgia, post-herpetic neuralgia, and diabetic neuropathy. The side effects are similar to those described below and there should be caution with concomitant use of anti-depressants. Given the risk-benefit associated with epilepsy, carbamazepine is used with caution during pregnancy; however, if it can be withdrawn when only used as an analgesic it should.

More recently, with better description and assessment of neuropathic pain, the drug.

Gabapentin and its analog **pregabalin** [both structural analogues of γ-aminobutyric acid (GABA)], has been shown to have efficacy, particularly in studies of FM (🕮 Chapter 18, p 489).

Gabapentin can be titrated from 300–3600 mg daily in divided doses; Pregabalin from 150–600 mg daily in divided doses.

The most common side effects include dizziness/light-headedness, oedema and weight gain, and sedation. Other concerns include ataxia, Stevens Johnson Syndrome, hepato-biliary and pancreatic pathology.

Both should be avoided during pregnancy and breastfeeding.

Muscle relaxants

Drugs such as baclofen, dantrolene, methocarbamol, and tizanidine usually sit within the realm of the neurologist and may be valuable in controlling muscle spasm and pain in conditions such as stroke and multiple sclerosis. Where indicated the rheumatologist should seek advice from a neurologist if spasm pain is considered to be the consequence of a neurological condition.

For the rheumatologist the most likely agent to consider is **diazepam**, a benzodiazepine. Given at doses of 2–5 mg tds for up to 14 days at any one time it can be helpful in alleviating acute severe pain associated with spasm, particularly across the neck and shoulder girdle, and the lumbar spine.

As with opioids care should be taken to counsel the patient over perceived risk of dependency, and prescription should be avoided if there are any concerns over potential abuse.

Benzodiazepines should be avoided in hepatic and renal impairment, pregnancy and breastfeeding.

Quinine sulphate is often used in doses of 200–300 mg to control nocturnal cramps. It should be prescribed with caution noting the following:

- Increased risk of atrial fibrillation, conduction defects, heart block particularly in the elderly (baseline and monitor ECG) during parenteral treatment.
- Avoid or halve the dose in hepatic and renal impairment.
- May be teratogenic (certainly in higher dosage) in the first trimester of pregnancy, but safe during breastfeeding.
- Contra-indicated in haemoglobinuria, myasthenia gravis, optic neuritis, and tinnitus.

Topical agents

The most common classes to be used (excluding opioid transcutaneous delivery by patch) include a variety of 'over the counter' preparations (rubefacients), NSAIDs [perhaps logical if there is superficial local pain (see above)] and capsaicin.

Capsaicin is licensed for the relief of post-herpetic neuralgia and diabetic neuropathy. The major problem is risk of severe burning sensation and irritation if contact is made with mucous membranes, including the lips and conjunctiva. Hand-washing after use should be meticulous.

Capsaicin is prescribed as a 45-g tube of 0.025% or 0.075% concentration, to be applied twice daily in the smallest of volume; literally a tiny amount squeezed onto the tip of the little finger and then rubbed in over the site of pain.

Glucocorticoids

Corticosteroid use could be considered ubiquitous in managing rheumatological conditions. They are powerful anti-inflammatories and range in use from short duration low and high dosage to gain control of a condition [including intra-articular (📖 Chapter 22, p 589)], through to prolonged and even life-long therapy.

It is not the intention of this section to go through each agent. The indications and common dosing regimens are discussed throughout Part II, under each specific disease condition.

Table 21.6 highlights the major and common cautions and concerns that should be monitored and discussed with the patient.

Patients should be encouraged to hold a steroid card or some form of alert bracelet, etc.

Table 21.6 Cautions and complications of glucocorticoids use

Caution	Comment
Endocrine/renal	Long-term use can lead to adrenal atrophy
Adrenal insufficiency	Abrupt withdrawal should be avoided
	Replacement (even higher dosing) should be given during surgery, intercurrent illness (especially associated vomiting).
Diabetes	Induction and exacerbation of hyperglycaemia
Hypokalaemia	
Infection	Corticosteroids are immunosuppressive—there is a theoretical risk of increase in general infections
	Live viral immunization should be avoided
	Exposure to chickenpox of measles leading to concern over significant infection should be managed with passive immunoglobulin
	May expose latent TB
Neuropsychiatric	Can induce mania, confusion, delirium, and suicidal thoughts—can occur early after starting corticosteroid (3–5 days on average) and take several weeks to resolve having discontinued therapy.
Weight gain	This may be either as a consequence of peripheral oedema or increased appetite—patients should be warned to be careful of this and to use tricks like drinks of water to reduce sense of hunger
Skin	Long-term use leads to atrophy and bruising
Eyes	Increased risk of cataracts and glaucoma
Cardiovascular	Induction and exacerbation of hypertension and congestive cardiac failure

Table 21.6 (Cont'd)

Caution	Comment
Peptic ulceration	
Bone and muscle	Induction and exacerbation of osteoporosis
	Growth retardation
	Myopathy
	Avascular necrosis
Pregnancy	No evidence of teratogenic effects; occasional neonatal adrenal suppression; better avoided, but can be used or continued if indicated—prednisone dose preferably not >10 mg/day.
Breastfeeding	*Breastfeeding:* drug should be avoided on theoretical grounds, especially if dose >7.5 mg/day prednisone or equivalent.

Specific drug interactions
- *All anti-hypertensives:* because of the tendency for corticosteroids to increase blood pressure they may antagonize the hypotensive effect of anti-hypertensives in any class.
- *Barbiturates and anti-epileptics:* increase the metabolism of corticosteroids.
- *Diuretics:* effect may be antagonized by corticosteroids.
- *Erythromycin and azoles:* may inhibit the metabolism of corticosteroids thus increasing their effect.
- *NSAIDs:* add to the risk of GI ulceration.
- *Methotrexate:* corticosteroids may increase the risk of bone marrow suppression.
- *Theophylline:* increases the risk of hypokalaemia.
- *Warfarin:* corticosteroids may increase or decrease the anti-coagulant effect.

(Non-biologic) disease-modifying anti-rheumatic drugs

- Non-biologic disease-modifying anti-rheumatic drugs (DMARDS) are a cornerstone in the arrest and remission of destructive inflammatory rheumatic disease. In Part II of this book reference is made to their use in controlling joint and end-organ disease in conditions such as rheumatic arthritis (RA), psoriatic arthritis, juvenile idiopathic arthritis (JIA), systemic lupus erythematosus (SLE), myositis, and vasculitis.
- Terminology can be confusing since the introduction of 'Biologics' as these, too, are DMARDs. For the purposes of this book we have used the traditional term 'DMARD' to apply to 'non-biological' agents, and the term 'Biologic' for the newer groups of agents.
- DMARDs are slow acting drugs that take 8–12 weeks to begin to demonstrate benefit, and even then possibly longer to achieve maximum benefit as the dose is escalated (typically over 6 months). Patients should always be informed of this, clarifying expectation and improving compliance.
- It is not uncommon for combinations of DMARDs to be used either by sequential 'step up' (adding one after the other over time) or 'step down' (starting typically with 2 or 3, and reducing to 1 over time). It is unlikely that more than 3 DMARDs would be used since the introduction of Biologics; UK guidance allows use of Biologics after failure of at least 2 DMARDs (see below).
- The most common drugs used are (in alphabetical order): azathioprine, hydroxychloroquine, leflunomide, methotrexate, and sulfasalazine; amongst these methotrexate is probably the drug of first choice for 50–60% of cases because it is considered the most appropriate one to initiate in the presence of moderate-severe erosive-joint disease in the more common conditions such as RA (🕮 Chapter 5, p 233).

Common concerns and themes

DMARDs are not without their toxicity and the protean complications and monitoring requirements can seem daunting. In the first part of this section Tables 21.7–21.10 describe common themes applicable to all DMARDs. Each DMARD will then be presented in alphabetical order with a description of dosing and specific concerns over monitoring and toxicity.

The common themes described below are:
- Advice on immunization and risk assessment of viral infection (Table 21.7).
- General monitoring regimen (Table 21.8).
- Common side-effects and initial action to be taken (Table 21.9).
- Use in pregnancy and breastfeeding (Table 21.10).
- All drugs should be used with caution in hepatic and renal impairment, blood dyscrasias (including suspected or known G6PD deficiency, and porphyria), recurrent infection, and in the elderly.

Table 21.7 Immunization and assessment of infection risk before commencing DMARDs

1 Patients on DMARDs must not receive live vaccine immunization (e.g. oral polio, BCG, MMR, yellow fever)

2 Patients should receive the pneumococcal vaccine

3 Annual flu vaccination is recommended

4 Patients exposed to chickenpox (who have no clear history of chicken pox in the past) or to shingles, should receive passive immunization using varicella zoster immunoglobulin (VZIG)

5 Patients should be screened for hepatitis B and C risk by history, and if required serum antibodies

6 Patients should be assessed for risk of HIV and tested if applicable

7 Patients should be assessed for risk of active/latent TB

Surgery and infective illness

DMARDs do not need to be discontinued before surgery. They are discontinued during severe infective illness if there is concern their immunosuppressant effect outweighs the risk of a disease flare.

If the surgeon wishes DMARDs to be stopped then, as a 'rule of thumb', it is reasonable to discontinue for 2 weeks before and up to 2 weeks after surgery.

It is not possible to predict the risk of a flare of inflammation during this period, although many patients report a level of tolerance for up to 4 weeks. Often steroids need to be given if there is a 'flare', potentially negating the benefit of having stopped the DMARD.

Co-administered NSAIDs

Concern is often expressed over the co-administration of DMARDs and NSAIDs. Toxicity monitoring is a fundamental responsibility when managing DMARDs. The general principles of monitoring introduction of DMARDs is described in Table 21.8; typically, this is intensive for 6–12 weeks and then settles to 3-monthly. This applies irrespective of concomitant use of NSAID. Perhaps more importantly the early intensive monitoring regimen should also apply when an NSAID is introduced in the patient already on a stable dose of DMARD.

Family planning, pregnancy, and breastfeeding

In general DMARDs should be stopped at least 3 months before (in men and women) trying to conceive; contraceptive methods are advised for the 3 months. Certainly, the majority of DMARDs should be stopped having fallen pregnant. Table 21.10 outlines specific regimens advised before trying to conceive, and which drugs to avoid during pregnancy and breastfeeding.

The one exception is leflunomide. In women this should have been stopped **2 years** before trying to conceive, or 'washed' out as described below.

Advice on use of analgesics and corticosteroids in pregnancy and breastfeeding is given in the sections above.

Table 21.8 Principles of monitoring. General rules may vary with local protocols/policy

Time line	Action
Pre-treatment assessment	FBC, U&E, LFTs
	CRP and ESR
	Urinalysis (protein)
	CXR (methotrexate)
	Blood pressure
	Exclude current infection
	Exclude unexplained rash/skin lesion
	Complete applicable disease activity assessment tools
	Visual acuity assessment (hydrochloroquine)
Early monitoring on treatment First 6–8 weeks	FBC and LFT every 2 weeks for 6–8 weeks except: • Hydroxycholoroquine (not required) • Gold (before every dose) • Sulfasalazine (every 4 weeks) • U&Es also for ciclosporin
6–8-week clinical review	FBC, U&E, LFTs
	CRP and ESR
	Urinalysis (protein)
	Blood pressure
	Exclude current infection
	Exclude unexplained rash/skin lesion
	Complete applicable disease activity assessment tools
8 weeks to 6 months If on stable dose	FBC and LFT every 4 weeks except: • Hydroxycholoroquine (not required) • Gold (before every dose) • Sulfasalazine (every 4 weeks) • Some drugs require close monitoring of U&Es and urinalysis—see ciclosporin
6-month clinical review	FBC, U&E, LFTs
	CRP and/or ESR (as part of assessment criteria)
	Urinalysis (protein)
	Blood pressure
	Exclude current infection
	Exclude unexplained rash/skin lesion
	Complete applicable disease activity assessment tools

Table 21.8 (Cont'd)

Time line	Action
6 months onward If on stable dose	FBC and LFT every 8–12 weeks Some drugs require close monitoring of U&E and urinalysis—see ciclosporin
12 month Clinical Review	FBC, U&E, LFTs CRP and ESR
(repeat 6 monthly if stable)	Urinalysis (protein) Blood pressure Exclude current infection Exclude unexplained rash/skin lesion Complete applicable disease activity assessment tools

General principles	• Return to the early monitoring protocol whenever increasing after a period of stable dosage, or when introducing another DMARD or an NSAID or other potentially toxic drug (by interaction) for the first time.
	• Any sequential negative change (3 recordings in a row) in biochemical or haematological indices should be reviewed irrespective of whether the count is inside the normal range.
	• If concern over toxicity a detailed history should include enquiry as to:
	  • over the counter preparations
	  • alcohol consumption
	  • any intercurrent illness (typically an infection)
	  • dosing error of DMARD

Sequential negative changes in monitoring tests

DMARDs should be re-assessed if there is any sequential negative change (3 recordings in a row) in biochemical or haematological indices, irrespective of whether the values have fallen inside the normal range.

Whenever there is concern over the potential toxicity of a DMARD a detailed history is required as to recent change in medication including:
• Over the counter preparations.
• Alcohol consumption.
• Any intercurrent illness (typically an infection).
• Dosing error of DMARD.

Malignancy

Many of these drugs are associated with an increased risk of lymphoma and skin malignancies. The possibility of these should always be part of the enquiry on clinical review, at least in the form of an enquiry over skin changes noticed and 'B' symptoms of weight loss and night sweats

Shared care information

It is essential that the patient receive written information and advice on these drugs, and that they and their primary care physician have access to correspondence from the prescribing clinician and results of monitoring whether this be by paper or electronic means. It is also essential that there is clarity over the roles and responsibilities of the prescribing and primary/community clinician, and the patient. How this is done varies in shared-care protocols, but the principles remain the same.

A detailed British Society for Rheumatology guideline on DMARD monitoring (2008) and a Quick Reference guide on monitoring (2009) can be found at: http://www.rheumatology.org.uk/resources/guidelines/bsr_guidelines.aspx

The information in Tables 21.9 and 21.10 is a broad general guideline. Detailed information can be obtained from national sites. Two examples are:

- British Society for Rheumatology. Available at: http://www.rheumatology.org.uk/resources/guidelines/bsr_guidelines.aspx
- American College of Rheumatology. Available at: http://www.rheumatology.org/wren/acrsearch.asp?zoom_query=DMARDmonitoring

The following section takes each (non-biological) DMARD in alphabetical order and describes drug specific considerations that have not been discussed in the section above.

Azathioprine

Azathioprine is prescribed for a number of autoimmune conditions, rheumatic, hepatic and gastro-intestinal, dermal, renal, and neurological. The typical dose is 0.5–2.5 mg/kg/day oral, increasing after 4–6 weeks to 2–3 mg/kg/day with an anticipated response within 6–12 weeks.

Specific cautions

Thiopurine methyl transferase (TPMT) deficiency:

- Many clinicians do not check this routinely, particularly if monitoring toxicity closely over the first 6–12 weeks.
- 99.7% of individuals will have high or intermediate TPMT levels. Measuring levels in this group does not predict risk of toxicity. Criteria for assigning risk of homozygous status are not available, although suspicion would arise if there were any family history of major adverse reaction to drugs.

Table 21.9 Common side effects to assess with every set of blood tests and every clinical review

Concern	Action
Abnormal AST/ALT on LFT	Only stop DMARD if enzyme level > twice upper limit of normal. As with all blood indices below, repeat weekly until normalized
Abnormal white blood cell	Only stop if WBC<3.0 × 10^9/L, neutropenia <1.5 × 10^9/L.
	Eosinophilia >0.5 × 10^9/L increased vigilance required
Low platelets	Only stop if platelets <100 × 10^9/L
Abnormal bruising	Check clotting and platelets, and withhold immediately
Abnormal MCV	MCV>110 fl, check serum folate, B12 & TSH.
	Note may be direct effect of azathioprine, methotrexate or sulfasalazine
Proteinuria	Exclude infection and treat
	If persistent, quantify, check U&Es, exclude haematuria and casts and consider a KUB ultrasound first before stopping agent if it is known to cause proteinuria.
	Note: the proteinuria may be a manifestation of worsening disease and stopping the DMARD may be appropriate
Rash	If mild, may respond to small drop in DMARD dose or leave alone and monitor.
	If moderate to severe—stop DMARD
Mucosal ulceration	If mild, may respond to small drop in DMARD dose or leave alone. Add folic acid (see methotrexate below) and monitor.
	If moderate to severe—stop
Hair loss	If mild, may respond to small drop in DMARD dose or leave alone and monitor
	If moderate to severe—stop, but not may not recover for 1 hair cycle, i.e. several months.
Hypertension	If mild rise, may respond to small drop in DMARD dose or leave alone and monitor
	If moderate to severe—treat hypertension first (see advice for ciclosporin on dose reduction)
Weight-loss	If mild rise, may respond to small drop in DMARD dose or leave alone and monitor
	If moderate to severe—stop DMARD
Breathless	Auscultate the chest and CXR
	Treat infection/cardiac failure, etc.
	If suspicion of pulmonary fibrosis stop treatment and arrange for further investigation (see methotrexate below).

(Continued)

Table 21.9 *(Cont'd)*

Concern	Action
General rule if stopping a DMARD	<ul><li>Repeat blood test after 1 and 2 weeks in first instance.</li><li>A detailed history is required as to recent change in medication including over the counter preparations, alcohol consumption, intercurrent illness, dosing error of DMARD.</li><li>Be prepared to cover inflammatory 'flare' with corticosteroid.</li><li>Any sequential change (3 recordings in a row) in biochemical or haematological indices should be reviewed irrespective of whether the count lies within the cut off points described above.</li><li>Once abnormalities return to normal the DMARD might be re-started at lower dose assuming efficacy in the first place or a new DMARD tried, in both cases returning to the 'early monitoring' phase and following through as in timeline in Table 21.7.</li></ul>

- Although measurement of TPMT is advised in many protocols, it is often impractical. Close monitoring in the first 6–12 weeks is imperative.
- However, in the homozygous state (0.3% of the population) it may be fatal—toxicity likely to appear in the first 6 weeks.
- In the heterozygous (10% of the population) this may be associated with delayed (up to 6 months), but usually reversible bone marrow toxicity.

Photosensitivity reaction—patients should be advised to wear sunscreens and protective covering.

Specific drug interactions
- *Allopurinol:* azathioprine dose should be reduced—recommended 0.25–0.5 mg/kg/day.
- *Angiotensin-converting enzyme (ACE) inhibitors:* co-prescription may exacerbate anaemia.
- *Anticonvulsants:* azathioprine may reduce absorption.
- *Aminosalicylates (mesal/olsal/sulfasalazine):* increase risk of bone marrow toxicity.
- *Ciclosporin:* azathioprine can decrease ciclosporin levels.
- *Co-trimoxazole and trimethoprim:* life-threatening bone marrow toxicity.
- *Warfarin:* azathioprine inhibits anticoagulant effects.

Ciclosporin

Although rarely used it is most typically encountered in PsA, RA, and JIA. It should be avoided in PSA if PUVA has been given (see below). It is dosed at 2.5 mg/kg/day in 2 divided doses for 6 weeks, and then may be increased at 4-weekly intervals in 25 mg increments up to a maximum dose of 4 mg/kg/day. A response is usually observed within 12 weeks.

Additional monitoring:

- Pre-monitoring (Table 21.8) should include fasting lipids, repeated 6-monthly and the drug discontinued if an uncontrollable significant rise occurs.
- Calculate creatinine clearance/GFR. A rise in creatinine >30% above baseline on 2 consecutive readings 7 days apart warrants stopping the drug and reassessing.
- It is essential that blood pressure monitoring be commenced at baseline. If uncontrollable hypertension occurs the drug should be stopped.
- Electrolyte balance should be checked every 2 weeks until stable dose achieved and then every 3 months with other routine monitoring (Table 21.8). If the potassium rises above the laboratory threshold the drug should be stopped and re-assessed [having ensured not consequent on other medication changes, e.g. diuretic (see below)].
- Specific cautions.
- Grapefruit (including juice) increases the bioavailability of ciclosporin. Grapefruit should be avoided for an hour before and after taking the drug.

Table 21.10 Disease modifying anti-rheumatic drugs in pregnancy and breastfeeding

Drug	Effects
Azathioprine	*Pregnancy*: no convincing evidence of teratogenic effects; occasional neonatal adrenal and white cell suppression. Risk-benefit assessment advised with dose reduction if possible. *Breastfeeding*: Avoid drug
Hydroxychloroquine	*Pregnancy*: adverse effects unlikely from limited data; termination not justified, drug can be continued. Risk-benefit assessment advised with dose reduction if possible. *Breastfeeding*: Avoid drug
Leflunomide	*Pregnancy and breastfeeding*: teratogenic—avoid drug **Note:** the drug has a long half-life. Rapid removal of the active metabolite can be achieved using washout with colestyramine 8 g tds or activated charcoal 50 g qds for 11 days. Blood concentrations should be checked twice, 14 days apart prior to conceiving (levels should be < 0.02 mg/L)
Methotrexate	*Pregnancy*: teratogenic and abortificient. Termination not mandatory. Long-term follow-up data lacking - Avoid drug. *Breastfeeding*: avoid drug
Mycophenolate mofetil	*Pregnancy*: Avoid drug *Breastfeeding*: Avoid drug **Note:** in family planning the drug should be discontinued for at least 6 weeks with contraception advised.
Sulfasalazine	*Pregnancy*: isolated report of foetal abnormalities, but limited data and no convincing reports of teratogenic effects; drug can be continued. *Breastfeeding*: inadequate data; probably safe if dose not >2 g/day. **Note:** can be prescribed to men, but may be transient and reversible oligospermia
Other DMARDs • Auranofin • Ciclosporin • Chlorambucil • Cyclophosphamide • Penicillamine • Sodium aurothiomalate	Avoid in pregnancy and breastfeeding

Specific drug interactions
- *Calcium channel blockers:* reduce dose of ciclosporin to 50%.
- *Colchicine:* should be avoided.
- *Diclofenac:* reduce the maximum dosage of diclofenac to 75 mg daily.
- *Digoxin:* measure levels and reduce dose accordingly—ciclosporin can increase serum levels.
- *Diuretics:* caution with electrolyte imbalance.
- *Hydroxychloroquine:* may increase plasma concentrations of ciclosporin.
- *PUVA:* avoid ciclosporin given significant increase risk of invasive squamous cell carcinoma.
- *Simvastatin:* avoid dosing above 10 mg/day.
- *St. John's Wort:* decreases ciclosporin activity.

Cyclophosphamide

This drug is usually reserved for severe autoimmune rheumatic conditions, and primarily for the remission induction of vasculitis.

It is dosed at 1–1.5 mg/kg/day orally and 500–1000 mg intravenous. Intravenous dosing is typically once every 4 weeks for up to 6 months after which (assuming remission is achieved) patients are often switched to azathioprine or methotrexate.

The introduction of biologics has meant that in many severe cases where once there might only have been cyclophosphamide, now there are viable, and potentially less toxic and more effective alternatives.

Specific cautions
- Gametogenesis is severely impaired and irreversible; patients should be counselled re storage of sperm/ova.
- Urothelial toxicity from the active metabolite Acrolein can cause haemorrhagic cystitis. Patients should be well hydrated before taking cyclophosphamide and for 24–48 h after iv administration.
- Mesna is given to reduce risk of urothelial toxicity; usual dosage 2 g before, and repeated 2 and 6 h after iv therapy. Common side-effects include nausea, vomiting, diarrhoea, arthralgia, fatigue, headache, tachycardia, and hypotension.

Specific drug interactions
- *Avoid clozapine:* increased risk of agranulocytosis.
- *Digoxin:* cyclophosphamide reduces absorption.
- *Phenytoin:* cyclophosphamide reduces absorption.

Gold (auranofin and sodium aurothiomalate)

- Gold is used in the management of RA and JIA. It is given as 3 mg
  2–3 times daily oral (auranofin — not licensed in the UK) or perhaps
  more often as a 50 mg im injection (sodium aurothiomalate).
- A test dose of 10 mg im sodium aurothiomalate should be given on the
  first occasion; thereafter 50 mg is given weekly until response achieved.
  Thereafter, the injection is given every 4 weeks. In children it should be
  dosed at 1 mg/kg up to a maximum of 50 mg.
- If no response is seen after a cumulative dose of 1 g (approx. 20 weekly
  doses) of sodium aurothiomalate, it should be discontinued.

Additional monitoring

FBC and urinalysis (for proteinuria) on each occasion before injection.

Specific cautions

- Both agents should be used with caution if there is a history of urticaria,
  eczema or inflammatory bowel disease.
- Both are contraindicated in severe renal or hepatic impairment,
  ulcerative colitis, history of marrow dysplasia, porphyria, exfoliative
  dermatitis, SLE, and pulmonary fibrosis/bronchiolitis.

Specific drug interactions

- Gold should not be given with penicillamine as it increases risk of
  toxicity.
- There is also an increased risk of anaphylaxis in patients also taking
  angiotensin-converting-enzyme inhibitors.

Hydroxychloroquine

Hydroxychloroquine (200–400 mg daily, oral) is an antimalarial drug often
encountered in the management of RA, JIA, and SLE, and as a 'steroid
sparing' agent.

It is important to note that it may exacerbate psoriasis and is contraindicated if maculopathy is present.

Additional monitoring

At baseline there should be an assessment of visual acuity. Enquire as
to any form of impairment that is not corrected by glasses. Near vision
testing should demonstrate the capacity to read small print N8 or N6
on an acuity chart. If there are concerns at baseline the patient should
be referred to an optometrist initially (possibly an ophthalmologist thereafter) and the drug withheld.

Once on the drug, patients should report any changes in visual acuity/
blurring; this would trigger re-assessment at any time and immediate
withdrawal of the drug until the nature of the problem is found.
Otherwise, visual acuity assessment should take place annually as per
baseline, preferably by an optometrist.

Specific drug interactions

- Hydroxychloroquine can increase the plasma concentration of digoxin,
  methotrexate, and ciclosporin.
- Avoid use with amiodarone, quinine, mefloquine, and quinolones for
  risk of hypersensitivity reaction.

Leflunomide

Leflunomide (10–20 mg daily) is used in RA and psoriatic arthritis (PsA), and often concomitant with methotrexate.

A loading dose of 100 mg daily for 3 days is suggested in the literature but often this causes gastrointestinal upset and most practitioners avoid it, starting at 10 mg and increasing to 20 mg after 6–12 weeks according to tolerability and efficacy.

It has a long half-life and therefore requires washout if severe toxicity is expected.

Rapid removal of the active metabolite can be achieved using colestyramine 8 g tds or activated charcoal 50 g qds for 11 days. Blood concentrations should be checked twice, 14 days apart prior to conceiving (levels should be <0.02 mg/L).

Specific cautions
- Hypertension.
- Pneumonitis acute allergic reaction.
- Women planning a family should have stopped leflunomide for 2 years (teratogenic) (men 3 months) before trying to conceive.

Specific drug interactions
- Risk of bone marrow toxicity increased by the co-use of leflunomide and methotrexate (note: they are nevertheless often used together for their synergy).
- Leflunomide can increase anticoagulation effect of warfarin, the hypoglycaemic effects of tolbutamide, and the concentration of phenytoin.

Methotrexate

- Methotrexate is the most commonly used DMARD.
- The typical dosage is 7.5–25 mg once a week.
- Regimens for commencing therapy may have slight variations, but typically begin at 5–7.5 mg per week and increase by 2.5–5 mg every 2 weeks for a period of 6–8 weeks, such that at the point of next assessment the dose is 10–20 mg. The typical maintenance dose is 10–25 mg once a week (occasionally split over 2 days if nausea is excessive).
- A lower dose and slower escalation should be considered in the elderly and frail.
- GI side effects may prohibit oral use. The drug can be given by intramuscular and subcutaneous route also, using the same dosing regimen.

Note: tablets should be taken whole, not crushed or chewed.

Note: tablets come in 2.5 and 10 mg sizes—it is recommended that only 2.5 mg tablets are prescribed to avoid confusion and risk of overdose. However, this is a conversation for the clinician, pharmacist, and patient as to which is the preferred prescribing pattern for the patient; most importantly this tablet size should then not be altered for risk of confusion.

The monitoring profile in Table 21.8 is typical of the introduction and management of methotrexate.

Folic acid (5 mg) is given to reduce side effects. Often this is prescribed once weekly (preferably the day after methotrexate), but may be increased to 6 days of the week avoiding the same day as methotrexate.

Indications for increasing the folic acid include:
• Raised MCV.
• Mildly deranged LFTs.
• Anaemia.
• Mucosal ulceration.
• Hair loss.

Emergency **Folinic acid** rescue (15–25 mg qds orally) is discussed in 📖 Chapter 24, p 609, but essentially should be given if any concern over toxicity (primarily pneumonitis and marrow suppression) and in overdose usually above a cumulative of 100 mg methotrexate. If serum levels can be measured it is advised to continue rescue until the levels fall below <0.1 μmol/L. In most cases the response is judged by the daily improvement in haematological indices.

Note: azathioprine and sulfasalazine may also impair folate metabolism. A growing literature suggests folic acid replacement should be considered with these drugs too.

Additional methotrexate monitoring

The role of liver biopsy and serum pro-collagen III testing remains unclear and does not form part of routine clinical practice in the UK.

When monitoring, the serum PIIINP should be measured a baseline and every 3 months on treatment. Indications for a liver biopsy would be either elevation of PIIINP pretreatment or 3 consecutive levels rise above a previous normal range over a 12-month period. The decision to stop therapy would be based on a risk-benefit assessment in each individual.

History should be taken at each visit for onset of shortness of breath and assessed for risk of pneumonitis/pulmonary fibrosis. Further investigation may require high-resolution CT and lung function tests detailing lung volume and gas transfer coefficients.

Specific drug interactions

• The anti-folate effect of drugs may increase the toxicity of methotrexate. Commonly used drugs include phenytoin, co-trimoxazole, and trimethoprim.
• Methotrexate concentration can be increased by NSAIDs, penicillin and tolbutamide.

Mycophenolate mofetil

Routinely used in organ transplantation, Mycophenolate has recently joined the armamentarium in the control of nephritis, myositis, and vasculitis.

It is given at 1–3 g/day orally in divided doses, starting at 500 mg daily for the 7 days, then 500 mg bd for 7 days, building sequentially by an additional 500 mg daily every 7 days over the ensuing weeks to an optimal/tolerable dose.

Additional monitoring
- Urinalysis at each visit to ensure no sterile haematuria.
- Enquiry as to skin lesions – increased risk of tumours.

Specific drug interactions
- Decreased absorption of the drug can occur with use of antacids (magnesium and aluminum hydroxide) and colestyramine.
- Increased concentration may arise with the use of probenecid and aciclovir.
- NSAIDs may add to nephrotoxic risk.

Sulfasalazine

- This drug tends to be used less than methotrexate, but most often in the context of RA, PsA, and AS.
- Like mycophenolate the dosage ranges from 500 mg to 3g/day typically starting at 500 mg/day for 7 days and increasing by an additional 500 mg daily every 7 days over the ensuing weeks to an optimal/tolerable dose.
- Patients should be warned that bodily fluids may turn a darker yellow/orange and not to be alarmed.
- The 'EN' formulation (Salazopyrin EN®) is better tolerated. It also comes in liquid form.

Specific caution
- Slow–acetylators of the drug may develop a drug-induced lupus-like syndrome. It is not considered necessary to an check acetylator phenotype unless suspicion is raised as a consequence of side-effects. Even then, the answer is academic as the drug will have been stopped.
- A history of hypersensitivity to sulfonamides/co-trimoxazole or aspirin would deter use of the drug.

Specific drug interactions
- Sulfasalazine in combination with azathioprine may potentiate the risk of bone marrow toxicity.
- Sulfasalazine may reduce the absorption of digoxin.

Biologic therapies

Anti-TNF-α therapy

- TNF-α is a potent pro-inflammatory cytokine; levels are elevated in autoimmune inflammatory conditions.
- At present, there are 4 agents available in the UK namely adalimumab (Humira®), etanercept (Enbrel®), certolizumab pegol (Cimzia®), and infliximab (Remicade®).
- Infliximab is a chimeric human–murine anti-TNFα monoclonal antibody, etanercept a recombinant human TNF receptor fusion protein, certolizumab pegol a pegylated Fab fragment of a fully humanized anti-TNF monoclonal antibody, and adalimumab a fully humanized complete anti-TNF-α monoclonal antibody.
- Infliximab is administered by slow iv infusion at 0, 2, 4, and every 4–8 weeks, thereafter depending on response.
- Etanercept is administered by sc injection and can now be given once (50 mg) instead of twice (25 mg) weekly.
- Certolizumab pegol is given by sc injection at a dose of 400 mg in weeks 0, 2, and 4, followed by a maintenance dose of 200 mg every 2 weeks.
- Adalimumab is given by sc injection every 2 weeks.
- With all the above anti-TNF-α agents, co-administration with methotrexate is recommended when tolerated as this has been shown to increase efficacy, and use with infliximab also reduces the production of anti-infliximab antibodies.
- There is evidence that patients may respond to a second anti-TNF α if there is inadequate response to a first therapy. In revised NICE guidelines (2010) for RA, a second anti-TNF-α agent is recommended only if rituximab (see below) has not been effective or is contra-indicated.[1]
- In the UK, NICE has published guidelines for the use of these drugs based on clinical efficacy, health-related quality of life and cost effectiveness. (Table 21.11)
- The efficacy of anti-TNF-α therapy in SLE is at present not clear. 16% of RA patients on these therapies develop double-stranded DNA antibodies, and 0.2% a transient lupus-like syndrome. A small, open label study has shown benefit in lupus nephritis, but further work needs to be done.
- Infliximab has been used in several scenarios off license for conditions such as Behçet's disease (📖 Chapter 18, p 489). There is no doubt from the already growing international case-study literature that these agents will be tried more and more often in complex inflammatory conditions, fuelled also by the availability of new agents ready for market such as golimumab, which has recently been licensed in the UK.

---

1 National Institute for Health and Clinical Excellence (2010). *Rheumatoid Arthritis—Drugs for Treatment after Failure of a TNF Inhibitor: Final Appraisal Determination.* June 2010. Available at: www.nice.org.uk/.

Table 21.11 Summary of UK NICE/BSR Guidelines for the use of the first anti-TNF-α therapy in RA (From NICE clinical guidance 79—Rheumatoid arthritis, and NICE Technology appraisal guidance 130)

1	Patients must satisfy 1987 ACR criteria for diagnosis of RA
2	A Disease Activity Score of >5.1 at 2 points, 1 month apart
3	Adequate trial of at least 2 standard DMARDs, one of which should be methotrexate. An adequate trial is defined as: • Treatment for at least 6 months, with at least 2 months at standard target dose (unless toxicity). • Treatment for <6 months where treatment was withdrawn due to intolerance or toxicity, normally after at least 2 months of therapeutic doses.
4	*Exclusion criteria:* pregnancy or breastfeeding. Active infection or high risk of infection. Malignant or pre-malignant states.
5	*Criteria for withdrawal of therapy:* adverse events or inefficacy.
6	An alternative anti-TNF-α therapy may be considered for patients in whom treatment is withdrawn due to an adverse event before the initial 6-month assessment of efficacy.

Cautions and monitoring

All the assessment and monitoring principles set out in Tables 21.7–21.9 apply to biologics as much as they do DMARDs, particularly the assessment of infection and malignancy risk:

• Pregnancy, breastfeeding, sepsis, and malignancy are exclusion criteria, although there have been many reports of successful pregnancies in patients on anti-TNF-α therapy.

• It is advisable to stop the drug at least 4 weeks before trying to conceive.

• Common reactions include headache, nausea, and injection-site reactions. Serious bacterial infections have been reported, and patients with active infection should have their treatment stopped. Patients at risk of recurrent infection should not use these drugs (e.g. in-dwelling urinary catheter, immunodeficiency states). Other reported side-effects include demyelination, worsening of heart failure, lupus-like syndromes, and blood dyscrasia.

• Reactivation of tuberculosis has been reported mainly in Infliximab and adalimumab patients (3–4 times increased risk compared with etanercept), and most commonly within 3 months of beginning of treatment. Patients should be assessed for TB risk.

• Guidelines for assessing risk and managing TB infection in patients due to start anti-TNF-α therapy have been published by the British Thoracic Society (www.brit-thoracic.org.uk). Use of anti-TNF-α therapy is not contraindicated but patients may require up to 6 months concomitant therapy with isoniazid.

- There remains concern about the long-term safety of these drugs, especially with regard to malignancy. It is well known that RA patients have a 2 times higher risk of increased risk of developing lymphoma compared with the general population. Debate continues as to whether reports of lymphoma in RA patients on anti-TNF-α therapy reflect a real drug effect or the known increased incidence of lymphoma in RA patients, but current evidence from the UK Registry suggests no increased in cadence of lymphoma in patients with RA on anti-TNF-α therapy compared with RA controls. No increased risk has been found with other types of malignancy.

At the time of this text going to press, the British Society for Rheumatology guideline group on anti-TNF-α therapy in RA ([] Chapter 5, p 233) is anticipated to publish detailed guidelines in late 2010. This will include recommendations for screening and managing infection and malignancy risk, peri-operative dosing, pregnancy, and lactation. Guidelines are anticipated as being available at: http://www.rheumatology.org.uk/resources/guidelines/bsr_guidelines.aspx.

B cell depletors

- There is increasing evidence that B cells play an important role in the pathogenesis of RA and other auto-immune conditions.
- Rituximab, a chimeric monoclonal antibody against human CD 20 that is present on developing B cells prior to the plasma cell stage. Administration of rituximab leads to rapid CD20 positive B cell depletion in the peripheral blood.
- Normal B cell repopulation (measured by monitoring the CD19 count) occurs within the next 3 months. Rituximab was first used in non-Hodgkins lymphoma. Randomized placebo-controlled trials have shown that in RF positive patients who have failed several DMARDs, a course of rituximab (2 infusions 2 weeks apart with corticosteroids) achieves a significant improvement in disease activity at 6 months compared to methotrexate alone. The time to next infusion regimen can range from 6 to 18 months, but has a mean of 9 months.
- There is concern about persistent hypogammaglobulinaemia after repeated courses. A recent systematic review has shown no increase in serious infections with rituximab.
- NICE has recommended rituximab to be used with methotrexate in the treatment of severe RA, where there has been an inadequate response to other DMARDs and at least one other anti-TNF-α therapy.
- Open-label studies in SLE have confirmed efficacy of rituximab, with benefits extending to 6 months. However, a recent randomized placebo-controlled trial failed to demonstrate that rituximab was beneficial to patients with moderate-to-severe SLE, although this could have been due to methodological issues and is still being investigated. Significant side-effects seen in this treatment group include infusion-related reactions and infection.

In addition, progressive multifocal leukoencephalopathy (PML) has been reported in association with Rituximab in a small number of patients. Patients should be counselled appropriately before commencing treatment. The monitoring profile is like that for anti-TNF-α therapy:

- A CD 19 count should be performed before administering rituximab. The observation of it falling at 6 weeks into therapy and then rising as the disease 'flares' is evidence in favour of efficacy and a means of predicting need for further treatment.
- As with anti-TNF-α therapy there is a growing international case-study literature suggesting benefit of this agent in other complex inflammatory conditions, for example, undifferentiated connective tissue disease with polymyositis.

Interleukin-1 receptor antagonists

- Interleukin-1 (IL-1) is a pro-inflammatory cytokine. Anakinra is an IL-1 receptor antagonist that competes with Il-1 for binding. The agent is given by daily sc injection. Randomized controlled trials have shown it is more effective than placebo. Side effects include injection-site reactions, blood dyscrasias, and infection.
- Anti-TNF-α therapies should not be used in conjunction, and clearance is reduced in renal impairment.
- Anakinra has not been approved by NICE for use in the UK.

Interleukin-6 inhibitors

Interleukin-6 is a potent pro-inflammatory cytokine with and high levels have been found in serum and synovial fluid of RA patients, and levels correlate with disease activity. Tocilizumab is a fully humanized anti-IL6 receptor antibody and is given by monthly intravenous infusion. Studies have shown that it is effective in controlling disease and limiting radiographic progression in RA patients in whom methotrexate and anti-TNF-α therapies have been ineffective or not tolerated. Non-inferiority studies are currently underway to determine the effectiveness and tolerability of sc tocilizumab.

NICE has recently approved its use after failure of anti-TNF-α therapy and B cell depletion (if applicable).

Lipids should be monitored 6-monthly given the association with drug-induced hyperlipidaemia.

CTLA4-Ig

Abatacept disrupts the CD80/86 co-stimulatory signal required for T-cell activation by competing with CD28 for binding. Abatacept is administered intravenously at weeks 0, 2, and 4 and then monthly thereafter, and is effective in patients who have previously failed methotrexate or anti TNF-α therapy. A recent systematic review has shown that the incidence of serious infections compared with placebo was equal.

The revised NICE guidance in 2010 has approved its use in patients who have had an inadequate response to a first anti-TNF-α therapy, and in whom rituximab has been ineffective or contraindicated.

Autologous haemopoietic stem cell transplantation

Haemopoietic stem cell transplantation (HSCT) is used to treat haematological diseases, but has been used in patients with severe refractory SLE. The procedure is effective in inducing remission, but is curative in <50%. Mortality is high and long-term effects are unknown. New autoimmune conditions have been reported after HSCT. It is currently used only in those with life-threatening SLE.

Other experimental agents (primarily under investigation in RA) are shown in Table 21.12.

Table 21.12 Experimental therapies for the treatment of rheumatoid arthritis

Target	Principle
Cell cycle inhibitor	Temsirolimus
Ion channel blockers	Receptor antagonists
Cytokine inhibition	Anti-IL-6 antibody
	Oral TNF inhibitor
	Anti-IL-15 monoclonal antibody
B cells	Humanized anti-CD-20 agents Anti-B cell stimulator protein (belimumab)
	Anti-BLyS/APRIL
	Anti TACI-Ig
Cell adhesion molecules	Humanized 4-1 and 4-7 monoclonal antibody (natalizumab)
Pro-inflammation	Fish/plant seed oils

Other medication

Iloprost

Iloprost is used in the management of severe Raynaud's with peripheral ischaemia and in pulmonary hypertension (PAH) (📖 Chapter 13, p 363). It is a synthetic analogue of prostacyclin PGI2 and works by dilating systemic and pulmonary arterial vascular beds.

It can be given in a nebulized form, but more often rheumatologists are familiar with giving it by iv route.

For pulmonary hypertension via nebulizer the first inhaled dose should be 2.5 mcg. If tolerated the dose should be increased to 5.0 mcg and given 3–4-hourly to gain 6–9 doses per day according to need, but no more than 45 mcg per day and no more often than 2 hourly.

For pulmonary hypertension by iv route in a stable patient, iloprost can be given at 2 mcg/h initially and increasing by 1 mcg/h every 12 h with a target dose of 12 mcg/h for the duration determined by a pulmonary vascular specialist.

In an emergency the rate is commenced at 2 mcg/h, but increased by 1 mcg every 15 min to a rate of 6 mcg/h after 1 h. Again, the usual target dose is then 12 mcg/h for a duration determined by a pulmonary vascular specialist.

Studies in critical ischaemia with Raynaud's recommend progressive increasing dose from 0.5 to 2 ng/kg/min (i.e. 2–8 mcg/h in an 70 kg adult) over a period of 6 h each day for up to 10 days with repeated cycles at regular intervals of 3 months as required.

Monitoring

This should include pulse, blood pressure, and oxygen saturation every 15 min for the first hour, every 30 min over the ensuing hours for a 6-h regimen in Raynaud's. For prolonged therapy in PAH the rate can move to every hour for 4 h then every 4 h thereafter.

Cautions—in each case aim to reduce dose first before stopping

- Hypotension.
- Headache.
- Jaw and limb pain.

Pooled intravenous immunoglobulin

There are very few approved indications for pooled IVIG. In rheumatology these include immune thrombocytopenic purpura (ITP), (SLE 📖 Chapter 10, p 321), dermatomyositis (📖 Chapter 14, p 385), and Kawasaki disease (📖 Chapter 15, p 405). Approval is occasionally gained for use in severe vasculitis usually associated with RA and SLE.

The typical dosing regimen is 400 mg/kg/day as a single infusion over 2–4 h as tolerated and for 5 days, or 1 g/kg/day for 2 days. This is repeated every 4–8 weeks for up to 6 months in the first instance according to efficacy.

IVIG can induce reactions in patients with IgA deficiency. The IgA level should be checked prior to the first treatment

Side effects occur in less than 5% of patients and most often within the 24 h after an infusion. These include headache, flushing, chills, myalgia, wheezing, tachycardia, lower back pain, nausea, and hypotension. If these occur during an infusion it should be slowed or stopped.

Most cases will respond to antihistamines and intravenous hydrocortisone if symptoms persist.

Other significant, but rare complications include acute renal failure, arteriovenous thrombosis, disseminated intravascular coagulation, transient serum sickness, transient neutropenia, aseptic meningitis, post-infusion hyperproteinaemia with pseudohyponatraemia, eczematous dermatitis, and alopecia.

Corticosteroid injection therapy

Anatomical drawings for each region of the body are found in 📖 Chapter 2, p 19.

Introduction

- Local anaesthetic and steroid injection into joints or soft tissues is a very effective treatment for localized pain and inflammation.
- Injection offers a local maximal anti-inflammatory effect with minimal systemic absorption.
- As a general rule it is recommended that any one joint should not be injected more than four times in 12 months and there are at least 6 weeks between injections.
- The indications for local steroid injection include:
  - reduction of inflammation in joints, entheses, tendon sheaths and bursa;
  - relief of pain from inflammatory ligament lesions;
  - relief of inflammation at sites of nerve compression;
  - reduce the size of nodules and ganglia;
  - relieve pain at trigger points.
- The contraindications are:
  - *Absolute*—
    — septic arthritis/sepsis;
    — febrile patient, cause unknown;
    — serious allergy to previous injection;
    — sickle cell disease;
  - *Relative*—
    — unknown cause of monoarthritis;
    — neutropenia, thrombocytopenia;
    — anticoagulation or bleeding disorder.
- Common agents used include:
  - hydrocortisone acetate; a short-acting, weak anti-inflammatory, useful for superficial lesions such as tendons and bursae. A dose of 25 mg is typical;
  - methylprednisolone acetate at 40 mg/ml;
  - prednisolone acetate, 25 mg/ml, and;
  - triamcinolone acetone, 10 and 40 mg/ml.

The latter three agents are long-acting synthetic steroids. Choice of strength of steroid remains empiric.

- Volume of agent varies:
  - small joints accept only a small volume; thus, for interphalangeal (ip), metacarpophalangeal (mcp), metatarsophalangeal (mtp), adhesive capsulitis (ac), and temperomandibular (tm), 0.5 mL of triamcinolone acetonide (10 mg) is appropriate;
  - all other joints should accept at least 1 mL;
  - there may be merit in diluting the steroid in sterile saline, to increase volume for better distribution in larger joints. Alternatively larger volume levobupivacaine (10 mL) is of value.

- Potential, although uncommon, side-effects include:
  - exacerbation of pain for 24–48 h;
  - septic arthritis and reactivation of TB;
  - tissue atrophy (less likely with hydrocortisone than others);
  - depigmentation of skin;
  - anaphylaxis;
  - nerve damage;
  - tendon rupture;
  - avascular necrosis;
  - cartilage damage;
  - soft-tissue calcification;
  - temporary exacerbation of hyperglycaemia in diabetes.

The general side-effects of glucocorticoids are discussed in 📖 Chapter 21, p 545.

Principles of injection techniques

The procedure need not necessarily be done in a sterile environment. However, there is a need to maintain an aseptic technique. Efficacy may be greater using US-guided injection; certainly efficacy may be greater using US-guided injection; certainly more accurate. US technique should only be performed by appropriately qualified clinicians.

- Mark the exact spot of needle insertion.
- Wash hands. Use sterile gloves for the procedure.
- Clean the skin with povidone-iodine and allow it to dry.
- Anaesthetize the skin (either with local anaesthetic or refrigerant alcohol spray). Children and some adolescents may require a light general anaesthetic given the procedure can be traumatic. An alternative is to use local anaesthetic gel pads (e.g. EMLA® patch).
- Insert a clean needle with empty syringe and aspirate back.
- Leave the needle in place, detach the syringe, and place the syringe containing steroid/local anaesthetic onto the end of a new needle.
- Insert needle into site to be injected.
- Pull back the syringe plunger again before injecting to confirm placement, ensuring the needle is not in a blood vessel.
- Introduction of steroid should be effortless. Resistance implies the end of the needle is in the wrong space. Stop if it causes more pain.
- On completion remove the syringe and needle and throw away the 'sharps'.
- Cover the injection site with clean gauze or bandage.
- Rest the joint for 24 h (consider up to 48 h for a weight-bearing joint), and re-emphasize possible side-effects and benefits.

The shoulder

The glenohumeral joint

- The approach may be anterior or posterior.
- The anterior route gives reliable access in patients with adhesive capsulitis. It is also better suited for aspiration of joint effusions.
- Palpate the coracoid process anteriorly and the acromion posteriorly. The injection is made just lateral to the coracoid with the needle pointing towards the acromion (Plate 3).
- The posterior route requires the clinician to palpate the spine of the scapula with the thumb to its lateral end where it bends forward as the acromion. With the forefinger then palpate the coracoid anteriorly. The line between finger and thumb then marks the position of the joint line.
- The needle is advanced from behind, 1 cm below the acromion, and towards the coracoid. There should be no resistance.
- By either approach this joint and capsule can be injected with larger volumes 10–20 mL local anaesthetic, particularly if there is a capsulitis as well as 40 mg Depo-Medrone®.
- Withdrawing the needle slightly and redirecting 30° upward will allow one to reach the rotator cuff with the same procedure!

Subacromial bursa

- The subacromial bursa is approached from the lateral side. To inject this space the arm is placed in a neutral position, hanging to the side, and the gap between the acromion and the humeral head is palpated.
- A small gauge needle is directed medially and slightly posterior and no deeper than 1–2 cm (Plate 4).
- Only small volume should be injected; 1 mL of triamcinolone acetate 25 mg, for example. The subacromial space is too small for larger volumes that may induce considerable pain.

Acromioclavicular joint

- The AC joint is located by following the clavical laterally. The joint is often tender to palpate.
- With the patient lying supine a small gauge needle with 0.5 mL of steroid is directed in to the joint, whilst palpating the joint line.

The elbow

Tennis elbow/lateral epicondylitis

- Lateral humeral epicondylitis is injected with the elbow resting on the examination table and flexed at 90°.
- This superficial injection is directed at 45° to the end of the common extensor tendon origin.
- A fair amount of pressure is required for this injection. It is often painful (Plate 5).
- This site will normally only tolerate a small volume 0.5–1 mL local anaesthetic plus 1–2 mL of steroid solution.
- If steroid fails, autologous blood may be tried. The NICE guidance on this procedure may be found at: http://www.nice.org.uk/guidance/IPG279.

Golfers elbow/medial epicondylitis

- The medial humeral epicondylitis is managed similarly to that above.
- The needle is directed to the flexor tendon origin. However, care should be taken to avoid the groove just behind the medial epicondyle—the site of the ulnar nerve.

Olecranon bursa

An olecranon bursa can be aspirated and injected superficially with minimal effort. Needle position is confirmed by the aspiration of fluid.

Elbow joint

- The elbow joint is most easily reached by a posterior approach.
- Place the thumb on the lateral epicondyle and the third finger on the olecranon. The groove between the two fingers identifies the joint line.
- Inject at 90° to the skin, just above and lateral to the olecranon.
- Alternatively, the radial head can be palpated (by feeling for it during forearm pronation/supination) and the needle sited tangentially just under the capsule (an antero-lateral approach).

The wrist and hand

Lesions of the wrist

Radiocarpal joint
- The radiocarpal joint is best felt with the patient's hand held palm down and the wrist in slight flexion. A triangular gap is felt between the radius and the carpal bones.
- The needle (small gauge) is pointed proximally and at 60°.
- 1 mL of steroid is usually the tolerated volume.

Carpal tunnel
- The carpal tunnel is injected on the palmar surface of the wrist in the first crease.
- If the palmaris tendon is present the injection should be sited just medial (i.e. closer to the 'little finger') to the midline, by about 1 cm, and towards the palm at 45°.
- There should be no resistance on injection or nerve pain (Plate 11).

Extensor pollicis brevis/abductor pollicis longus
De Quervain's tenosynovitis should be injected at the point of maximal tenderness, advancing the needle through the tendon sheath along the line of the tendon rather than at 90° to the tendon.

The hand
- The small joints of the hand will normally only accept 0.5–1 mL of injected fluid.
- It is important to remember that the joint line of an mcp is about 1 cm distal to the crest of the knuckle.
- The approach to a pip is from the lateral side.
- PIPs and dips are often difficult to inject. Accuracy of needle placement within a joint space might be improved by using US guidance.

The hip and peri-articular lesions

Hip joint

Hip injection is not a routine outpatient procedure, and aspiration and injection under US or fluoroscopic guidance is recommended.

Trochanteric bursa

- Trochanteric bursitis or enthesitis at the greater trochanter can be injected with the patient lying on their good side.
- The site of injection should be chosen based on the point of maximal tenderness.
- The injection site can be very deep and to reduce the risk of fat atrophy from a 'blind approach', it is reasonable to try using hydrocortisone first.
- Injection failure should raise the possibility of poor needle position or a different diagnosis, e.g. gluteus medius muscle tear at its insertion or pain referred from a lumbosacral disorder.

Other

- Meralgia paraesthetica occurs as a consequence of lateral cutaneous nerve entrapment (🕮 Chapter 2, p 19) as it traverses the fascia 10 cm below and medial to the anterior superior iliac spine. If this spot can be clearly demarcated because of localized tenderness, steroid injection has a greater chance of success.
- The ischial tuberosities are located deep in the medial side of the buttocks. The overlying bursae can become inflamed, causing pain on sitting. These tender points can be injected. The differential diagnosis is enthesitis or possibly coccidynia.
- The coccyx can be palpated centrally (with the patient prone or lying on their side). This site is also amenable to local anaesthetic and steroid injections.
- Adductor apophysitis occurring from a sports injury can be injected simply although it can be difficult to access.
- An inflamed symphysis pubis is best injected under US guidance.

The knee and peri-articular lesions

The knee joint

- The most common technique for injection of the knee joint involves either the lateral or medial retropatellar approach.
- A wide gauge needle is most appropriate given aspiration of synovial fluid is often also required for symptom relief and diagnostics.
- 40 mg Depo-Medrone® and 2–5 mL of 1–2% lidocaine are typical dosages.
- For the lateral approach palpate the patella and mark a line on the lateral edge of the patella at the point between its upper and middle third.
- Then mark a point 1–2 cm below this point. This is the needle site.
- Access to the joint space may be improved by depressing the medial aspect of the patella, tipping it up laterally.
- The needle is advanced at 90° to the skin surface tangentially under patella and between the patella and the femoral condyle (Plate 18).
- The entry site for the medial approach is at the midline of the patella, with the needle advanced under the patella and towards the suprapatellar pouch.
- In both techniques, aspiration as the needle is inserted will reveal fluid as soon as the capsule is entered, so:
  - reducing the risk of forcing the needle too far forward causing cartilage damage;
  - allowing aspiration of large volumes of synovial fluid before injecting steroid;
  - confirming correct positioning of the needle before injecting steroid.

Knee peri-articular injections

- Prepatellar bursitis, painful ligaments, and trigger points around the knee may all respond to local steroid and anaesthetic.
- Popliteal cysts can be directly aspirated and injected but owing to the risk of damaging superficial neurovascular structures, should be done under US guidance.
- See 📖 Chapter 2, p 19 for anatomical positioning of the anserine bursa, a common site for soft tissue inflammation.

The ankle and foot

Ankle and tarsal tunnel

- The ankle joint is located most easily with the patient supine on a couch. The joint line can be palpated just lateral to the extensor digitorum tendon as it crosses the ankle crease. The needle is initially advanced downwards over the talus (Plate 19a).
- Tendon sheaths and the tarsal tunnel (Plate 19b) can also be injected; the latter is injected under the flexor retinaculum between the calcaneum and the medial malleolus.

Plantar faciitis

- Painful points under the heel (plantar fasciitis) should be injected from the medial side after carefully localizing the position of maximal pain (Plate 19c).
- Never inject through the sole of the foot.
- Some clinicians will numb the area by local anaesthetic to the posterior tibial nerve, in the tarsal tunnel (Plate 19b).

Small joints of the feet

- The mtps are injected from the lateral side having felt the joint line by flexing and extending the joint.
- Care should be taken as these joints have a greater than normal risk of infection after the procedure.

Complementary and alternative medicine in rheumatology

Introduction

The popularity of complementary and alternative medicine (CAM) among people with chronic diseases including arthritis is widely recognized.[1] Up to one-third of arthritis sufferers have received CAM from CAM practitioners and CAM use prevalence has been reported at between 30–100% of patients with rheumatic disease.[2,3] Among the most popular are dietary approaches, herbalism, and acupuncture.[4,5] From formal studies to date, few appear to have any more than a placebo effect.[6] That said, many have recognized anti-inflammatory and/or immunomodulatory activity, and potential antidepressant and pain modulatory mechanisms (Table 23.1).[7,8]

The prevalence of CAM use for chronic arthritis and pain chiefly mirrors that in other chronic diseases and appears to be consistent across Western populations.

CAM is very popular despite a paucity of data. There may be no universal explanation as to why patients use CAMs; perhaps, simply, the 'power' of the placebo effect. Gender, age, income, education, degree of underlying psychological stress, and desire to regain 'greater self-control' may all influence use.

Published suggestions for CAM use also include dissatisfaction with conventional medicine or the belief that a philosophy associated with a particular CAM is desirable and aligns with the patient's own philosophy.

To be able to work as closely as possible with their patient on the management of a condition, the clinician needs an appreciation of such therapies.

1 Cheung CK, Wyman JF, Halcon LL (2007). Use of complementary and alternative therapies in community-dwelling older adults. *J Altern Complement Med* **9**: 997–1006.

2 Resch KL, Hills, Ernst E (1997). Use of complementary therapies by individuals with 'arthritis'. *Clin Rheumatol* **16**: 391–5.

3 Ernst E (1998). Usage of complementary therapies in rheumatology: a systematic review. *Clin Rheumatol* **17**: 301–5.

4 Ernst E (2004). Musculoskeletal conditions and complementary/alternative medicine. *Best Pract Res Clin Rheumatol* **18**: 539–56.

5 Weiner DK, Ernst E (2004). Complementary and alternative approaches to the treatment of persistent Musculoskeletal pain. *Clin J Pain* **20**: 244–55.

6 Ernst E (2010). Homeopathy: what does the 'best' evidence tell us? *Med J Aust* **192**: 458–60.

7 Setty AR, Sigal LH (2005). Herbal medications commonly used in the practice of rheumatology: mechanisms of action, efficacy, and side effects. *Semin Arthritis Rheum* **34**: 773–84.

8 Efthimiou P, Kukar M (2010). Complementary and alternative medicine use in rheumatoid arthritis: proposed mechanism of action and efficacy of commonly used modalities. *Rheumatol Int* **30**: 571–86.

Herbal remedies (phytotherapy)[1]

- The likely mechanism of effect of most agents is on eicosanoid metabolism inhibiting either cyclooxygenase or lipoxygenase pathways (Table 23.1).
- Most efficacy studies illustrate methodological flaws—notably the failure to power studies sufficiently given small differences in outcome vs. placebo. Risk–benefit profiles are generally unknown.
- Adverse reactions similar to those from conventional medicines can occur and include allergy and drug interactions.
- In most countries few legal controls exist to ensure quality of herbal medicine constituents and no legislative 'medicine development' framework exists to reliably ensure safety and efficacy.

Phytodolor

This is a standardized extract of *Populus tremula* marketed for rheumatic pain. Reviews suggest studies overall show a pain reduction effect in patients with osteoarthritis (OA, 📖 Chapter 6, p 259) compared with placebo.

St. John's wort (*Hypericum perforatum*)

- St. John's wort has been shown in relatively robust trials to improve mild depression. This may relate to its effect on inhibiting synaptosomal uptake of 5-HT, dopamine, normetanephrine, glutamate, and GABA.
- Response patients with arthritis or chronic pain may be due to improvements in mood, pain perception or coping strategies.
- St. John's wort increases the activity of cytochrome P450 3A4, which is responsible for the metabolism of many drugs. Concomitant administration results in decreased serum levels of ciclosporin and digoxin. St. John's Wort also decreases the anticoagulant of warfarin, and patients may require dose adjustment as a result.

Gamma linoleic acid (GLA)

- GLA is a plant seed-oil derived unsaturated fatty acid, which suppresses production of Il-1β. It is contained in many different plant seed oils (e.g. blackcurrant seed oil).
- Compared with placebo, 2.8 g/d GLA significantly improves symptoms and signs of active RA over 6 months.[2] However, virtually all plant-seed oil preparations that contain GLA are likely to be taken at lower daily doses than those shown to be effective.

Devil's claw (*Harpagophytum procumbens*)

- This may work by inhibiting cyclooxygenase or iNO synthase in joint tissues or by suppressing matrix metalloproteinase production.
- At 60–100 mg/day, *Harpagophytum* extract (harpagoside) has moderate but significant effects on back and joint pain associated with OA.[3]

1 Soeken KL, Miller SA, Ernst E (2003). Herbal medicines for the treatment of rheumatoid arthritis: a systematic review. *Rheumatology* **42**: 652–9.

2 Zurier RB, Rossetti RG, Jacobson EW, *et al.* (1996). Gamma-linolenic acid treatment of rheumatoid arthritis. A randomized placebo-controlled trial. *Arth Rheum* **39**: 1808–17.

3 Gagnier JJ, Chrubasik S, Manheimer E (2004). Harpgophytum procumbens for osteo-carthritis and low back pain: a systematic review. *BMC Complement Altern Med* **4**: 13–23.

Table 23.1 Mechanism of action of herbal remedies commonly used to manage musculoskeletal complaints

Agent	Mechanism
Gamma linolenic acid	Competitive inhibitor of PGE2, leukotrienes and induction of IL-1
Harpagophytum procumbens (Devil's claw)	Inhibits COX and iNO synthetase
Hypericum perforatum (St John's wort)	Inhibits re-uptake of serotonin, dopamine, glutamate and GABA
Ocimum spp.	Antihistamine, anti-serotonin, and anti-prostaglandin
Tanacetum parthenium	Inhibits production of TNF-α and interferon gamma, and decrease T-cell adhesion
Tripterygium wilfordii	Blocks up-regulation of pro-inflammatory genes influencing production of TNF-α, interferon gamma, COX2, and iNO synthetase
Uncaria tomentosa Urtica diocia	Inhibit TNF-α production
Zingiber officinale	Inhibits production of TNF-α, prostaglandins, and leukotrienes

Physical and 'hands on' therapies

Acupuncture

- Acupuncture is commonly used to treat neck and back pain and is easily incorporated into primary care consultations.
- Meta-analyses suggest short-term efficacy for low back pain,[1] but no overall effect for neck pain.[2]
- Controversy exists among acupuncturists as to adequacy of acupuncture techniques used for back pain in published trials.
- No convincing evidence exists to suggest acupuncture should be advised for long-term relief of symptoms in OA or RA.
- Serious complications of acupuncture exist (e.g. pneumothorax, hepatitis B, spinal cord injury, infection) but are rare. Complications may be under-reported.[3,4]

Tai Chi

- In RA, Tai Chi has been shown to increase plantar flexion range and is associated with a higher level of participant enjoyment.
- Trials have shown few benefits in terms of outcome measures. It appears not to exacerbate RA,[5] and may help with fibromyalgia and joint hypermobility syndrome.

Reflexology

- This is one of the most frequently used CAMs.
- From the few controlled trials taken together, results do not suggest there is any specific long-term therapeutic effect.

Spinal manipulation

- Of the most rigorous sham-controlled studies of manipulation (for any indication of back pain) none showed benefit compared with placebo.
- Review suggests that about 50% of patients have side-effects though these are chiefly mild or transient.[6,7]
- Reliable estimates of the incidence of serious adverse effects do not exist. Reported effects include vertebral arterial dissection, strokes, disc herniation, spinal fracture, cauda equina syndrome and worsening of undisclosed spinal inflammatory conditions (e.g. AS/SpA, discitis).

---

1 Ernst E, White AR (1998). Acupuncture for backpain: a meta-analysis of randomized controlled trials. *Arch Intern Med* **158**: 2235–41.

2 White AR, Ernst E (1999). A systematic review of randomized controlled trials of acupuncture for neck pain. *Rheumatology* **38**: 143–7.

3 Ernst E, White AR (1998). Life-threatening adverse reactions after acupuncture? A systematic review. *Pain* **71**: 123–6.

4 Ernst E (2006). Acupuncture—a critical appraisal. *J Intern Med* **259**(2): 125–37.

5 The Cochrane library. Issue **4**. 2004.

6 Ernst E (2001). Prospective investigations into the safety of spinal manipulation. *J Pain Symptom Manage* **21**: 238–42.

7 Ernst E, Canter PH (2006). A systematic review of systematic reviews of spiral manipulation. *J R Soc Med* **99**(4): 192–6.

Homeopathy

Homeopathy stems from the belief that tiny quantities of substances have a holistic therapeutic effect. There remains debate as to whether homeopathy is genuinely more effective than placebo and whether conventional randomized studies are a relevant way of evaluating its effect.

Nevertheless homeopaths are among the most frequently visited CAM practitioners by patients with arthritis.

- Meta-analyses of therapeutic trials might suggest the clinical effects of homeopathic remedies cannot be fully explained by placebo effects alone.[1] However, the most robust methodological studies do not show any positive effects compared with placebo.[2,3]
- There is some evidence that short-term improvement in RA symptomsis superior to placebo.[4] A more robust methodological study, however, suggested no symptomatic improvement in RA over 3 months in patients stabilized on DMARDs and NSAIDs.[5]
- Summarizing four RCTs of homeopathy use in OA, there appears to be a positive effect though firm conclusions cannot be reached.[6]
- One of the most frequently used homeopathic remedies is *Arnica montana*. A systematic review of its effects[7] suggests there's no proof of its effect.
- Preparations of *Echinacea* are believed by some to have immunomodulatory properties. Although this is a traditional treatment for a variety of ailments, some CAM practitioners advise that patients with autoimmune diseases avoid this supplement.

1 Linde K, Melchart D (1998). Randomized controlled trials of individualized homeopathy: a state-of-the-art review. *J Altern Complement Med* **4**: 371–88.

2 Ernst E, Pittler MH (1998). Efficacy of homeopathic arnica: a systematic review of placebo-controlled clinical trials. *Arch Surg* **133**: 1187–90.

3 Ernst E (1998). Are highly dilute homeopathic remedies placebos? *Perfusion* **1**: 291–2.

4 Jonas WB, Linde K, Ramirez G (2000). Homeopathy and rheumatic disease. *Rheum Dis Clin* **26**: 117–23.

5 Fisher P, Scott DL (2001). A randomized controlled trial of homeopathy in rheumatoid arthritis. *Rheumatology* **40**: 1052–5.

6 Long L, Ernst E (2001). Homeopathic remedies for the treatment of osteoarthritis: a systematic review. *Br Homeopath J* **90**: 37–43.

7 Ernst E, Pittler MH (1998). Efficacy of homeopathic arnica: a systematic review of placebo-controlled clinical trials. *Arch Surg* **133**: 1187–90.

Other complementary and alternative medicines

Magnet therapy

- In one randomized study, patients wearing a magnet bracelet experienced reduction of hip and knee pain associated with osteoarthritis when compared to patients wearing dummy bracelets.[1] However, another study has indicated that wrist magnets and copper bracelets are ineffective in relieving pain, stiffness, and impaired function in OA.[2]
- Overall, studies have not adequately demonstrated the effect of magnet therapy on pain relief to be any greater than placebo effect.[3]

Dietary supplements

- Glucosamine and chondroitin sulphate supplements have long been used for the treatment of osteoarthritis, but the results of clinical trials have been mixed, and its use is falling out of favour.
- Curcumin (turmeric) has anti-inflammatory properties, and may have some beneficial effects on arthritis.
- Other commonly used supplements by patients with arthritis and pain include cod liver oil, fish oil tablets, vitamins, and selenium.
- Although there is little available scientific evidence to support any recommendations regarding dietary modification, this form of intervention remains popular.

Hypnotherapy

- This is of long-standing interest in controlling pain.
- In studies, hypnotherapy has been shown to be effective at controlling anxiety.
- There is some evidence for efficacy in fibromyalgia patients.

Stress management/relaxation therapy

- Stress has been associated with an increased risk of sudden death, delay in wound healing, and higher rates of infection.
- Yoga, acupuncture, and meditation may improve quality of sleep, and decrease perceived stress, fatigue, and depression.
- Various studies suggest short-term benefit for patients with RA, but proof of the effects on measures of disease in the long term are lacking.
- Methodological deficiencies in studies and absence of cost-effectiveness data suggests no firm conclusion can be drawn about the role of therapy in specific individuals or disease groups.

1 Harlow T, Greaves C, White A, *et al.* (2004). Randomised controlled trial of magnetic bracelets for relieving pain of osteoarthritis in the hip and knee. *Br Med J* **18**: 1450–4.

2 Richard SJ, Brown SR, Campion PD, *et al.* (2009). Therapeutic effects of magnetic and copper bracelets in osteoarthritis. *Complement Therap Med* **17**: 249.

3 Pittler MH (2008). Static Magnets for reducing pain. *Focus Altern ComplimentTherap* **13**: 5.

Spiritual healing
- A 'therapeutic experience' transmitted by a therapist's touch, non-touch, prayer, or 'mental healing'.
- Examples include therapeutic touch, reiki, distance healing, and intercessional prayer.
- There's some evidence that 'therapeutic touch' done by nurses can reduce anxiety in hospital patients. No data exist that compare this with talking to/informing patients about their condition.

Other
- Electrical stimulation increases grip strength in RA patients with hand muscle atrophy. Pulsed electrical stimulation can help knee OA symptoms. Data is weaker for an effect on pain from neck OA.
- Thermotherapy for RA—including wax and Faradic baths, hot and ice packs—have brief positive effects without causing harm.[1]
- Balneotherapy may be effective for the treatment of RA and low back pain.[2] Trial methodology has been poor, however—trials have generally not studied relevant outcomes.

Further information
National Centre for Complementary and Alternative Medicine (NCCAM).
   Available at: http://nccam.nih.gov
MD Anderson Complementary/Integrative Medicine.
   Available at: http://www.mdanderson.org/departments/CIMER
Arthritis Foundation—*Arthritis Today* Supplement Guide.
   Available at: http://www.arthritis.org/at-supplement-guide.php
Mayo Clinic: 'Take a break to meditate.'
   Available at: http://mayoclinic.com/health/meditation/MM00623

1 Robinson V, Brosseau L, Casimiro L, *et al.* (2001). Thermotherapy for treating rheumatoid arthritis. *Cochrane Database System Rev* Issue **4**: CD002826.

2 Pittler MH, Karagulle MZ, Karagulle M, Ernst E (2006). Spa therapy and balneotherapy for treating low back pain: meta-analysis of randomized trials. *Rheumatology* **45**: 880–4.

Rheumatological emergencies

For acute skin and cardiac pathologies see 📖 Chapter 4, p 193.
For vertebral fracture see 📖 Chapter 20, p 525.

Septic arthritis

Infection in a joint can progress rapidly and cause destruction of tissues and permanent deformity and disability. When septic arthritis is suspected, investigations should be prompt, appropriate antibiotics should be started without delay, and, where feasible, infected tissue should be removed. The epidemiology of infections is discussed in ☐ Chapter 17, p 473.

Suspecting infection

- Septic arthritis is not common, but is more likely to occur in patients with established joint disease, with prosthetic joints, or with co-morbidities, such as diabetes, chronic renal disease, or immunosuppression.

Patients may not appear systemically unwell:
- The main differential diagnosis in adults is crystal arthritis (☐ Chapter 7, p 269).
- Staphylococcal and streptococcal infections are the most common; septic arthritis from *H. influenzae* type b is no longer seen due to vaccinations. Gonococci cause almost 30% of cases in children >11 years.

Immediate management of adult joint sepsis

See Table 24.1.
- Immobilize the joint and provide adequate analgesia.
- Take blood for full blood count (FBC), U&E and creatinine, liver function tests (LFT), erythrocyte sedimentation rate (ESR), C-reactive protein (CRP), and cultures.
- Manage sepsis as appropriate and rule out infective endocarditis (especially in iv drug user (IVDU) or in those with known cardiac valve disease).
- Drain the joint completely (use at least an 18-gauge needle, since the fluid is viscous) and send the sample of joint fluid for Gram stain, culture, and for polarized light microscopy (LM). If the polarized LM is positive and cultures negative after 48 h then consider a diagnosis of a crystalline arthropathy.
- If fluid is obtained, it should be sent for culture, since identification of an organism is most likely to change management.
- Joint fluid with a white blood cell count >50 000/mm^3 (mainly neutrophils) and a glucose <400 mg/L is highly suggestive of infection.
- Gonococcus is the most common cause of monoarthritis in a young, sexually-active adult; women during menstruation may be at particular risk. Disseminated gonococcal infection may present as a clinical triad of pustular skin lesions, tenosynovitis, or migratory arthralgias. The cutaneous manifestations are fleeting and are not required to make this diagnosis.

Table 24.1 Initial choice of antibiotics for septic arthritis based on Gram stain in adults. All antibiotics are given iv initially

Gram's stain result	Probable pathogen	Antibiotic choice
Gram-positive cocci clusters	Staph. aureus (meticillin resistance suspected)	Vancomycin (1 g bd),
	Staph. epidermis	Vancomycin (1 g bd)
	Streptococci	Benzylpenicillin (2.5 million U qds)
Pairs and chains (urinary, biliary, bowel)	Enterococci	Benzylpenicillin (2.5 million U qds) [or ampicillin (2 g iv qds)]+ gentamicin (3-5 mg/kg od)
Gram-negative cocci (haemorrhagic rash, meningitis)	N. gonorrhoeae	Ceftriaxone (1 g iv bd)
	N. meningitides	Benzylpenicillin (2.5–5 million U qds)
Gram-negative bacilli	Enterobacteriaceae	Ciprofloxacin (400 mg iv bd)
		Cefotaxime (2 g tds)
	Pseudomonas spp.	Ceftazidime (2 g tds) + gentamicin 5mg/kg iv q 24 h
Polymicrobial		Clindamycin (600 mg iv tds) + ciprofloxacin (400 mg iv bd)
No organisms seen (healthy young adult)	N. gonorrhoeae	Ceftriaxone (1–2 g bd)
(older adult, underlying disease)	Staphylococci	Vancomycin and cefotaxime
(intravenous drug abuser)	Streptococci	
	Enterobacteriaceae	
	Staphylococci	Vancomycin and ceftazidime
	Pseudomonas spp.	
	Enterobacteriaceae	

Source: Reprinted with modification from Parker RH. Acute bacterial arthritis. In: D. Schlossberg (ed.) Orthopedic Infections. New York: Springer-Verlag, 1998, p. 74.

- For a non-gonococcal septic arthritis, consult orthopaedics early to consider arthroscopic washout of knee, hip, or shoulder, and contact microbiology to arrange a Gram stain of joint fluid and set up cultures/ special tests for atypical organisms (especially for a septic arthritis resistant to empiric antibiotics).
- Empiric antibiotic treatment in the absence of a positive Gram stain in adults in a straightforward clinical scenario should be iv vancomycin 1 g bd due to the risk of methicillin-resistant S. aureus. For the elderly or immunocompromised patients, a third generation cephalosporin (e.g. ceftriaxone 1 g iv qds) should be added, given the possibility of gram-negative infection (Table 24.1).

- If pseudomonas is suspected—IVDU may be at particular risk—an iv cephalosporin should be used with an aminoglycoside (e.g. gentamicin 3–5 mg/kg iv)

Specific management in children

Prompt iv antibiotic therapy is essential (Fig. 24.1). Initially, treat according to the most likely organism for age: <3 months cover *S. aureus*, group B strep, and Gram-negative bacteria; for those 3 months to 2 years cover *S. aureus* and *S. pneumoniae*. Older children should be treated for staphylococcal and streptococcal infections, as in adults.

Post-immediate management of septic arthritis

- Review analgesia regularly.
- Rule out multiple foci of infection.
- Discontinue any immunosupressants, but consider stress-dose steroids if the patient is systemically unwell and has received chronic steroids.
- Adjust antibiotics according to culture sensitivities and in discussion with an infectious disease specialist.
- For affected weight-bearing joints keep non-weight-bearing until there is obvious improvement in pain and swelling, and you are confident the patient is on appropriate antimicrobials.
- Physical therapists should be involved early to help passive mobilization of joint before patient weight-bears.
- The evidence for routine duration of antibiotic course is not strong and the regime should be individualized. Common protocols include iv antibiotics for 1–2 weeks and a further oral course for 2–4 weeks.

Reasons for no/poor improvement

- Consider that you may have the wrong diagnosis: think about crystals, rheumatoid arthritis (RA, see 📖 Chapter 5, p 233), and SpA monoarthritis (📖 Chapter 8, p 281).
- Consider that the infection has been successfully treated, but that the slow progress is owing to super-added crystal-induced or reactive autoimmune arthritis, foreign body, or background disease (e.g. RA).
- The antimicrobials may not be covering the infection. Consider multiple infecting organisms (re-culture), atypical organisms (e.g. *M. marinum*, Lyme, fungal).

Gonococcal septic arthritis

- Cultures can be initially negative. If suspected re-culture blood but also urethra, cervix (80–90% positive), rectum, pharynx, pustules, and joint fluid. Send urine for gonococcal (GC) nucleic acid detection.
- Use iv ceftriaxone 1 g qds for 1 week (as >5% organisms are penicillin-resistant) then cefixime 400 mg bd for 1–2 weeks.
- Because of increasing resistance, treatment with ciprofloxacin is no longer advisable.
- Consider empiric therapy for *Chlamydia* with doxycycline 100 mg for 7 days or one dose of azithromycin 1 g, and concurrent testing for HIV and syphilis.
- All sexual partners should receive one dose of ceftriaxone 125 mg im and empiric treatment for *Chlamydia*.

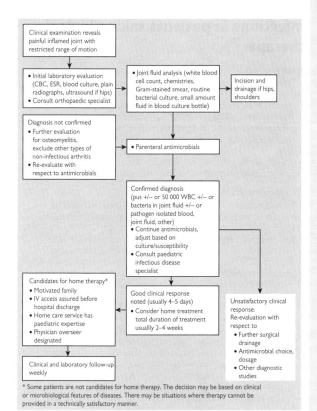

Fig. 24.1 Management of suspected septic arthritis in the child.
Reproduced with the permission of Oxford University Press from Isenberg D, *et al.* (eds) (2004) *Oxford Textbook of Rheumatology* 3rd edn.

Infections in patients taking biologic therapy

Background

- Over the last 5 years, immunosuppressants that specifically inhibit the actions of TNF-α, IL-6 and deplete B-cells have become widely used to treat multiple rheumatic diseases (📖 Chapter 21, p 545).
- The risk of infections is increased with biologic use, although probably greater with anti TNF-α agents than other classes. Patients with a history of serious infections should not be treated with this class of drug.
- Patients are at particular risk for tuberculosis (TB), histoplasmosis, listeriosis, and other opportunistic infections.

Characteristics of infections

- Patients receiving treatment with a biologic therapy should be monitored closely for signs of infection, which should be evaluated aggressively.
- Disseminated fungal and viral infections can occur (Table 24.2).
- Re-activation of latent infections may be a particular problem.
- Reports of TB occurring with biological treatments make the following precautions prudent:
  - patients for latent TB should be screened prior to initiation of therapy;
  - patients who travel to endemic areas and health care workers should be considered high risk;
  - screening should include intradermal injection of PPD, and consideration of chest radiograph given the possibility of anergy;
  - induration of ≥ 5 mm should be considered a positive response for most patients with rheumatic disease;
  - patients with a positive PPD should receive oral isoniazid 300 mg daily for 9 months (or alternate appropriate regimen).
- Reactivation of TB should be considered in febrile patients and those not screened for TB before biologic treatment.
- Latent histoplasmosis should be considered in patients from endemic regions or history of potential exposure (e.g. caving/potholing, construction)
- The risk and severity of infections may be increased in those also taking other immunosuppressants, typically methotrexate (MTX) or steroids.
- Patients may need a longer than normal course of antibiotics and need careful re-assessment before re-starting therapy.

Table 24.2 The range of organisms and type of infections reported with biologics

Organisms		Nature of infection
Bacteria	M. tuberculosis	Disseminated
		Pulmonary
	Atypical mycobacteria	
	Listeriosis	Septicaemia
		Septic arthritis
		Meningitis
	Staphylococcus	Septicaemia
		Cavitating pneumonia
	Salmonella	Septicaemia
		Septic arthritis
	Moraxella	Septic arthritis
	Actinobacillus	Septic arthritis
	Nocardia	Respiratory tract
Viruses	Varicella	Disseminated
	H. simplex	Severe
	Hepatitis B/C	Reactivation
	CMV	Disseminated
Fungi/yeasts	Candida	Septicaemia
	Cryptococcus	Pneumonia
	Aspergillosis	Disseminated
	Sporotrichosis	Skin
	Pneumocystis	Disseminated
	Histoplasmosis	Pneumonia
		Disseminated
Parasites	Leishmaniasis	Visceral

Acute systemic lupus erythematosus

Acute systemic lupus erythematosus (SLE) will manifest either as a flare in patients with an established diagnosis or as the first presentation of the disease. Declining C3 and increasing dsDNA titres may predict acute disease flares in some patients. The reader is referred to 📖 Chapter 10, p 321 for SLE and 📖 Chapter 11, p 343 for antiphospholipid syndrome and catastrophic (APS).

Diagnosing systemic lupus erythematosus in an acute medical context

- Consider SLE as a diagnosis in all young and middle-aged women who present with a history of joint pain, photosensitive rash, or pleuritic chest pain.
- Raynaud's phenomenon and recurrent mouth ulcers are non-specific, but may also appear in association with SLE.
- As labs usually do not test for ANA, C3/C4 and other serologies urgently, these tests may not be available when making an initial diagnosis of SLE.
- Inflammatory markers such as the ESR or CRP may not be a reliable indicator of SLE activity.
- Although pericardial effusions are common with SLE, they are generally trivial. Cardiac tamponade is found in less than 1% of patients with SLE. Since the effusion tends to reflect the overall disease state, generally treatment of the underlying disease is adequate to resolve the effusion. Rarely, therapeutic pericardiocentesis may be required.

Acute systemic lupus erythematosus nephritis (adults)

- Check the BP accurately, creatinine, blood urea, electrolytes, send urine for culture, a spot urine protein/creatinine ratio (as an estimate of proteinuria) and US the renal tract to rule out post-renal obstruction.
- Quantification of urinary protein and creatinine grades severity of the renal lesion and guides management approach (Fig. 24.2).
- Control BP. Often a diuretic, ACE inhibitor, or beta blocker are required.
- Biopsy can inform treatment decisions. Treatment will generally include steroids and oral mycophenolate mofetil (titrate to 1–1.5 g bd) or iv cyclophosphamide (0.75 g/m^2 iv monthly).
- Steroid-induced osteoporosis and cardiovascular risk should be managed from the outset. Consider getting the following done early: DEXA scan, ECG, and fasting lipid panel.
- Daily calcium (1000–1500 mg) and vitamin D (800 IU) should be administered to all patients receiving steroids.
- There is a need to counsel patients about infertility, malignancy, and haemorrhagic cystitis risks, the dose schedules (e.g. MESNA), monitoring (FBC at day 10 after and prior to iv pulse) and pneumocystis prophylaxis chemotherapy (e.g. dapsone; Fig. 24.2).

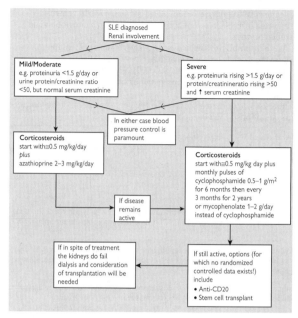

Fig. 24.2 The management of adult renal SLE: treatment algorithm. Corticosteroid doses are prednisolone equivalents.

Reproduced with the permission of Oxford University Press from Isenberg D, et al. (eds) (2004) *Oxford Textbook of Rheumatology* 3rd edn.

Acute SLE involving heart and lung (adults)

- Cardiac and isolated pulmonary manifestations of SLE are rare and in many patients with SLE, acute cardiac and pulmonary features may be due to other common conditions (Table 24.3)
- CRP elevation may reflect infection or significant pleuropericardial SLE. Lupus pericarditis alone without evidence of cardiac compromise can be treated with NSAIDs and prednisone 20–40 mg od for 2–4 weeks with subsequent steroid taper.
- If not due to cardiac failure, acute dyspnoea in SLE may be due to intercurrent infection, pneumonitis, pulmonary vasculitis, pulmonary embolism, pulmonary hypertension, or dyspnoea from the pain of pleural serositis.
- Cyclophosphamide should be considered for severe or life-threate manifestations of SLE.

Acute haematological manifestations of systemic lupu erythematosus (adults)

- Many patients with SLE are Coomb's positive without having s haemolysis (and do not need treating as such).

- Features of haemolysis include fever, shivers, pyrexia, anaemia, elevated bilirubin in serum and urine, low serum haptoglobins and reticulocytosis.
- Acute thrombocytopaenia is a relatively frequent presentation.
- If severe, both haemolytic anaemia (Hb <7 mg/dL) and thrombocytopaenia (platelets <25 000) require high dose prednisone 60–80 mg/day and intravenous immunoglobulin therapy.

Table 24.3 Important aspects in management of acute cardiopulmonary manifestations of SLE in adults

Initial clinical cardiac assessment	ECG, blood for CK, troponin T, echo
Initial lung assessment should include:	ABGs, CXR, spirometry, HRCT chest, VQ scan
Consider pulmonary embolus	Consider empirical anticoagulation early and check for lupus anticoagulant, APL antibodies, and complete thrombophilia screen.
Pulmonary vasculitis (very rare)	*Features:* severe dyspnoea, CXR abnormal. Requires ICU and respiratory physician support and consider plasma exchange.
Interstitial lung disease	Requires high-dose steroids and either AZA (up to 2.5 mg per kg/day) or cyclophosphamide has less chance side-effects as iv regime, e.g. 0.5–1 g every 2 weeks ×6 then maintenance doses every 3 months reviewed every 6 months.
Antiphospholipid syndrome	PE-associated with APL syndrome in SLE requires lifelong anticoagulation.
Specific therapies	
Steroids	Assuming non-viral infections excluded or treated most cardiopulmonary SLE features respond to oral prednisone 0.5–1 mg/kg/day. Consider methylprednisolone 1g iv × 3 days if clinical situation extreme.
Mycophenolate	Mycophenolate mofetil (0.5 mg bd initially increasing after 1–2 weeks to 1–1.5 g bd) can be considered if AZA or cyclophophamide contraindicated or patient intolerant. It is increasingly being used instead of cyclophosphamide for inducing remission in lupus nephritis.
Anti-CD20	Though evidence minimal, rituximab (anti-CD20) 1 g infusion repeated after 2 weeks may be considered if other immunosupressants contraindicated or patient intolerant.
Bone protection	All patients treated with steroids require daily calcium (1 g) and vitamin D (800 IU). Most should also get bisphosphonate initially—withdrawn if DEXA scan shows good BMD with all T scores >−1.5

Paediatric systemic lupus erythematosus —acute nephritis

- The most common lesion is diffuse proliferative GN (30–45% cases) (Fig. 24.3).
- One-third have hypertension which may need aggressive management.
- All have microscopic haematuria and proteinuria >3 mg/kg/day. Most have >25 mg/kg/d proteinuria. However up to a third may have serum albumin >35 g/L and about 50% maintain GFR >100 mL/min/1.73 m^2.
- Prognosis and therapy of nephritis is guided by the active ISN-grade pathological lesion and chronicity index; thus biopsy is important.
- Management includes high dose steroids and cyclophosphamide 750 mg/m^2 iv per month for 6–12 months.
- In acute fulminant renal disease consider plasmapheresis.

Paediatric systemic lupus erythematosus—acute haematological manifestations

- Overt haemolysis occurs in <10%, thrombocytopaenia in 15–45%.
- Bleeding is uncommon.
- Most with thrombocytopaenia respond to steroids. IVIG can be used.
- A high index of suspicion is needed to diagnose catastrophic APS. It is characterized by multiple organ thromboses and microangiopathic changes.
- All cases require working closely with hematologists as highly informed interpretation of detailed serial coagulation studies are required.
- The treatment of haematological manifestations of SLE is shown in Fig. 24.4.

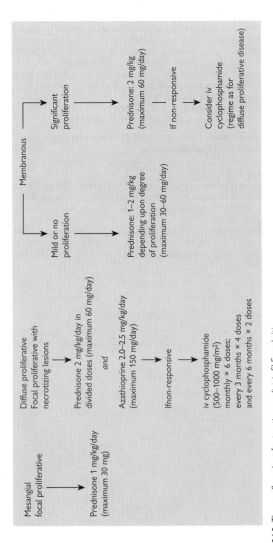

Fig. 24.3 Therapy flow chart for treating paediatric SLE nephritis.
Reproduced with the permission of Oxford University Press from the *Oxford Textbook of Rheumatology* 3e, edited by Isenberg, David et al. (2004)

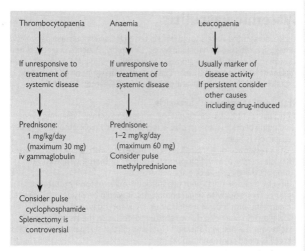

Fig. 24.4 Flow chart for treating paediatric haematological manifestations of SLE.
Reproduced with the permission of Oxford University Press from Isenberg,
David *et al.* (eds) (2004) *Oxford Textbook of Rheumatology* 3rd edn.

Systemic vasculitis

A severe vasculitis flare should be treated aggressively because permanent damage from tissue ischaemia may occur rapidly. Patients diagnosed with pulmonary capillaritis or glomerulonephritis will typically benefit from treatment with pulse steroids. The specific management of each type of vasculitis is outlined in relevant sections of 📖 Chapter 15, p 405.

Giant cell (temporal) arteritis

- Because giant cell arteritis (GCA) can lead to cranial ischaemic events including blindness and stroke, it is important to treat empirically when suspicion is high.
- The prevalence of giant cell arteritis increases with age. Visual changes, jaw claudication, and diplopia in the setting of B-type symptoms all support the diagnosis of giant cell arteritis.
- Empiric therapy starts with prednisone 1 mg/kg/d for 1 month; if the patient presents with visual complaints, it would be prudent to initiate treatment with methylprednisolone 1 g iv for 3 days.
- Daily aspirin has been demonstrated to decrease the risk of cranial ischaemic events, and should be used as part of standard therapy unless there is clear contraindication.
- Treatment should not be delayed; biopsy is diagnostically useful up to 2 weeks after steroid therapy is initiated.
- To optimize yield, temporal artery biopsy should be bilateral, with samples at least 1.5 cm in length.

'Severe' vasculitis

- Patients with active vasculitis can quickly develop manifestations that threaten life or the function of a vital organ. These patients are sometimes referred to as having 'severe' vasculitis.
- Severe manifestations of the small vessel vasculitides include pulmonary haemorrhage (or capillaritis) and glomerulonephritis. Severe manifestations of medium vessel vasculitis include mononeuritis multiplex (e.g. foot drop/wrist drop) or mesenteric angina/ischaemia.
- When glomerulonephritis is suspected, renal biopsy can be very useful to confirm the diagnosis.
- Severe vasculitis is generally treated with pulse methylprednisolone 1 g iv for 3 days, followed by prednisone 1 mg/kg/day.
- Most patients with severe vasculitis will also be treated with cyclophosphamide 1.5–2.0 mg/kg/day. Lower doses should be used in the elderly or in patients with renal insufficiency.
- Cyclophosphamide places patients at risk for *Pneumoncystis* infection, and appropriate chemoprophylaxis should be instituted. Cyclophosphamide should be administered in the morning in a single dose to minimize risk of haemorrhagic cystitis.

- In patients who are at high risk for infection, treatment with intravenous immunoglobulin or plasmapheresis may be appropriate.
- In patients who continue to decline despite immunosuppression, serious consideration should be given to the possibility that the patient has an infection mimicking a vasculitis flare.

Scleroderma crises

Renal crisis

- This may manifest as an acute or subacute hypertensive crisis, usually within the first four years after diagnosis of diffuse scleroderma (dcSScl). It can be the presenting feature of SScl (📖 Chapter 13, p 363).
- An abrupt increase in BP >150/85 and new renal insufficiency are consistent with this diagnosis.
- Other manifestations include what would be expected with hypertensive emergency, such as micro-angiopatic haemolytic anaemia, encephalopathy, and hypertensive retinopathy.

Acute SScl renal crisis management

- ACE inhibitors are the cornerstone of management of renal crisis. The patient should be treated with escalating doses of captopril until blood pressure is brought under control. Angiotensin II receptor blockers (ARB) and calcium channel blockers can be added sequentially if captopril is inadequate.
- Fast drops in blood pressure should be avoided, as low perfusion pressures in abnormal renal vessels may worsen renal failure.
- Consult nephrology about hemodialysis if necessary.
- Prompt initial treatment often leads to re-establishment of good renal function.

Pulmonary hypertension

- Primary pulmonary arterial hypertension (PAH) occurs as a complication of lcSSc, although it can also occur in dcSScl (both as a primary feature and secondary to pulmonary fibrosis).
- Echocardiography can be used to screen for PAH; an RVSP >40 mmHg is suggestive, but the diagnosis must be confirmed by right heart catheterization.
- Decompensated PAH presents with subacute onset of signs and symptoms consistent with right heart failure, including peripheral oedema and dyspnoea.

Management of acute SScl-related PAH

- Patients with rapidly decompensating heart failure secondary to pulmonary arterial hypertension should be treated with supplemental oxygen, diuresis, and continuous iv prostacyclin.
- Diuretics decrease right ventricular preload, and can lead to significant symptomatic relief.
- A large pulmonary embolism can also result in rapidly worsening of pulmonary arterial hypertension, and should be considered in the appropriate setting.
- Management of subacute PAH associated with SScl is discussed elsewhere.

Methotrexate-induced pneumonitis

This is rare, but it can occur in any patient given MTX. Reports suggest the incidence ranges from <0.5% to 7% of patients (variation due to definition of condition). It is probably much rarer in children/adolescents compared with adults. Life-threatening pneumonitis requiring hospital admission probably occurs in <1% patients taking MTX. It is thought that mild pneumonitis resolves on drug withdrawal alone.

Patients at risk

- Most patients suffering from pneumonitis do so within the first few months of starting MTX or after a significant dose change.
- In patients on stable-dose MTX, blood levels may change in the setting of progressive renal insufficiency or low levels of folate.
- Consider the diagnosis in all patients on MTX with acute onset of dry cough, dyspnoea, headache, and fever.
- The differential diagnosis lies between chest infection, acute pulmonary oedema, or acute interstitial lung disease associated with the underlying condition.

Immediate management of severe toxicity.

- Stop MTX.
- Optimal therapy for methotrexate-induced pneumonitis has not been well defined. Folinic acid (15–25 mg po qds) may reverse methotrexate toxicity.
- Anecdotally, steroids accelerate recovery; in cases of severe decompensation, it is reasonable to treat with methylprednisolone 1 g iv for 3 days, followed by prednisone 1 mg/kg/d. Prednisone can be tapered over the subsequent 1–6 months, depending on disease severity.
- The remainder of management should be focused on identifying alternate causes for respiratory compromise (e.g. BAL and high resolution CT to exclude infection) and supportive care (e.g. supplemental oxygen, consideration of transfusion if anaemia is present).
- Most patients with methotrexate-induced lung injury will recover, but may have chronic lung damage as a result.

Index

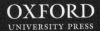